Food IS Medicine

THE SCIENTIFIC EVIDENCE

....

VOLUME ONE

Brian R. Clement, PhD, NMD, LN

....

HIPPOCRATES PUBLICATIONS
SUMMERTOWN, TENNESSEE
AN IMPRINT OF BOOK PUBLISHING COMPANY

Published by

Hippocrates Publications

a division of Book Publishing Company

P.O. Box 99

Summertown, TN 38483

888-260-8458

www.bookpubco.com

ISBN 978-1-57067-274-3

18 17 16 15 14   2 3 4 5 6 7 8 9

Library of Congress Cataloging-in-Publication Data

Clement, Brian R., 1951-

  Food is medicine : the scientific evidence / Brian R. Clement.

    p. cm.

  Includes bibliographical references and index.

  ISBN 978-1-57067-274-3 (pbk.)

  1. Diet therapy. 2. Nutrition. 3. Vegetarianism. 4. Naturopathy. I. Title.

  RM216.C57645 2011

  615.8'54--dc23

                        2011036094

Printed on recycled paper

Book Publishing Company is a member of Green Press Initiative. We chose to print this title on paper with 30% post consumer recycled content, processed without chlorine, which saved the following natural resources:

- 10 trees
- 293 pounds of solid waste
- 4,621 gallons of water
- 1,025 pounds of greenhouse gases
- 4 million BTU of energy

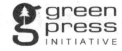

For more information on Green Press Initiative, visit www.greenpressinitiative.org. Environmental impact estimates were made using the Environmental Defense Fund Paper Calculator. For more information visit www.papercalculator.org.

Table of Contents

Introduction

Food IS Medicine: The Scientific Evidence represents my three-volume contribution to public education about the nutritional science of how disease prevention and increased longevity can be achieved by proper food choices.

During the past several decades, my work in the health field has focused on the fundamental role that nutrition and unprocessed, unheated, plant-based foods play in the process of disease recovery and prevention. Directing the Hippocrates Health Institute has afforded me the opportunity to conduct clinical research that has produced persuasive evidence to support the words of Hippocrates, the ancient Greek and father of Western medicine, "Let food be thy medicine and medicine be thy food."

Modern health science at some point in the 20th century estranged itself from a simple and practical truth—natural, organic fruits and vegetables in their raw state possess disease prevention and healing properties. Forgetting that the human body's cells require continuous nourishment to function and thrive has been one of the most abominable mistakes made in Western medicine's attempts at providing health care.

During the Institute's early days in the mid-20th century, we were enigmas in the world of futuristic science. We saw little support for our basic concepts and our prescription for healthy lifestyles coming from within the nutritional science departments of academia or among conventionally trained physicians.

As the 1980s drew to a close, there was a slight shift in the research community's traditional apathy about nutrition. Then the 1990s revived serious interest until now, well into the 21st century, there have been tens of thousands of medical science studies performed worldwide that affirm the results of our own half-century of clinical research.

We can now present in one place the collected wealth of science data that clearly demonstrates in fact that the most important ingested medicine comes from the very food we consume. We are giving this important information to you in a three-volume series highlighting the most noteworthy and provocative studies we have amassed.

This may well be the most comprehensive database ever assembled showing the health benefits of specific foods and nutrients, and the dangers to health posed by other foods, based on a chronological listing of relevant scientific medical studies.

Volume One comprises five chapters covering the following topics: phytochemicals in food and their health-creating properties; the importance of nutrient synergies to human health; the health benefits of calorie restrictive diets and fasting; the nutrient retention and health benefits of raw foods as opposed to cooked or processed; the nutrient superiority of organic fruits and vegetables to non-organic.

Volume Two is titled *Edible Plant Foods, Fruits, and Spices from A to Z: Evidence for Their Healing Properties,* and features more than fifty fruits, vegetables and spices, from marine algae to wheatgrass, listing hundreds of research studies that have affirmed their usefulness in treating or preventing dozens of health problems from cancer and diabetes to hypertension, ulcers, and wound healing.

Volume Three highlights the extensive scientific data showing the disease-causing unhealthy foods, from meat and dairy products to sugar and other additives, along with their toxin-producing cooking practices, and how they are often the underlying culprits in sparking health problems in people of all ages.

Although *Food IS Medicine* does not resemble a typical book written in a conversational manner, it is easy-to-read science portrayed in a way that both the layperson or consummate food and nutrition professional can appreciate. The key finding of each study is summarized. These studies are presented chronologically so the reader can grasp the evolution of findings and theories about the health impacts of various nutrients and foods. Tens of thousands of scientific medical studies conducted over a period of eight decades in dozens of countries were examined to bring you the most important three thousand or so in these three volumes.

Let us hope that this contribution once and for all silences the skeptics and ultimately helps to change the dietary patterns of future generations. Not many years ago, a colleague of mine remarked, "We are digging our grave with a knife and fork." The overwhelming data presented in these three volumes supports that analogy 100 percent.

CHAPTER ONE

The General Health Benefits of Phytochemicals in Foods

THROUGHOUT HUMAN HISTORY, our species has instinctually known that food was not only for sustenance, but had the power to protect and enhance health. Much of the evidence for this idea, which took root in ancient cultures, was intuitive or based on observations of what animals in the wild ate when sick. It was also grounded in observations about the results of long-term trial and error as generations of humans experimented with foods and herbs to tap their healing powers.

In the late 18th century, British ships began carrying citrus fruit on ocean voyages for sailors to consume. It was hoped that the fruit would prevent deadly scurvy. It did. No one knew at the time that a substance in citrus fruit, vitamin C, was responsible for this preventative effect. It wasn't until vitamin C was actually "discovered," which is to say isolated, in a laboratory in 1933 that the intuition and observations of the 18th-century British mariners were affirmed by science.

Knowledge about the "invisible" substances within fruits and vegetables that enhance human health took another giant leap forward in 1948 when scientists gave us the first evidence of a new type of chemistry found in plants, later called phytonutrients, or phytochemicals. Plants produce phytochemicals in response to the threat of insects and disease during the crop growing cycle, a process that is shortened and diluted when farmers add pesticides and insecticides to their crops. While phytochemicals are not necessary to the human body for its normal metabolic functioning (vitamins are necessary), they would be shown to have critical roles to play in preventing or healing human illness and disease.

During the early 1980s, the National Cancer Institute chemoprevention program began investigating the role that phytochemicals may play in human health. Seven general families of these nutrients were eventually identified. Within each of the seven groupings, thousands of individual phytochemical agents would be isolated by various teams of researchers worldwide.

Although this exciting finding was a profound and critical event in our understanding of nutrition, further and deeper work on the importance of phytochemicals to health was not fully engaged until the 1990s. From this point forward, biology has been inundated with one phytonutrient after another being discovered and traced to the effect they have on disease prevention and healing.

There is no doubt that this ever-emerging science has become the most important conducted throughout the history of nutritional biology. How wondrous it is to know that plants with origins dating back millions of years afford humans a powerful medicine that helps to maintain our balance and health. Well before the human species began spreading globally, nature had created an organic and natural antidote for our future disease-creating lifestyles.

Phytochemicals play well-documented roles in protecting human health, as revealed by the results of test tube and animal experiments, human epidemiological data, and human clinical trials. These connections are further solidified by the stories told by people who have successfully employed phytochemicals to address health and healing challenges.

Among hundreds of seemingly miraculous healing success stories involving phytochemicals that have been brought to my attention is that of Majlis Tooming Akesson of Stockholm, Sweden. She was diagnosed with breast cancer in 1992 at the age of 45 and had a mastectomy. Eleven years later she was diagnosed with liver cancer that had spread to her back and hip. In November 2003, her oncologist's prognosis was that she would probably not survive beyond Christmas.

While in the hospital, Majlis recalled having read about Ann Wigmore of Boston and how she had overcome cancer by consuming wheatgrass, greens, and other live foods. So Majlis asked her husband to bring her a thermos of wheatgrass juice, spinach soup, and green kale soup each day, instead of consuming the hospital food she was being offered. Her health began to undergo dramatic improvements and she was released from the hospital after only five days.

She continued a diet high in phytochemical nutrients from raw foods and her cancer went into remission. Seven years after being told that she had only a few months to live, she remains not only alive but vigorously and vitally so. "After nearly eighteen years of fighting for my health, I feel like I am 40-years old again," she told me.

Phytochemical nutrients may also play a role in regenerating fertility. One of many such cases that I'm aware of involves Jennifer Aiello, who wanted to have a child at age 44. But after three miscarriages she was told by physicians that she had chromosomal abnormalities, which made it unlikely that she could ever give birth to a healthy baby.

Jennifer tells her story this way: "I was devastated. My dream of having a child didn't seem possible. But I said to myself there has to be a way to make my body healthier or even to do something to improve the egg quality." She decided to try a raw vegetable diet with its high-density phytochemical nutrient content. She also gave up coffee, meat, sugar, and dairy products.

Within weeks of adopting this new dietary lifestyle, Jennifer became pregnant. "Nine months later," she relates, "I had what I wanted most in life: a baby girl. Not only is she beautiful, she is super healthy, and at birth, she weighed 8 pounds, 8 ounces. She is very alert and smart. At every checkup, the pediatrician remarks about how she is so healthy."

Every new leaf turned in the search for natural, plant-based health remedies reveals stunning and profound information about how raw, plant-based foods can protect us from all known disorders. This nutritional powerhouse carries the potential to alleviate the majority of human diseases and maladies. Rather than spend billions on research that attempts to synthetically replicate isolated chemicals from nature, wouldn't it be more prudent and cost-effective to simply educate and encourage people to consume what nature has provided us already?

With that said, I now present the first chapter of *Food IS Medicine*, detailing the scientific medical studies on phytochemicals that support the idea of natural food as the most important medicine on earth.

Major Phytochemicals in Foods

Phenolic compounds

- **Monophenols**
  - Apiole – *parsley*
  - Carnosol – *rosemary*
  - Carvacrol – *oregano, thyme*
  - Dillapiole – *dill*
  - Rosemarinol – *rosemary*

- **Flavonoids (polyphenols)** – *red, blue, purple pigments*
  - Flavonols
    - Quercetin – *red and yellow onions, tea, apples, cranberries, buckwheat, beans*
    - Gingerol – *ginger*
    - Kaempferol – *strawberries, gooseberries, cranberries, peas, cabbage, brocolli, and other members of the Brassicate family, chives*
    - Myricetin – *grapes, walnuts*
    - Resveratrol – *grape skins and seeds, nuts, peanuts*
    - Rutin – *citrus fruits, buckwheat, parsley, tomatoes, apricots, rhubarb, tea*
    - Isorhamnetin
  - Flavanones
    - Hesperidin – *citrus fruits*
    - Naringenin – *citrus fruits*
    - Silybin – *blessed milk thistle*
    - Eriodictyol
  - Flavones
    - Apigenin – *chamomile, celery, parsley*
    - Tangeritin – *tangerine and other citrus peels*
    - Luteolin

- Flavan-3-ols
  - Catechins – *white tea, green tea, black tea, grapes, apple juice, lentils, black-eyed peas*
  - (+)-Catechin
  - (+)-Gallocatechin
  - (-)-Epicatechin
  - (-)-Epigallocatechin
  - (-)-Epigallocatechin gallate (EGCG) – *green tea*
  - (-)-Epicatechin 3-gallate
  - Theaflavin – *black tea*
  - Theaflavin-3-gallate – *black tea*
  - Theaflavin-3'-gallate – *black tea*
  - Theaflavin-3,3'-digallate – *black tea*
  - Thearubigins
- Anthocyanins (flavonals) and Anthocyanidins – *many red, purple or blue fruits and vegetables*
  - Pelargonidin – *bilberries, raspberries, strawberries*
  - Peonidin – *bilberries, blueberries, cherries, cranberries, peach*
  - Cyanidin – *red apples and pears, bilberries, blackberries, blueberries, cherries, cranberries, peaches, plums, hawthorn, loganberries*
  - Delphinidin – *bilberries, blueberries*
  - Malvidin – *bilberries, blueberries*
  - Petunidin
- Isoflavones (phytoestrogens)
  - Daidzein (formononetin) – *soybeans, alfalfa sprouts, red clover, chickpeas, peanuts, other legumes*
  - Genistein (biochanin A) – *soybeans, alfalfa sprouts, red clover, chickpeas, peanuts, other legumes*
  - Glycitein – *soybeans*
- Dihydroflavonols
- Chalcones
- Coumestans (phytoestrogens)
  - Coumestrol – *red clover sprouts, alfalfa sprouts, soybeans, peas, brussels sprouts*

- **Phenolic acids**
  - Ellagic acid – *walnuts, strawberries, cranberries, blackberries, guava, grapes*
  - Gallic acid – *tea, mangoes, strawberries, rhubarb, soybeans*
  - Salicylic acid – *peppermint, licorice, peanut, wheat*
  - Tannic acid – *nettles, tea, berries*
  - Vanillin – *vanilla beans, cloves*
  - Capsaicin – *chiles*
  - Curcumin – *turmeric, mustard*
- **Hydroxycinnamic acids**
  - Caffeic acid – *burdock, hawthorn, artichokes, pears, basil, thyme, oregano, apples*
  - Chlorogenic acid – *echinacea, strawberries, pineapple, sunflower seeds, blueberries*
  - Cinnamic acid – *aloe*
  - Ferulic acid – *oats, rice, artichokes, oranges, pineapples, apples, peanuts*
  - Coumarin – *citrus fruits, maize*
- **Lignans (phytoestrogens)** – *seeds (flax, sesame, pumpkin, sunflower seeds, poppy), whole grains (rye, oats, barley), bran (wheat, oat, rye), fruits (particularly berries) and vegetables*
  - Silymarin – *artichokes, milk thistle*
  - Matairesinol – *flaxseed, sesame seed, rye bran and meal, oat bran, poppy seeds, strawberries, black currants, broccoli*
  - Secoisolariciresinol – *flaxseeds, sunflower seeds, sesame seeds, pumpkins, strawberries, blueberries, cranberries, zucchini, black currants, carrots*
  - Pinoresinol and lariciresinol – *sesame seed, cabbage, brocolli, and other members of the Brassica family*
- **Tyrosol esters**
  - Tyrosol – *olive oil*
  - Hydroxytyrosol – *olive oil*
  - Oleocanthal – *olive oil*
  - Oleuropein – *olive oil*

- **Stilbenoids**
  - Resveratrol – *grapes, peanuts*
  - Pterostilbene – *grapes, blueberries*
  - Piceatannol – *grapes*
- **Punicalagins** – *pomegranates*

Terpenes (isoprenoids)

- **Carotenoids (tetraterpenoids)**
  - Carotenes - *orange pigments*
    - α-Carotene – *to vitamin A, in carrots, pumpkins, maize, tangerines, oranges*
    - β-Carotene – *to vitamin A, in dark, leafy greens and red, orange, and yellow fruits and vegetables*
    - γ-Carotene
    - δ-Carotene
    - Lycopene – *Vietnam gac, tomatoes, grapefruit, watermelons, guava, apricots, carrots*
    - Neurosporene
    - Phytofluene – *star fruit, sweet potatoes, oranges*
    - Phytoene – *sweet potatoes, oranges*
  - Xanthophylls - *yellow pigments*
    - Canthaxanthin – *paprika*
    - Cryptoxanthin – *mangoes, tangerines, oranges, papayas, peaches, avocados, peas, grapefruit, kiwifruit*
    - Zeaxanthin – *wolfberries, spinach, kale, turnip greens, maize, red bell peppers, pumpkins, oranges*
    - Astaxanthin – *microalgae, yeast*
    - Lutein – *spinach, turnip greens, romaine lettuce, red peppers, pumpkins, mangos, papayas, oranges, kiwifruit, peaches, squash, legumes, cabbage, brocolli, and other members of the Brassica family, prunes, sweet potatoes, honeydew melons, rhubarb, plums, avocados, pears*
    - Rubixanthin – *rose hips*
- **Monoterpenes**
  - Limonene – *oils of citrus, cherries, spearmint, dill, garlic, celery, maize, rosemary, ginger, basil*
  - Perillyl alcohol – *citrus oils, caraway, mints*

- **Saponins** – *soybeans, beans, other legumes, maize, alfalfa*
- **Lipids**
    - Phytosterols – *almonds, cashews, peanuts, sesame seeds, sunflower seeds, whole wheat, maize, soybeans, many vegetable oils*
        - Campesterol - *buckwheat*
        - Beta sitosterol – *avocados, rice bran, wheat germ, corn oils, fennel, peanuts, soybeans, hawthorn, basil, buckwheat*
        - Gamma sitosterol
        - Stigmasterol – *buckwheat*
    - Tocopherols (vitamin E)
    - Omega-3,6,9 fatty acids – *dark, leafy greens, grains, legumes, nuts*
        - Gamma-linolenic acid – *evening primrose, borage, black currant*
- **Triterpenoid**
    - Oleanolic acid - *American pokeweed, honey mesquite, garlic, java apples, cloves, and many other Syzygium species*
    - Ursolic acid - *apples, basil, bilberries, cranberries, elder flowers, peppermint, lavender, oregano, thyme, hawthorn, prunes*
    - Betulinic acid - *Ber tree, white birch, tropical carnivorous plants Triphyophyllum peltatum and Ancistrocladus heyneanus, Diospyros leucomelas (a member of the persimmon family), Tetracera boiviniana, the jambul (Syzygium formosanum), and many other Syzygium species*
    - Moronic acid - *Rhus javanica (a sumac), mistletoe*

Betalains

- **Betalains**
    - Betacyanins
        - betanin - *beets*
        - isobetanin - *beets*
        - probetanin - *beets*
        - neobetanin - *beets*
    - Betaxanthins (non-glycosidic versions)
        - Indicaxanthin - *beets, Sicilian prickly pear*
        - Vulgaxanthin - *beets*

Organosulfides

- **Dithiolthiones (isothiocyanates)**
  - Sulphoraphane – *cabbage, brocolli, and other members of the Brassica family*
- **Thiosulphonates (allium compounds)**
  - Allyl methyl trisulfide – *garlic, onions, leeks, chives, shallots*
  - Diallyl sulfide – *garlic, onions, leeks, chives, shallots*

Indoles, glucosinolates

- **Indole-3-carbinol** – *cabbage, kale, brussels sprouts, rutabagas, mustard greens*
- **Sulforaphane** - *broccoli family*
- **3,3'-Diindolylmethane** or DIM - *broccoli family*
- **Sinigrin** - *broccoli family*
- **Allicin** - *garlic*
- **Alliin** - *garlic*
- **Allyl isothiocyanate** - *horseradish, mustard, wasabi*
- **Piperine** - *black pepper*
- **Syn-propanethial-S-oxide** - *cut onions*

Other organic acids

- **Oxalic acid** – *oranges, spinach, rhubarb, tea and coffee, bananas, ginger, almonds, sweet potatoes, bell peppers*
- **Phytic acid** (inositol hexaphosphate) – *cereals, nuts, sesame seeds, soybeans, wheat, pumpkins, beans, almonds*
- **Tartaric acid** – *apricots, apples, sunflower seeds, avocados, grapes*
- **Anacardic acid** - *cashews, mangoes*

(*Source*: http://en.wikipedia.org/wiki/List_of_phytochemicals_in_food)

Medical Conditions Addressed by Phytochemicals

Aging

Berries: improving human health and **healthy aging***, and promoting quality life—a review.* Paredes-Lopez O, Cervantes-Ceja ML, Vigna-Perez M, Hernandez-Perez T. Plant Foods Hum Nutr. 2010 Sep;65(3):299-308. **Key Finding**: "Berries are rich sources of a wide variety of phytochemicals. The isolation and characterization of compounds that may delay the onset of aging is receiving intense research attention. Some berry phenolics are being associated with this functional performance."

Curcumin, inflammation, **ageing and age-related diseases***.* Sikora E, Scapagnini G, Barbagallo M. Immun Ageing. 2010 Jan 17;7(1):1. **Key Finding**: "Ageing is manifested by the decreasing health status and increasing probability to acquired age-related disease such as cancer, Alzheimer's disease, atherosclerosis, metabolic disorders and others. They are likely caused by low grade inflammation driven by oxygen stress and manifested by the increased level of pro-inflammatory cytokines. It is believed that ageing is plastic and can be slowed down by **caloric restriction** as well as by some nutraceuticals. Accordingly, slowing down ageing and postponing the onset of age-related diseases might be achieved by blocking the NF-kappaB-dependent inflammation. In this review we consider the possibility of the spice curcumin, a powerful antioxidant and anti-inflammatory agent possibly capable of improving the health status of the elderly."

Emerging role of polyphenolic compounds in the treatment of neurodegenerative diseases: A review of their intracellular targets. Ramassamy C. Eur J Pharmacol. 2006 Sep;545(1):51-64. **Key Finding: "Aging** is the major risk factor for neurodegenerative diseases such as **Alzheimer's** and **Parkinson's**. A large body of evidence indicates that oxidative stress is involved in the pathophysiology of these diseases. Oxidative stress can induce neuronal damages, modulate intracellular signaling, ultimately leading to neuronal death by apoptosis or necrosis. Thus antioxidants have been studied for their effectiveness in reducing these deleterious effects and neuronal death in many in vitro and in vivo studies. Increasing number of studies demonstrated the efficacy of polyphenolic antioxidants from fruits and vegetables to reduce or to block neuronal death."

Green tea and the skin. Hsu S. J Am Acad Dermatol. 2005 Jun;52(6):1049-59. **Key Finding:** "Plant extracts have been widely used as topical applications for wound-healing, anti-aging, and disease treatments. This article summarizes the findings of studies using green tea polyphenols as chemopreventive, natural healing, and **anti-aging** agents for human skin, and discusses possible mechanisms of action."

Flavonols, flavones, flavanones, and human health: epidemiological evidence. Graf BA, Milbury PE, Blumberg JB. J Med Food. 2005 Fall;8(3):281-90. **Key Finding:** "Observational studies that have examined polyphenolic flavonoids and reductions in the risk of **age-related chronic diseases** are reviewed. The requirement for caution in interpreting these studies is discussed with regard to the limited information available on the bioavailability and biotransformation of these flavonoids. As the totality of the available evidence on these flavonoids suggests a role in the prevention of cancer and cardiovascular disease, further research is warranted, particularly in controlled clinical trials."

***Aging**, exercise, and phytochemicals: promises and pitfalls.* Ji LL, Peterson DM. Ann NY Acad Sci. 2004 Jun;1019:453-61. **Key Finding:** "In vitro and in vivo studies have demonstrated convincingly that dietary supplementation of phytochemicals has beneficial effects against certain types of pathogenesis, disease, cancer, and aging. There is evidence that these effects are related to the ability of phytochemicals to promote the antioxidant defense system and reduce oxidative stress and damage in the cell."

Potential impact of strawberries on human health: a review of the science. Hannum SM. Crit Rev Food Sci Nutr. 2004;44(1):1-17. **Key Finding:** "Individual compounds in strawberries have demonstrated **anticancer** activity in several different experimental systems, blocking initiation of carcinogenesis, and suppressing progression and proliferation of tumors. Preliminary animal studies have indicated that diets rich in strawberries may also have the potential to provide benefits to the **aging brain**."

*Natural extracts as possible protective agents of **brain aging**.* Bastianetto S, Quirion R. Neurobiol Aging. 2002 Sep-Oct;23(5):891-97. **Key Finding:** "These results support the hypothesis that dietary intake of natural substances may be beneficial in normal aging of the brain."

Anitoxidant *health effects of aged garlic extract.* Borek C. J Nutr. 2001 Mar;131(3s):1010S-5S. **Key Finding:** "Although additional observations are warranted in humans, compelling evidence supports the beneficial health effects attributed to aged garlic extract, i.e., reducing the risk of **cardiovascular disease, stroke, cancer and aging**, including the oxidant-mediated brain cell damage that is implicated in **Alzheimer's disease**."

*Neurobehavioral aspects of antioxidants in **aging**.* Cantuti-Castelvetri I, Shukitt-Hale B, Joseph JA. Int J Dev Neurosci. 2000 Jul-Aug;18(4-5):367-81. **Key Finding:** This paper reviews studies concerning the influence of antioxidants on age-related reactive oxygen species-induced behavioral changes in humans and animals. The antioxidants reviewed may have synergistic effects among them.

*Membrane and receptor modifications of oxidative stress vulnerability in **aging**. Nutritional considerations.* Joseph JA, Denisova N, Fisher D, et al. Ann NY Acad Sci. 1998 Nov 20;854:268-76. **Key Finding:** "Results indicated that these diets were effective in preventing oxidative stress-induced decrements in several parameters (e.g., nerve growth factor decreases), suggesting that although there may be increases in OS vulnerability in aging, phytochemicals present in antioxidant-rich foods may be beneficial in reducing or retarding the functional central nervous system deficits seen in aging or oxidative insult."

*Nutrition, **cancer**, and **aging**.* Dreosti IE. Ann NY Acad Sci. 1998 Nov 20;854:371-7. **Key Finding:** "Several other well-established anticancer dietary strategies, which include increased fiber intake and the consumption of more fruits and vegetables, have not been studied extensively in relation to aging, although many of the phytochemicals considered important as chemopreventive agents for cancer may well contribute to delaying the aging process."

Reversals of age-related declines in neuronal signal transduction, cognitive, and motor behavioral deficits with blueberry, spinach, or strawberry dietary supplementation. Joseph JA, Shukitt-Hale B, Denisova NA, et al. J Neurosci. 1999 Sep 15;19(18):8114-21. **Key Finding:** "These findings suggest that, in addition to their known beneficial effects on **cancer and heart disease**, phytochemicals present in antioxidant-rich foods may be beneficial in reversing the course of **neuronal and behavioral aging**."

*Oxidants, antioxidants, and the degenerative diseases of **aging**.* Ames BN, Shigenaga MK, Hagen TM. Proc Natl Acad Sci. 1993 Sep 1;90(17):7915-22. **Key Finding:** "Metabolism, like other aspects of life, involves tradeoffs. Oxidant by-products of normal metabolism cause extensive damage to DNA, protein, and lipid. We argue that this damage (the same as that produced by radiation) is a major contributor to aging and to degenerative diseases of aging such as cancer, cardiovascular disease, immune-system decline, brain dysfunction, and cataracts. Antioxidant defenses against this damage include ascorbate, tocopherol, and carotenoids. Dietary fruits and vegetables are the principal source. Low dietary intake of fruits and vegetables doubles the risk of most types of **cancer** and also markedly increase the risk of **heart disease** and **cataracts**."

Allergies

Extract of Perilla frutescens enriched for rosmarinic acid, a polyphenolic phytochemical, inhibits seasonal allergic rhinoconjunctivitis in humans. Takano H, Osakabe N, Sanbongi C, et al. Exp Biol Med. 2004 Mar;229(3):247-54. **Key Finding:** "Extract of Perilla frutescens enriched for rosmarinic acid can be an effective intervention for mild seasonal allergic rhinoconjunctivitis at least partly through inhibition of PMNL infiltration into the nostrils. Use of this alternative treatment for SAR might reduce treatment costs for **allergic** diseases."

Alzheimer's disease

*Oxidative stress and **Alzheimer's disease**: dietary polyphenols as potential therapeutic agents.* Darvesh AS, Carroll RT, Bishayee A, Geldenhuys WJ, Van der Schyf CJ. Expert Rev Neurother. 2010 May;10(5):729-45. **Key Find-

ing: Oxidative stress has been strongly implicated in the pathophysiology of neurodegenerative disorders such as Alzheimer's. This article reviews the antioxidant potential of polyphenolic compounds such as anthocyanins from berries, catechins and theaflavins from tea, curcumin from turmeric and resveratrol from grapes.

Protective effects of piceatannol against beta-amyloid-induced neuronal cell death. Kim HJ, Lee KW, Lee HJ. Ann NY Acad Sci. 2007 Jan;1095:473-82. **Key Finding:** "Piceatannol has a structure homologous to resveratrol and is an anti-inflammatory and antiproliferative stilbene derived from plants. Beta-amyloid is a main component of senile plaques in **Alzheimer's disease** that induces neuronal cell death. These results suggest that piceatannol blocks Abeta-induced accumulation of reactive oxygen species, thereby protecting PC12 cells from oxidative stress."

Emerging role of polyphenolic compounds in the treatment of neurodegenerative diseases: A review of their intracellular targets. Ramassamy C. Eur J Pharmacol. 2006 Sep;545(1):51-64. **Key Finding:** "**Aging** is the major risk factor for neurodegenerative diseases such as **Alzheimer's** and **Parkinson's** diseases. A large body of evidence indicates that oxidative stress is involved in the pathophysiology of these diseases. Oxidative stress can induce neuronal damages, modulate intracellular signaling, ultimately leading to neuronal death by apoptosis or necrosis. Thus antioxidants have been studied for their effectiveness in reducing these deleterious effects and neuronal death in many in vitro and in vivo studies. Increasing number of studies demonstrated the efficacy of polyphenolic antioxidants from fruits and vegetables to reduce or to block neuronal death."

Protective effects of quercetin and vitamin C against oxidative stress-induced neurodegeneration. Heo HJ, Lee CY. J Agric Food Chem. 2004 Dec 15;52(25):7514-7. **Key Finding:** "We observed that quercetin decreased oxidative stress-induced neuronal cell membrane damage more than vitamin C. These results suggest that quercetin, in addition to many other biological benefits, contributes significantly to the protective effects of neuronal cells from oxidative stress-induced neurotoxicity, such as **Alzheimer's disease**."

Anitoxidant health effects of aged garlic extract. Borek C. J Nutr. 2001 Mar;131(3s):1010S-5S. **Key Finding:** "Although additional observations are warranted in humans, compelling evidence supports the beneficial health effects attributed to aged garlic extract, i.e., reducing the risk of **cardiovascular disease, stroke, cancer and aging**, including the oxidant-mediated brain cell damage that is implicated in **Alzheimer's disease**."

Antimicrobial/Antiviral

Wild and commercial mushrooms as source of nutrients and nutraceuticals. Barros L, Cruz T, Baptista P, Estevinho LM, Ferreira IC. Food Chem Toxicol. 2008 Aug;46(8):2742-7. **Key Finding:** Experiments were performed in wild and commercial species of mushrooms to analyze nutrient and phytochemical levels. Commercial species seemed to have higher concentrations of sugars, while wild species had higher contents of alpha-Tocopherol. Wild also had a higher content of phenols but a lower content of ascorbic acid than commercial species. There was no difference found in the **antimicrobial** properties of wild and commercial species.

Antiviral activity of phytochemicals: a comprehensive review. Naithani R, Huma LC, Holland LE, et al. Mini Rev Med Chem. 2008 Oct;8(11):1106-33. **Key Finding:** In this review, descriptions are provided of different phytochemical **antiviral** agents and a summary is made of the viral interactions in various biological assays, and how these agents inhibit viral reproduction.

*Phytochemicals for **bacterial** resistance—strengths, weaknesses and opportunities.* Gibbons S. Planta Med. 2008 May;74(6):594-602. **Key Finding:** "This review covers some of the opportunities which currently exist to exploit plants for their natural products as templates for new antibacterial substances."

Inhibitory effects of various plant polyphenols on the toxicity of Staphylococcal alpha-toxin. Choi O, Yahiro K, Morinaga N, Miyazaki M, Noda M. Microb Pathog. 2007 May-Jun;42(5-6):215-24. **Key Finding:** "We found hop bract tannin and apple condensed tannin to exert inhibitory effects on alpha-toxin cytotoxicity. Inhibition of alpha-toxin was dose dependent, suggesting that these polyphenols may be a useful adjunct to current treatments for alpha-toxin catalyzed **Staphylococcal infectious diseases.**"

Evaluation of the antimicrobial effects of several isothiocyanates on Helicobacter pylori. Haristoy X, Fahey JW, Scholtus I, Lozniewski A. Planta Med. 2005 Apr;71(4):326-30. **Key Finding:** "Our data indicate that isothiocyanates have a potent **antibacterial** effect against H. pylori and these naturally occurring phytochemicals might have potential as novel therapeutic agents for H. pylori eradication."

Antimicrobial *and chemopreventive properties of herbs and spices.* Lai PK, Roy J. Curr Med Chem. 2004 Jun;11(11):1451-60. **Key Finding:** "A growing body of research has demonstrated that the commonly used herbs and spices such as garlic, black cumin, cloves, cinnamon, thyme, allspices, bay leaves, mustard and rosemary, possess antimicrobial properties that, in some cases, can be used therapeutically. Other spices, such as saffron, turmeric, green or black tea, and flaxseed do contain potent phytochemicals, including carotenoids, curcumins, catechins, and lignin, which provide significant protection against **cancer.**"

Health effects of vegetables and fruit: assessing mechanisms of action in human experimental studies. Lampe JW. Am J Clin Nutr. 1999 Sep;70(3 Suppl):4755-4905. **Key Finding:** "Phytochemicals can have complementary and overlapping mechanisms of action, including modulation of detoxification enzymes, stimulation of the immune system, reduction of platelet aggregation, modulation of **cholesterol** synthesis and hormone metabolism, reduction of **blood pressure**, and **antioxidant, antibacterial, and antiviral** effects. Although these effects have been examined primarily in animal and cell-culture models, experimental dietary studies in humans have also shown the capacity of vegetables and fruit and their constitutents to modulate some of these potential disease-preventive mechanisms."

Antiviral *assays on phytochemicals: the influence of reaction parameters.* Hudson JB, Graham EA, Towers GH. Planta Med. 1994 Aug;60(4):329-32. **Key Finding:** "We found that the activities of several known antiviral phytochemicals were profoundly affected by the presence of serum components, but in different ways. The reactions were also strongly affected by the order of incubation of the components: virus, compound, serum, and light. The antiviral effects were not influenced significantly by temperature."

Therapeutic potential of plant photosensitizers. Hudson JB, Towers GH. Pharmacol Ther. 1991;49(3):181-222. **Key Finding:** "Many bioactive phytochemicals have been shown in recent years to be photosensitizers, i.e. their toxic activities against **viruses, micro-organisms,** insects or cells are dependent on or are augmented by light of certain wavelengths. The main classes of photosensitizers reviewed here are polyyines, furanyl compounds, beta-carbolines and other alkaloids, and complex quinines."

Antioxidation

*A novel dietary supplement containing multiple phytochemicals and vitamins elevates hepatorenal and **cardiac antioxidant** enzymes in the absence of significant serum chemistry and genomic changes.* Bulku E, Zinkovsky D, et al. Oxid Med Cell Longev. 2010 Mar-Apr;3(2):129-44. **Key Finding**: "A novel dietary supplement composed of three well-known phytochemicals, namely, Salvia officinalis (sage) extract, Camellia sinensis (oolong tea) extract, and Paullinia cupana (guarana) extract, and two prominent vitamins (thiamine and niacin) was designed to provide nutritional support by enhancing metabolism and maintaining healthy weight and energy. The present study evaluated the safety of this dietary supplement and assessed changes in target organ antioxidant enzymes (liver, kidneys and heart), serum chemistry profiles and organ histopathology in Fisher 344 rats. Results suggest that dietary supplement exposure produces normal serum chemistry coupled with elevated antioxidant capacity and does not adversely influence any of the vital target organs. This study reiterates the potential benefits of exposure to a pharmacologically relevant **combination of phytochemicals** compared to a single phytochemical entity."

The phytochemical composition and antioxidant actions of tree nuts. Bolling BW, McKay DL, Blumberg JB. Asia Pac J Clin Nutr. 2010;19(1):117-23. **Key Finding**: "Most tree nuts provide an array of phytochemicals that may contribute to the health benefits attributed to this whole food. A limited number of human studies indicate these nut phytochemicals are bioaccessible and bioavailable and have **antioxidant** actions in vivo."

Are the health attributes of lycopene related to its antioxidant function? Erdman JW, Ford NA, Lindshield BL. Arch Biochem Biophys. 2009 Mar 15;483(2):229-35. **Key Finding:** "We conclude that there is an overall shortage of supportive evidence for the 'antioxidant hypothesis' as lycopene's major in vivo mechanism of action. Our laboratory has postulated that metabolic products of lycopene, the lycopenoids, may be responsible for some of lycopene's reported bioactivity."

Regulation of cellular signals from nutritional molecules: a specific role for phytochemicals, beyond antioxidant activity. Virgilli F, Marino M. Free Radic Biol Med. 2008 Nov 1;45(9):1205-16. **Key Finding:** "We summarize the current knowledge of the mechanisms by which specific molecules of nutritional interest, and in particular, polyphenols, play a role in cellular response and in preventing pathologies."

Phytochemicals of apple peels: isolation, structure elucidation, and their antiproliferative and antioxidant activities. He X, Liu RH. J Agric Food Chem. 2008 Nov 12;56(21):9905-10. **Key Finding:** "Most tested flavonoids and phenolic compounds had high antioxidant activity when compared to ascorbic acid and might be responsible for the antioxidant activities of apples. These results showed apple peel phytochemicals have potent antioxidant and antiproliferative activities."

Effect of antioxidant phytochemicals on the hepatic tumor promoting activity of 3,3',4,4'-tetrachlorobiphenylI (PCB-77). Tharappel JC, Lehmler HJ, Srinivasan C, Roberston LW, Spear BT, Glauert HP. Food Chem Toxicol. 2008 Nov;46(11):3467-74. **Key Finding:** "These findings show that none of the antioxidant phytochemicals produced a clear decrease in the promoting activity of PCB-77," which may induce oxidative stress in the liver.

Nutrients and phytochemicals: from bioavailability to bioefficiency beyond antioxidants. Holst B, Williamson G. Curr Opin Biotechnol. 2008 Apr;19(2):73-82. **Key Finding:** Phytochemicals are 'lifespan essentials' to maintain health and body functions throughout the adult life. "Major mechanisms involved in chronic, age-related diseases include the oxidant/antioxidant balance, but the latest research indicates indirect effects of dietary bioactives in vivo and adaptive responses in addition to direct radical scavenging."

Protective effect of dietary phytochemicals against arsenite induced genotoxicity in mammalian V79 cells. Roy M, Sinha D, Mukherjee S, Paul S, Bhattacharya RK. Indian J Exp Biol. 2008 Oct;46(10):690-7. **Key Finding:** "During repair experiments the phytochemicals enhanced recovery of DNA damage (from arsenic exposure) and ellagic acid gave promising results. The results indicated that natural phytochemicals may have the efficacy in reducing arsenic induced genotoxicity, in scavenging ROS and in enhancing the process of DNA repair."

Antioxidant *properties of sour cherries (Prunus cerasus L.): role of colorless phytochemicals from the methanolic extract of ripe fruits.* Piccolella S, Fiorentino A, Pacifico S, D'Abrosca B, Uzzo P, Monaco P. J Agric Food Chem. 2008 Mar 26;56(6):1928-35. **Key Finding:** Three fruit crude extracts were found to "exercise a massive and dose-increasing antioxidative capacity." Twenty secondary metabolites were isolated for the first time. Flavonoids and quinic acid derivatives were found to be the more antioxidative substances.

Phytochemicals of foods, beverages and fruit vinegars: chemistry and health effects. Shahidi F, McDonald J, Chandrasekara A, Zhong Y. Asia Pac J Clin Nutr. 2008;17(Suppl 1):380-2. **Key Finding:** Processing of phytochemicals in plants and fruits, including fermentation, may alter the chemical nature and efficacy of their phenolic constitutents. Fruit vinegars often contain acetic acid, citric, malic, lactic, and tartaric acids and some phenolics produced by fermentation. "The beneficial health effects of fruit vinegars may in part be related to the process-induced changes in their phenolics and generation of new **antioxidative** phenolics during fermentation."

DNA repair phenotype and dietary antioxidant supplementation. Guarnieri S, Loft S, Riso P, et al. Br J Nutr. 2008 May;99(5):1018-24. **Key Finding:** "Phytochemicals may protect cellular DNA by direct **antioxidant** effect or modulation of the DNA repair activity. We investigated the repair activity towards oxidized DNA in human mononuclear blood cells in two placebo-controlled antioxidant intervention studies. In conclusion, nutritional status, DNA repair activity and DNA damage are linked, and beneficial effects of antioxidants might only be observed among poorly nourished subjects with high levels of oxidized DNA damage and low repair activity."

*Anthocyanins induce the activation of phase II enzymes through the **antioxidant** response element pathway against oxidative stress-induced apoptosis.* Shih PH, Yeh CT, Yen GC. J Agric Food Chem. 2007 Nov 14;55(23):9427-35. **Key Finding:** "Our data suggest that natural anthocyanins are recommended as chemopreventive phytochemicals and could stimulate the antioxidant system to resist oxidant-induced injury. And, more important, the promoting effect of anthocyanins on ARE-regulated phase II enzyme expression seems to be a critical point in modulating the defense system against oxidative stress."

Polyphenolic phytochemicals—just antioxidants or much more? Stevenson DE, Hurst RD. Cell Mol Life Sci. 2007 Nov;64(22):2900-16. **Key Finding:** "We summarize the current knowledge of the intake, bio-availability and metabolism of polyphenolics, their **antioxidant effects**, regulatory effects on signaling pathways, neuro-protective effects and regulatory effects on energy metabolism and gut health."

A review of the interaction among dietary antioxidants and reactive oxygen species. Seifried H,. Anderson DE, Fisher EI, Milner JA. J Nutr Biochem. 2007 Sep;18(9):567-79. **Key Finding:** "Reactive oxygen species have been linked to **cancer** and **cardiovascular disease**, and antioxidants have been considered promising therapy for prevention and treatment of these diseases, especially given the tantalizing links observed between diets high in fruits and vegetables (and presumably **antioxidants**) and decreased risks for cancer."

Carotenoids and human health. Rao AV, Rao LG. Pharmacol Res. 2007 Mar;55(3):207-16. **Key Finding:** "Recent interest in carotenoids has focused on the role of lycopene in human health. Unlike some other carotenoids, lycopene does not have pro-vitamin A properties. Because of the unsaturated nature of lycopene it is considered to be a potent **antioxidant** and a singlet oxygen quencher. This article reviews carotenoids in general and lycopene in particular for their role in human health."

***Antioxidant** phytochemicals in hazelnut kernel (Corylus avellana L.) and hazelnut byproducts.* Shahidi F, Alasalvar C, Liyana-Pathirana CM. J Agric Food Chem. 2007 Feb 21;55(4):1212-20. **Key Finding:** "Generally, extracts of hazelnut byproducts (skin, hard shell, green leafy cover, and tree leaf) exhibited stronger activities than hazelnut kernel at all concentrations tested. Extracts of hazelnut skin showed superior antioxidative efficacy and higher phenolic content as compared to other extracts. These results suggest that hazelnut byproducts could potentially be considered as an excellent and readily available source of natural antioxidants."

Dietary botanical diversity affects the reduction of oxidative biomarkers in women due to high vegetable and fruit intake. Thompson HJ, Heimendinger J, Diker A, et al. J Nutr. 2006 Aug;136(8):2207-12. **Key Finding:** "The objective of this study was to determine whether the botanical diversity of high vegetables and fruit diets alters the response in oxidative biomarkers for lipid peroxidation and DNA oxidation. Two diets were developed. The high botanical diversity diet included foods from the 18 botanical families that induced a reduction in oxidative damage or lipids or DNA. The low botanical diversity diet emphasized 5 of these botanical families. A total of 106 women completed the study. Only the high botanical diversity diet induced a significant reduction in DNA oxidation. Both the high and low diets were associated with a reduction in lipid peroxidation. These findings indicate that botanical diversity plays a role in determining the bioactivity of high vegetable/fruit diets and that smaller amounts of many phytochemicals may have greater beneficial effects than larger amounts of fewer phytochemicals."

Pre-exposure to a novel nutritional mixture containing a series of phytochemicals prevents acetaminophen-induced programmed and unprogrammed cell deaths by enhancing BCL-XL expression and minimizing oxidative stress in the liver. Ray SD, Patel N, Shah N, Naggori A, Nagvi A, Stohs SJ. Mol Cell Biochem. 2006 Dec;293(1-2):119-36. **Key Finding:** "We proposed that the additive and synergistic effects of phytochemicals in fruits and vegetables are responsible for these potent **antioxidant** and **anticancer** activities, and that the benefit of a diet rich in fruits and vegetables is attributed to the complex mixture of phytochemicals present in plants. Our investigation suggests that a mixture containing an assortment of phytochemicals/nutraceuticals may serve as a much more powerful blend in preventing drug or chemical-induced organ injuries than a single phytochemical or nutraceutical entity."

Antioxidant *activities and anthocyanin content of fresh fruits of common fig (Ficus carica L.)* Solomon A, Golubowicz S, Yablowicz Z, et al. J Agric Food Chem. 2006 Oct 4;54(20):7717-23. **Key Finding:** "Six commercial fig varieties differing in color (black, red, yellow and green) were analyzed for total polyphenols, total flavonoids, antioxidant capacity and amount and profile of anthocyanins. Extracts of darker varieties showed higher contents of phytochemicals compared to lighter colored varieties. Fruits skins contributed most of the above phytochemicals and antioxidant activity compared to the fruit pulp."

Neurohormetic phytochemicals: Low-dose toxins that induce adaptive neuronal stress responses. Mattson MP, Cheng A. Trends Neurosci. 2006 Nov;29(11):632-9. **Key Finding:** "Neurohormetic phytochemicals such as resveratrol, resveratrol, sulforaphanes and curcumin might protect **neurons** against injury and disease by stimulating the production of **antioxidant** enzymes, neurotorphic factors, protein chaperones and other proteins that help cells to withstand stress. "

Cranberry phytochemicals: Isolation, structure elucidation, and their antiproliferative and antioxidant activities. He X, Liu RH. J Agric Food Chem. 2006 Sep 20;54(19):7069-74. **Key Finding:** "These results showed cranberry phytochemical extracts have potent **antioxidant** and antiproliferative activities."

Neoplastic transformation of BALB/3T3 cells and cell cycle of HL-60 cells are inhibited by mango (Mangifera indica L.) juice and mango juice extracts. Percival SS, Talcott ST, Chin ST, Maliak AC, Lounds-Singleton A, Pettit-Moore J. J Nutr. 2006 May;136(5):1300-4. **Key Finding:** "In this study, whole mango juice and juice extracts were screened for **antioxidant** and **anticancer** activity. Incubation of HL-60 cells with whole mango juice and mango juice fractions resulted in an inhibition of the cell cycle in the G(0) G(1) phase. A fraction of the eluted mango juice with low peroxyl radical scavenging ability was most effective in arresting cells in the G(0)G(1) phase."

Effect of apple extracts on NF-kappaB activation in human umbilical vein endothelial cells. Davis PA, Polagruto JA, Valacchi G, et al. Exp Biol Med. 2006 May;231(5):594-8. **Key Finding:** "We suggest that flavonoid-rich apple extract downregulates NF-kappaB signaling and that this is indicative of an **antioxidant** effect of the flavonoids present."

In vivo investigation of changes in biomarkers of oxidative stress induced by plant food rich diets. Thompson HJ, Heimendinger J, Gillette C, et al. J Agric Food Chem. 2005 Jul 27;53(15):6126-32. **Key Finding:** "An oxidative effect was observed primarily in individuals whose oxidative end points at baseline were above the median for the study population. These findings imply that increasing exogenous antioxidant exposure may primarily benefit individuals with elevated levels of oxidative stress. Null findings do not necessarily indicate than an **antioxidant** compound lacks in vivo activity."

*Some essential phytochemicals and the **antioxidant** potential in fresh and dried persimmon.* Jung ST, Park YS, Zachwiela Z, et al. Int J Food Sci Nutr. 2005 Mar;56(2):105-13. **Key Finding:** "Both fresh and dried persimmon possess high contents of bioactive compounds and have a high antioxidant potential, though the content of total polyphenols in fresh persimmon was higher than in dried fruit."

Synergy among Phytochemicals within Crucifers: Does It Translate into Chemoprotection? Wallig M., Heinz-Taheny K., Epps D., Gossman T. J Nutr. Dec. 2005; 135(12 Suppl):2972S-2977S. **Key Finding:** Two derivatives, indole-3-carbinol and 1-cyano-2-hydroxy-3-butene (crambene) have been shown in rats to induce a synergistic enhancement of **detoxification** enzyme activity. High combination dietary doses also demonstrated enhanced protection from short-term carcinogenicity using aflatoxin B1.

Phytochemicals in broccoli transcriptionally induce thioredoxin reductase. Hintze KJ, Wald K, Finley JW. J Agric Food Chem. 2005 Jul 13;53(14):5535-40. **Key Finding:** "These data suggest that sulforaphane accounts for most of the **antioxidant r**esponse element-activated transcriptional induction of antioxidant genes by broccoli."

8-Isoprostane F2alpha excretion is reduced in women by increased vegetable and fruit intake. Thompson HJ. Heimendinger J. Sedlacek S. Haegele A. Diker A. O'Neill C. Meinecke B. Wolfe P. Zhu Z. Jiang W. Am J Clin Nutr. 2005 Oct;82(4):768-76. **Key Finding:** "An 8-week dietary intervention was conducted to test the hypothesis that increased vegetable and fruit consumption decreases **oxidative stress.** A significant reduction in the excretion of 8-iso-PGF2alpha was induced by the run-in diet and the high-vegetable fruit diet."

*Phenolics as potential **antioxidant** therapeutic agents: mechanisms and actions.* Soobrattee MA, Neergheen VS, Luximon-Ramma A, Aruoma OI, Bahorun T. Mutat Res. 2005 Nov 11;579(1-2):200-13. **Key Finding:** "Plant-derived phenolics represent good sources of natural antioxidants, however, further investigation on the molecular mechanism of action of these phytochemicals is crucial to the evaluation of their potential as prophylactic agents."

Major phytochemicals in apple cultivars: contribution to peroxyl radical trapping efficiency. Vanzani P, Rossetto M, Rigo A, et al.. J Agric Food Chem. 2005 May 4;53(9):3377-82. **Key Finding:** "Forty-one samples of apples (peel plus pulp) obtained from eight cultivars were examined for concentration of some important phytochemicals and for **antioxidant** activity. The antioxidant efficiency of the apple extracts and of representative pure compounds for each group of phytochemicals (five major polyphenolic groups) was measured. The antioxidant efficiency calculated on the basis of the contribution of the pure compounds was lower than the antioxidant efficiency of the apple extracts. The higher efficiency of apples appears to be strictly related to the overwhelming presence of oligomeric proanthocyanidins."

Chlorophyll, chlorophyllin, and related tetrapyrroles are significant inducers of mammalian phase 2 cytoprotective genes. Fahey JW, Stephenson KK, Dinkova-Kostova AT, Egner PA, Kensler TW, Talalay P. Carcinogenesis. 2005 Jul;26(7):1247-55. **Key Finding:** Plant chlorophylls and carotenoids, which play central roles in photosynthesis, have the ability to induce mammalian phase 2 proteins that protect cells against **oxidants** and electrophiles. "One of the most potent inducers was isolated from chlorophyllin, a semisynthetic water-soluble chlorophyll derivative. Although chlorophyll itself is low in inducer potency, it may nevertheless account for some of the disease-protective effects attributed to diets rich in green vegetables because it occurs in much higher concentrations in those plants than the widely studied phytochemicals."

Isolation and structure identification of grape seed polyphenols and its effects on oxidative damage to cellular DNA. Fan PH, Lou HX. Yao Xue Xue Bao. 2004 Nov;39(11):869-75. **Key Finding:** "That polyphenols investigated were shown to be good cellular DNA oxidative damage-preventing phytochemicals at lower concentration could be used to explain the nutrient effect of grape seed polyphenols measured at a certain degree. At the same time, higher concentration of polyphenols can induce **oxidative damage**, suggesting that dose is one factor to determine the nutrient effects."

Major flavonoids in grape seeds and skins: antioxidant capacity of catechin, epicatechin, and gallic acid. Yilmaz Y, Toledo RT. J Agric Food Chem. 2004 Jan 28;52(2):255-60. **Key Finding:** "The results indicated that dimeric, trimeric, oligomeric, or polymeric procyanidins account for most of the superior **antioxidant** capacity of grape seeds."

*Varietal differences in phenolic content and **antioxidant** and antiproliferative activities of onions.* Yang J., Meyers KJ., Van der Heide J., Liu RH. J Agric Food Chem. 2004 Nov 3;52(22):6787-93. **Key Finding:** "The proliferation of HepG(2) and Caco-2 cells was significantly inhibited in a dose-dependent fashion after exposure to the Western Yellow, shallots, New York Bold, and Northern Red extracts of onion. Western Yellow, shallots, and New York Bold exhibited the highest antiproliferative activity against HepG(2) cells and New York Bold and Western Yellow exhibited the highest antiproliferative activity against Caco-2 cells. However, the varieties of Western White, Peruvian Sweet, Empire Sweet, Mexico, Texas 1015, Imperial Valley Sweet, and Vidalia demonstrated weak antiproliferative activity against both HepG(2) and Caco-2 cells. These results may influence consumers toward purchasing onion varieties exhibiting greater potential health benefits."

*Effects of polyphenols from grape seeds on **oxidative** damage to cellular DNA.* Fan P, Lou H. Mol Cell Biochem. 2004 Dec;267(1-2):67-74. **Key Finding:** "In this study, eleven phenolic phytochemicals from grape seeds were purified by gel chromatography and high performance liquid chromatography. Collectively, these data suggest that procyanidin B4, catechin, and gallic acid were good antioxidants; at low concentrations they could prevent oxidative damage to cellular DNA. But at higher concentration, these compounds may induce cellular DNA damage, taking catechin for example, which explained the irregularity of dose-effect relationship."

Health benefits of fruit and vegetables are from additive and synergistic combinations of phytochemicals. Liu RH. Am J Clin Nutr. 2003 Sep;78(3 Suppl): 517S-520S. **Key Finding:** "We propose that the additive and synergistic effects of phytochemicals in fruit and vegetables are responsible for their potent **antioxidant** and anticancer activities, and that the benefit of a diet rich in fruit and vegetables is attributed to the complex mixture of phytochemicals present in whole foods."

*Phenolic **antioxidants** attenuate hippocampal **neuronal** cell damage against kainic acid induced excitotoxicity.* Parihar MS, Hemnani T, J Biosci. 2003 Feb;28(1):121-8. **Key Finding:** "In the present study we examined whether medicinal plant extracts protect neurons against excitotoxic lesions induced by kainic acid in female Swiss albino mice. The finding of this study has suggested that phytochemicals present in plant extracts mitigate the effects of excitotoxicity and oxidative damage in hippocampus and this might be accomplished by their antioxidative properties."

Protective effect of resveratrol on beta-amyloid-induced oxidative PC12 cell death. Jang JH, Surh YJ. Free Radic Biol Med. 2003 Apr 15;34(8):1100-10. **Key Finding:** "In this study we have investigated the effects of resveratrol on beta-amlyoid-induced **oxidative** cell death in cultured rat PC12 cells. Resveratrol attenuated beta-amyloid-induced cytotoxicity, apoptotic features, and intracellular ROI accumulation."

*The **antioxidant** responsive element (ARE) may explain the protective effects of cruciferous vegetables on **cancer**.* Finley JW. Nutr Rev. 2003 Jul;61(7):250-4. **Key Finding:** "Most studies show that phytochemicals in crucifers upregulate many detoxification enzyme systems in the animal that consumes them. Recent reports of the molecular events involved in the activation of a gene promoter called the antioxidant responsive element have begun to provide clues as to how a single substance may induce a battery of many genes."

Quercetin, a flavonoid antioxidant, prevents and protects against ethanol-induced oxidative stress in mouse liver. Molina MF, Sanchez-Reus I, Inglesias I, Benedi J.

Biol Pharm Bull. 2003 Oct;26(10):1398-402. **Key Finding:** "Pre-treatment of quercetin may protect against ethanol-induced oxidative stress by directly quenching lipid peroxides and indirectly by enhancing the production of the endogenous **antioxidant** GSH. There was no protective effect on post-treatment with quercetin."

*Tea catechins and polyphenols: health effects, metabolism, and **antioxidant** functions.* Higdon JV, Frei B. Crit Rev Food Sci Nutr. 2003;43(1):89-143. **Key Finding:** "In humans, modest transient increases in plasma antioxidant capacity have been demonstrated following the consumption of tea and green tea catechins. The effects of tea and green tea catechins on biomarkers of oxidative stress, especially oxidative DNA damage, appear very promising in animal models, but data on biomarkers of in vivo oxidative stress in humans are limited. Larger human studies examining the effects of tea and tea catechin intake on biomarkers of oxidative damage to lipids, proteins, and DNA are needed."

Green tea polyphenols prevent toxin-induced hepatotoxicity in mice by down-regulating inducible nitric oxide-derived prooxidants. Chen JH, Tipoe GL, Liong EC, et al. Am J Clin Nutr. 2004 Sep;80(3):742-51. **Key Finding:** "Green tea polyphenols reduce the severity of liver injury in association with lower concentrations of lipid peroxidation and proinflammatory nitric oxide-generated mediators. Green tea polyphenols can be a useful supplement in the treatment of **liver disease**."

Polyphenolic flavonoids differ in their antiapoptotic efficacy in hydrogen peroxide-treated human vascular endothelial cells. Choi YJ, Kang JS, Park JH, Lee YJ, Choi JS, Kang YH. J Nutr. 2003 Apr;133(4):985-91. **Key Finding:** "Quercetin and (-)epigallocatechin gallate qualify as potent **antioxidants** and are effective in preventing endothelial apoptosis caused by oxidants, suggesting that flavonoids have differential antiapoptotic efficacies."

Effects of phenol-depleted and phenol-rich diets on blood markers of oxidative stress, and urinary excretion of quercetin and kaempferol in healthy volunteers. Kim HY, Kim OH, Sung MK. J Am Coll Nutr. 2003 Jun;22(3):217-23. **Key Finding:** "These results suggest that polyphenol-rich diets may decrease the risk of **chronic diseases** by reducing oxidative stress."

Antioxidant *and antiproliferative activities of common vegetables.* Chu YF, Sun J, Wu X, Liu RH. J Agric Food Chem. 2002 Nov 6;50(23):6910-6. **Key Finding:** "In this study, 10 common vegetables were selected on the basis of consumption per capita data in the U.S. Broccoli possessed the highest total phenolic content, followed by spinach, yellow onion, red pepper, carrot, cabbage, potato, lettuce, celery, and cucumber. Red pepper had the highest total antioxidant activity, followed by broccoli, carrot, spinach, cabbage, yellow onion, celery, potato, lettuce and cucumber. Antiproliferative activities were also studied in vitro using human liver cancer cells. Spinach showed the highest inhibitory effect, followed by cabbage, red pepper, onion, and broccoli."

The effect of wild blueberry (Vaccinium angustifolium) consumption on postprandial serum ***antioxidant*** *status in human subjects.* Kay CD, Holub BJ. Br J Nutr. 2002 Oct;88(4):389-98. **Key Finding:** "The consumption of wild blueberries, a food source with high in vitro antioxidant properties, is associated with a diet-induced increase in ex vivo serum antioxidant status. It has been suggested that increasing the antioxidant status of serum may result in the reduced risk of many chronic degenerative diseases."

Antioxidant *and antiproliferative activities of raspberries.* Liu M, Li XQ, Weber C, Lee CY, Brown J, Liu RH. J Agric Food Chem. 2002 May 8;50(10):2926-30. **Key Finding:** "The antioxidant activity of the raspberry was directly related to the total amount of phenolics and flavonoids found in the raspberry. No relationship was found between antiproliferative activity and the total amount of phenolics/flavonoids found in the same raspberry."

Flavonoid phytochemicals regulate activator protein-1 signal transduction pathways in endometrial and kidney stable cell lines. Frigo DE, Duong BN, Melnik LI, et al. J Nutr. 2002 Jul;132(7):1848-53. **Key Finding:** "This work suggests that phytochemicals affect multiple signaling pathways that converge at the level of transcriptional regulation. The ability of flavonoids to regulate MAPK-responsive pathways in a selective manner indicates a mechanism by which phytochemicals may influence human health and disease."

Antioxidant *and antiproliferative activities of common fruits.* Sun J, Chu YF, Wu X, Liu RH. J Agric Food Chem. 2002 Dec 4;50(25):7449-54. **Key**

Finding: "This study was designed to investigate the profiles of total phenolics, including both soluble free and bound forms in common fruits, by applying solvent extraction, base digestion, and solid-phase extraction methods. Cranberry had the highest total phenolic content, followed by apple, red grape, strawberry, pineapple, banana. peach, lemon, orange, pear, and grapefruit. Cranberry had the highest total antioxidant activity followed by apple, red grape, strawberry, peach, lemon, pear, banana, orange, grapefruit and pineapple. Cranberry showed the highest antiproliferation activity followed by lemon, apple, strawberry, red grape, banana, grapefruit, and peach."

Antioxidant *health effects of aged garlic extract.* Borek C. J Nutr. 2001 Mar;131(3s):1010S-5S. **Key Finding:** "Although additional observations are warranted in humans, compelling evidence supports the beneficial health effects attributed to aged garlic extract, i.e., reducing the risk of **cardiovascular disease, stroke, cancer and aging**, including the oxidant-mediated brain cell damage that is implicated in **Alzheimer's disease**."

Disparate effects of similar phenolic phytochemicals as inhibitors of oxidative damage to cellular DNA. Kelly MR, Xu J, Alexander KE, Loo G. Mutat Res. 2001 May 10;485(4):309-18. **Key Finding:** Nordihydroguaiaretic acid (NDGA) and curcumin are two phenolic phytochemicals with similar molecular structures. This study evaluated the capacities of NDGA and curcumin to function as antioxidants in inhibiting oxidative damage to DNA. "It is concluded that NDGA has **antioxidant** activity but curcumin has proxidant activity in cultured cells based on their opposite effects on DNA."

Effects of epigallocatechin gallate and quercetin on ***oxidative*** *damage to cellular DNA.* Johnson MK, Loo G. Mutat Res. 2000 Apr 28;459(3):211-8. **Key Finding:** "The aims of this study were to assess the free radical-scavenging activities of several common phenolic phytochemicals, and then the effects of the most potent phenolic phytochemicals on oxidative damage to DNA in cultured cells. Epigallocatechin gallate EGCG scavenged the stable free radical, alpha, alpha-diphenyl-beta-picrylhydrazyl most effectively, while quercetin was about half as effective. Genistein, daidzein, hesperetin and naringenin did not scavenge appreciably."

Cytotoxicity, genotoxicity and oxidative reactions in cell-culture models: modulatory effects of phytochemicals. O'Brien NM, Woods JA, Aherne SA, O'Callaghan YC. Biochem Soc Trans. 2000 Feb;28(2):22-6. **Key Finding:** "Our research examines modulatory effects of phytochemicals on cytotoxicity, genotoxicity and **oxidative** reactions in cell systems. First, the potential benefits of flavonoids are demonstrated. Secondly, we illustrate the use of cellular models to study oxysterol-induced toxicity. Oxysterols are generated during the cooking and processing of foods and may be produced endogenously by the oxidation of membrane lipids."

*A diet high in whole and unrefined foods favorably alters lipids, **antioxidant** defenses, and **colon function**.* Bruce B, Spiller GA, Klevay LM, Gallagher SK. J Am Coll Nutr. 2000 Feb;19(1):61-7. **Key Finding:** "This study compared the effects of a phytochemical-rich diet versus a refined-food diet on lipoproteins, antioxidant defense and colon function. A diet abundant in phytochemical-rich foods beneficially affected lipoproteins, decreased need for oxidative defense mechanisms and improved colon function."

*Role of **antioxidant** lycopene in **cancer** and **heart disease**.* Rao AV, Agarwal S. J Am Coll Nutr. 2000 Oct;19(5):563-9. **Key Finding:** "Serum and tissue lycopene levels have been inversely related with chronic disease risk, such as cancer and cardiovascular disease. Although the antioxidant properties of lycopene are thought to be primarily responsible for its beneficial properties, evidence is accumulating to suggest other mechanisms such as modulation of intercellular gap junction communication, hormonal and immune system and metabolic pathways may also be involved."

Nutritional antioxidants as therapeutic and preventive modalities in exercise-induced muscle damage. Goldfarb AH. Can J Appl. Physiol. 1999 Jun;24(3):249-66. **Key Finding:** This paper reviews the role of isoflavonoids and some phytochemicals and their **antioxidant** properties in the prevention of oxidative stress and muscle damage.

*Tissue injury by **reactive oxygen species** and the protective effect of flavonoids.* De Groot H, Rauen U. Fundam Clin Pharmacol. 1998;12(3):249-55. **Key Finding:** "Reactive oxygen species contribute to a great variety of diseases.

Flavonoids are benzo-gamma-pyrone derivatives of plant origin found in various fruits and vegetables but also in tea and in red wine. Some of the flavonoids, such as quercetin and silibinin, can effectively protect cells and tissues against the deleterious effects of reactive oxygen species."

Relative bioavailability of the **antioxidant** *flavonoid quercetin from various foods in man.* Hollman PC, Van Triip JM, Buysman MN, et al. FEBS Lett. 1997 Nov 24;418(1-2):152-6. **Key Finding:** "We fed nine subjects a single large dose of onions, which contain glucose conjugates of quercetin, apples, which contain both glucose and non-glucose quercetin glycosides, or pure quercetin-3-rutinoside, the major quercetin glycoside in tea. Plasma levels were then measured. Bioavailability of quercetin from apples and of pure quercetin rutinoside was both 30% relative to onions. Peak levels were achieved less than 0.7 h after ingestion of onions, 2.5 h after apples and 9 h after the rutinoside. Half-lives of elimination were 28 h for onions and 23 h for apples. We conclude that conjugation with glucose enhances absorption from the small gut. Because of the long half-lives of elimination, repeated consumption of quercetin-containing foods will cause accumulation of quercetin in blood."

Actions of Carotenoids in Biological Systems. Krinsky NI. Annu Rev Nutr 1993 Jul; 13:561-587. **Key Finding:** This review discusses the evidence to date for carotenoid actions in vitro and in vivo **antioxidant,** antimutagenesis, protection against genotoxicity and malignant transformation, and its **anticarcinogenic** role.

Arthritis

Green tea protects rats against autoimmune **arthritis** *by modulating disease-related immune events.* Kim HR, Rajaiah R, Wu QL, et al. J Nutr. 2008 Nov;138(11):2111-6. **Key Finding:** "We investigated whether polyphenolic compounds from green tea can afford protection against autoimmune arthritis and also examined the immunological basis of this effect using the rat adjuvant arthritis model of human rheumatoid arthritis. Green tea induced changes in arthritis-related immune responses. We suggest further systematic exploration of dietary supplementation with polyphenolic green tea compounds as an adjunct nutritional strategy for the management of **rheumatoid arthritis.**"

Anti-inflammatory and anti-arthritic effects of Yucca schidigera: a review. Cheeke PR, Piacente S, Oleszek W. J Inflamm (Lond). 2006 Mar 29;3:6. **Key Finding:** "Yucca schidigera is a medicinal plant native to Mexico. Yucca phenolics are anti-oxidants and free-radical scavengers, which may aid in suppressing reactive oxygen species that stimulate inflammatory responses. Based on these findings, further studies on the anti-arthritic effects of Yucca schidigera are warranted."

Vegetarian diets: what are the advantages? Leitzmann C. Forum Nutr. 2005;(57):147-56. **Key Finding:** "In most cases, vegetarian diets are beneficial in the prevention and treatment of certain diseases, such as **cardiovascular disease, hypertension, diabetes, cancer, osteoporosis, renal disease and dementia**, as well as **diverticular disease, gallstones, and rheumatoid arthritis.**"

Divergent responses of chondrocytes and endothelial cells to shear stress: Cross-talk among COX-2, the phase 2 response, and apoptosis. Healy ZR, Lee NH, Gao X, et al. Proc Natl Acad Sci. 2005 Sept 27;102(39):14010-5. **Key Finding:** Compounds in edible plants that boost production of phase 2 enzymes have been isolated in this study. These beneficial enzymes seem to prevent the activation of the inflammatory COX-2 enzyme that triggers inflammation in joints. This finding may help to develop therapeutic strategies for **arthritic disorders**.

Asthma

*Dietary intake of flavonoids and **asthma** in adults.* Garcia V, Arts IC, Sterne JA, Thompson RL, Shaheen SO. Eur Respir J. 2005 Sep;26(3):449-52. **Key Finding:** "No evidence was found for a protective effect of three major subclasses of dietary flavonoids on asthma. They were catechins, flavonols and flavones. It is possible that other flavonoids or polyphenols present in apples may explain the protective effect of apples on obstructive lung disease."

Food and nutrient intakes and **asthma** *in young adults.* Woods RK, Walters EH, Raven JM, et al. Am J Clin Nutr. 2003 Sep;78(3):414-21. **Key Finding:** "Apples and pears appeared to protect against current asthma. Intervention studies using whole foods are required to ascertain whether such modifications of food intake could be beneficial in the prevention or amelioration of asthma."

Flavonoid intake and risk of chronic diseases. Knekt P, Kumpulainen J, Jarvinen R, et al. Am J Clin Nutr. 2002 Sep;76(3):560-68. **Key Finding:** "The total dietary intakes of 10,054 men and women were determined with a dietary history method. Persons with higher quercetin intakes had lower mortality from ischemic **heart disease**. The incidence of **cerebrovascular disease** was lower at higher kaempferol, naringenin, and hesperetin intakes. Men with higher quercetin intakes had a lower **lung cancer** incidence and men with higher myricetin intakes had a lower **prostate cancer** risk. **Asthma** incidence was lower at higher quercetin, naringenin, and hesperetin. A trend toward a reduction in risk of **type 2 diabetes** was associated with higher quercetin and myricetin intakes."

Dietary antioxidants and **asthma** *in adults: population-based case-control study.* Shaheen SO, Sterne JA, Thompson RL, Songhurst CE, Margetts BM, Burney PG. Am J Respir Crit Care Med. 2001 Nov 15;164(10 Pt 1):1823-8. **Key Finding:** "Apple consumption was negatively associated with asthma. The associations between apple and red wine consumption and asthma may indicate a protective effect of flavonoids."

Atherosclerosis

Dietary flavonoids as antioxidants. Terao J. Forum Nutr. 2009;61:87-94. **Key Finding:** "Our in vivo study using high cholesterol-fed rabbits also showed accumulation of quercetin metabolites in aortic tissue, and inhibition of deposition of cholesteryl ester hydroperoxide. It is evident that quercetin metabolites are distributed in human **atherosclerotic le-**

sions, particularly the macrophage-derived foam cell. The specific target should therefore be taken into account when evaluating the antioxidant activity of dietary flavonoids in vivo."

Dietary soy protein isolate ameliorates atherosclerotic lesions in apolipoprotein E-deficient mice potentially by inhibiting monocyte chemoattractant protein-1 expression. Nagarajan S, Burris RL, Steward BW, Wilkerson JE, Badger TM. J Nutr. 2008 Feb;138(2):332-7. **Key Finding:** "Collectively, these findings suggest that the reduction in **atherosclerotic lesions** observed in mice fed the soy-based diet is mediated in part by inhibition of MCP-1 that could result in reduced monocyte migration, an early event during atherogenesis."

Comparative effects of quercetin and its predominant human metabolites on adhesion molecule expression in activated human vascular endothelial cells. Tribolo S, Lodi F, Connor C, et al. Atherosclerosis. 2008 Mar;197(1):50-6. **Key Finding:** "These results indicate that both quercetin and its metabolites, at physiological concentrations, can inhibit the expression of key molecules involved in monocyte recruitment during the early stages of **atherosclerosis**."

*Cranberry and blueberry: evidence for protective effects against **cancer** and vascular diseases.* Neto CC. Mol Nutr Food Res. 2007 Jun;51(6):652-64. **Key Finding:** "Growing evidence from tissue culture, animal, and clinical models suggests that the flavonoid-rich fruits of the North American cranberry and blueberry have the potential ability to limit the development and severity of certain cancers and vascular diseases including **atherosclerosis, ischemic stroke**, and neurodegenerative diseases of aging. Cranberry and blueberry constitutents are likely to act by mechanisms that counteract oxidative stress, decrease inflammation, and modulate macro-molecular interactions and expression of genes associated with disease processes."

Nobiletin, a citrus flavonoid, suppresses phorbol ester-induced expression of multiple scavenger receptor genes in THP-1 human monocyte cells. Eguchi A, Murakami A, Ohigashi H. FEBS Lett. 2006 May 29;580(13):3321-8. **Key Finding:** "Our results suggest that nobiletin is a promising phytochemical for regulating **atherosclerosis** with reasonable action mechanisms."

*Dealcoholized red wine containing known amounts of resveratrol suppresses **atherosclerosis** in hypercholesterolemic rabbits without affecting plasma lipid levels.* Wang Z, Zou J, Cao K, Hsieh TC, Huang Y, Wu JM. Int J Mol Med. 2005 Oct;16(4):533-40. **Key Finding:** "To determine whether resveratrol has alcohol-independent effects, we compared cardioprotective properties of dealcoholized Chinese red wine with alcohol containing Chinese red wine having comparable amounts of resveratrol using a hypercholesterolemic rabbit model and resveratrol as a reference. Our study shows that animals given dealcoholized red wine exhibited cardio-active effects comparable to those of animals orally administered resveratrol, and suggests that wine polyphenolics, rather than alcohol present in red wine, suffice in exerting cardioprotective properties. The results also provide support for the notion that resveratrol and phytochemicals in red wine can suppress atherosclerosis without affecting plasma lipid levels."

Flavones mitigate tumor necrosis factor-alpha-induced adhesion molecule upregulation in cultured human endothelial cells: role of nuclear factor-kappa B. Choi JS, Choi YJ, Park SH, Kang JS, Kang YH. J Nutr. 2004 May;134(5):1013-9. **Key Finding:** This study examined the effect of the flavones luteolin and apigenin on adhesion of THP-1 monocytes to the intracellular cell adhesion molecule-1 (ICAM-1) and E-selectin, and nuclear appearance and DNA binding activity of NF-kappa B were determined. The flavones may hamper initial **atherosclerotic** events involving endothelial CAM induction.

The action of dietary phytochemicals quercetin, catechin, resveratrol and naringenin on estrogen-mediated gene expression. Ratna WN, Simonelli JA. Life Sci. 2002 Feb 15;70(13):1577-89. **Key Finding:** "To determine whether dietary phytochemicals purported to prevent hormone-dependent **breast and prostate cancers, and atherosclerosis**, acted via the estrogen-cell-signaling pathway, roosters were administered increasing doses up to 1 mmole/kg of resveratrol, quercetin, catechin, or naringenin parenternally and tested for hepatic expression of E-RmRNASF. Besides estrogen, the expression of E-RmRNASF in the liver was stimulated by resveratrol and catechin, indicating these agents to be estrogenic. A lack of E-Rm-RNASF expression was seen with the roosters treated with the naringenin or quercetin."

*Flavonoids protect LDL from oxidation and attenuate **atherosclerosis**.* Fuhrman B, Aviram M. Curr Opin Lipidol. 2001 Feb;12(1):41-8. **Key Finding:** "Plant flavonoids, as potent natural antioxidants that protect against lipid peroxidation in arterial cells and lipoproteins, significantly attenuate the development of atherosclerosis."

Phytoestrogens and human health effects: weighing up the current evidence. Humfrey CD. Nat Toxins. 1998;6(2):51-9. **Key Finding:** "Epidemiological studies suggest that foodstuffs containing phytoestrogens may have a beneficial role in protecting against a number of chronic diseases and conditions. For cancer of the **prostate, colon, rectum, stomach and lung,** the evidence is most consistent for a protective effect resulting from a high intake of grains, legumes, fruits and vegetables. Dietary intervention studies indicate that in women soya and linseed may have beneficial effects on the risk of **breast cancer** and may help to alleviate **postmenopausal symptoms**. For **osteoporosis**, tentative evidence suggests phytoestrogens may have similar effects in maintaining **bone density**. Soya also appears to have beneficial effects on blood lipids which may help to reduce the risk of **cardiosvascular disease** and **atherosclerosis**. Generally, however, little evidence exists to link these effects directly to phytoestrogens; many other components of soy and linseed are biologically active in various experimental systems and may be responsible for the observed effects in humans."

Attention deficit hyperactivity disorder

*Nutritional and environmental approaches to preventing and treating **autism** and **attention deficit hyperactivity disorder** (ADHD): a review.* Curtis LT, Patel K. J Altern Complement Med. 2008 Jan-Feb;14(1):79-85. **Key Finding:** "Numerous studies have reported that supplemental nutrients such as omega-3 fatty acids, vitamins, zinc, magnesium, and phytochemicals may provide moderate benefits to autism/ADHD patients."

Autism

*Nutritional and environmental approaches to preventing and treating **autism** and **attention deficit hyperactivity disorder** (ADHD): a review.* Curtis LT, Patel K. J Altern Complement Med. 2008 Jan-Feb;14(1):79-85. **Key Finding:** "Numerous studies have reported that supplemental nutrients such as omega-3 fatty acids, vitamins, zinc, magnesium, and phytochemicals may provide moderate benefits to autism/ADHD patients."

Cancer (in general, alimentary, bladder, breast, cervical, colon, gastric, hepatocellular carcinoma, laryngeal, leukemia, liver, lung, non-Hodgkin's lymphoma, neck, oral, ovarian, pancreatic, prostate, renal, skin, stomach)

***Cancer** prevention with natural compounds.* Gullett NP, Ruhul Amin AR, Bayraktar S, et al. Semin Oncol. 2010 Jun;37(3):258-81. **Key Finding**: "Phytochemicals have great potential in cancer prevention because of their safety, low cost, and oral bioavailability. In this review, we discuss potential natural cancer preventive compounds and their mechanisms of action."

Recent trends and advances in berry health benefits research. Seeram NP. J Agric Food Chem. 2010 Apr 14;58(7):3869-70: **Key Finding**: "Recent advances have been made in our scientific understanding of how berries promote human health and prevent chronic illnesses such as some **cancers, heart disease, and neurodegenerative diseases.** Berry bioactives encompass a wide diversity of phytochemicals."

***Antioxidative and antigenotoxic** properties of vegetables and dietary phytochemicals: the value of genomics biomarkers in molecular epidemiology.* de Kok TM, de Waard P, Wilms, LC, van Breda SG. Mol Nutr Food Res. 2010 Feb;54(2):208-17. **Key Finding**: "There is considerable evidence that consumption of fruits and vegetables may contribute to the prevention of cancer. Both human and animal studies demonstrated that vegetable intake modulates gene expression in the gastrointestinal tract of many genes involved in biological pathways in favor of cancer risk prevention.

The use of genomics techniques appears to be a promising approach to establish mechanistic pathways involved in chemoprevention by phytochemicals, particularly when genetic variability is taken into account."

*Reduced **cancer risk** in **vegetarians**: an analysis of recent reports.* Lanou AJ, Svenson B. Cancer Manag Res. 2010 Dec 20;3:1-8. **Key Finding**: "Most large prospective observational studies show that vegetarian and vegan diets are at least modestly cancer protective (10%-12% reduction in overall cancer risk) although results for specific cancers are less clear. A broad body of evidence links specific plant foods and plant constitutents such as phytochemicals to a reduced risk of cancer diagnosis and recurrence. Also, research links the consumption of meat, especially red and processed meats, to increased risk of several types of cancer."

Antimutagenic effects of lycopene and tomato puree. Polivkova Z, Smerak P, Demova H, Houska M. J Med Food. 2010 Dec;13(6):1443-50. **Key Finding**: "Results indicate that lycopene, a tomato carotenoid, has antimutagenic effects, although the effects are lower than that of tomato puree, which contains a complex mixture of bioactive phytochemicals. The antimutagenic effect is connected with the chemopreventive role of lycopene, tomatoes, and tomato products in the prevention of **carcinogenesis.**"

Bioactive compounds in cranberries and their biological properties. Cote J, Cailet S, Doyon G, Sylvain JF, Lacroix M. Crit Rev Food Sci Nutr. 2010 Aug;50(7):666-79. **Key Finding**: "Numerous phytochemicals are present in cranberries – the anthoycanins, the flavonols, the flaven-3-ols, the proanthocyanidins, and the phenolic acid derivatives. The presence of these phytochemicals appears to be responsible for the cranberry property of preventing many diseases and infections, including **cardiovascular diseases, various cancers, and infections** involving the urinary tract, dental health, and Helicobacter pylori-induced stomach ulcers and cancers."

Diet-Derived Phytochemicals: From Chemoprevention to Cardio-Oncological Prevention. Ferrari N, Tosetti F, De Flora S, et al. Curr Drug Targets. 2010 Dec 15. [Epub ahead of print] **Key Finding**: "There is now increasing evidence that some phytochemicals can be protective for the heart, having the potential to reduce cancer, **cardiovascular disease** and even anti-cancer drug-induced cardiotoxicity."

Curcumin in cancer chemoprevention: molecular targets, pharmacokinetics, bioavailability, and clinical trials. Shehzad A, Wahid F, Lee YS. Arch Pharm. 2010 Sep;343(9):489-99. **Key Finding**: "Sufficient data has been shown to advocate phase II and phase III clinical trials of curcumin for a variety of cancer conditions including **multiple myeloma, pancreatic, and colon cancer**."

*Perspectives for **cancer** prevention with natural compounds.* Amin ARM, Kucuk O, Khuri FR, Shin DM. J Clin Oncol. 2009 June 1; 27(16):2712-25. **Key Finding:** "In this review, we discuss promising natural chemopreventive compounds, their molecular targets, and their mechanisms, which may help the further design and conduct of preclinical and clinical trials."

***Anticancer** and chemopreventing natural products: some biochemical and therapeutic aspects.* Karikas GA. J BUON. 2010 Oct-Dec;15(4):627-38. **Key Finding**: "More than 1,000 different phytochemicals are already proved to possess interesting chemopreventing activities. Effectiveness of chemopreventing agents reflects their ability to counteract certain upstream signals that leads to genotoxic damage, redox imbalances and other forms of cellular stress. Chemoprevention by edible phytochemicals is now considered to be an inexpensive, readily applicable, acceptable and accessible approach to cancer control and management."

*Nutrition and the prevention and treatment of **cancer**: association of cytochrome P450 CYP1B1 and the role of fruit and fruit extracts.* Ware WR. Integr Cancer Ther. 2009 Mar;8(1):22-8. **Key Finding:** One potential mechanism for fruits and vegetables to assist in cancer prevention involves the cytochrome P450 enzyme CYP1B1, which appears to be a universal cancer marker overexpressed in cancer cells. A few case histories have been published that use specially designed fruit extracts with demonstrated cytotoxic metabolic products and these reports provide initial confirmation of the potential of exploiting this enzyme for cancer therapy.

Flavonoids inhibit the AU-rich element binding of HuC. Kwak H, Jeong KC, Chae MJ, Kim Sy, Park WY. BMB Rep. 2009 Jan 31;42(1):41-6. **Key**

Finding: Screening of 52 natural compounds identified 14 candidate compounds that displayed potent inhibitory activity in **tumorigenesis.**

Nuclear factor-kappa B links carcinogenic and chemopreventive agents. Ralhan R, Pandey MK, Aggarwal BB. Front Biosci. 2009 Jun 1;1:45-60. **Key Finding:** "Suppression of NF-kappa B activation by the phytochemicals present in fruits and vegetables provides the molecular basis for their ability to prevent **cancer.** The current review discusses in detail numerous agents such curcumin, resveratrol, silymarin, catechins and others as potential chemopreventive agents."

Phytochemicals of cranberries *and cranberry products: characterization, potential health benefits, and processing stability.* Pappas E, Schaich KM. Crit Rev Food Sci Nutr. 2009 Oct;49(9):741-81. **Key Finding**: "Emerging evidence is elucidating how non-nutrient phytochemicals underlie the health promotion afforded by fruits and vegetables. This review focuses on the American cranberry compiling a comprehensive list of its known phytochemical components. Evidence for protection from several **bacterial pathogens, cancer, cardiovascular disease, and inflammation** is compelling, while **neuroprotection and anti-viral activity** also have begun to draw new consideration."

Interindividual differences in response to plant-based diets: implications for ***cancer risk.*** Lampe JW. Am J Clin Nutr. 2009 May;89(5):15535-15575. **Key Finding:** "Genetic polymorphisms in enzymes that metabolize phytochemicals may account in part for variation in disease risk and also have to be considered in the context of other aspects of human genetics, gut bacterial genetics, and environmental exposures."

Modulation of CXCR4, CXCL12, and tumor cell invasion potential in vitro by phytochemicals. Hsu EL, Chen N, Westbrook A, et al. J Oncol. 2009:491985. Epub 2009 Mar 24. **Key Finding:** "Our data suggest a novel mechanism for the protective effects of phytochemicals against **cancer** progression and indicate that in combination, these compounds may prove even more efficacious."

Chemoprevention with phytochemicals targeting inducible nitric oxide synthase. Murakami A. Forum Nutr. 2009;61:193-203. **Key Finding:** A regulated low level of nitric oxide production in the body is essential for maintaining homeostasis. "This review highlights the molecular mechanisms underlying endotoxin-induced NOS expression in macrophages and also focuses on promising natural agents that may be useful for anti-inflammation and anticarcinogenesis strategies."

Phytochemicals as modulators of neoplastic phenotypes. Ding H, Tauzin S, Hoessli DC. Pathobiology. 2009;76(2):55-63. **Key Finding:** "Despite important gaps in our knowledge regarding how phytochemicals interfere with cellular function in vivo, effective chemopreventive measures have shown that phytochemicals can be utilized to prevent **cancer,** and possibly to treat cancer patients as well. We review how phytochemicals exert their beneficial effects at the cellular level."

Phytochemicals that counteract the cardiotoxic side effects of ***cancer*** *chemotherapy.* Piasek A, Baroszek A, Namiesnik J. Postepy Hig Med Dosw. 2009 Apr 17;63:142-58. **Key Finding:** "Although to date only a limited number of investigations have been carried out, their results suggest that dietary intervention with antioxidants found in edible plants may be a safe and effective way of alleviating the toxicity of anticancer chemotherapy and preventing heart failure."

Natural antioxidants: therapeutic prospects for ***cancer*** *and* ***neurological diseases****.* Mates JM, Segura JA, Alonso FJ, Marquez J. Mini Rev Med Chem. 2009 Aug 1. [Epub ahead of print] **Key Finding:** This review provides "an updated revision of the function of some natural compounds having main roles in antioxidant function. We will point on some phytochemicals working at two outstanding targets, tumour cells and neurons."

Metabolic regulation and redox activity as mechanisms for angioprevention by dietary phytochemicals. Tosetti F, Noonan DM, Albini A. Int J Cancer. 2009 Nov 1;125(9):1997-2003. **Key Finding:** "We discuss recent findings on the metabolic effects of several phytochemicals with **anticancer** properties. The different molecular targets shared by these compounds seem to converge on crosstalking signaling networks involved in controlled energy metabolism through a redox-regulated code."

*Molecular basis for **cancer** chemoprevention by green tea polyphenol EGCG.* Tachibana H. Forum Nutr. 2009;61:156-69. **Key Finding:** "This article reviews some of the reported mechanisms and possible targets for the action of EGCG. We especially focus on the current understanding of the signaling pathway for physiologically relevant EGCG through the 67LR for cancer prevention."

Epigallocatechin-3-gallate reduces DNA damage induced by benzo[a]pyrene diol epoxide and cigarette smoke condensates in human mucosa tissue cultures. Baumeister P, Reiter M, Kleinsasser N, Matthias C, Harreus U. Eur J Cancer Prev. 2009 Jun;18(3):230-5. **Key Finding:** "Data suggest a **cancer** preventive potential of epigallocatechin-3-gallate as demonstrated on a subcellular level. An additional mechanism of tea catechin action is revealed by using a primary mucosa culture model."

*Dietary intake of selected flavonols, flavones, and flavonoid-rich foods and risk of **cancer** in middle-aged and older women.* Wang L, Lee IM, Zhang SM, et al. Am J Clin Nutr. 2009 Mar;89(3):905-12. **Key Finding:** "A total of 3,234 incident cancer cases were identified during 11.5 years of follow-up among 38,408 women. Intake of individual flavonoids (quercetin, kaempferol, and myricetin) and flavones (apigenin and luteolin) was assessed from food-frequency questionnaires. Our results do not support a major role of 5 common flavonols and flavones or selected flavonoid-rich foods in cancer prevention."

*The effect of genistein aglycone on cancer and **cancer** risk: a review of in vitro, preclinical, and clinical studies.* Taylor CK, Levy RM, Elliot JC, Burnett BP. Nutr Rev. 2009 Jul;67(7):398-415. **Key Finding:** "The recent increased intake of soy foods and supplements in the American diet has raised concerns about the possible estrogen-like effects of natural isoflavones and possible promotion or propagation of estrogen-sensitive cancers. These concerns are primarily based on in vitro and roden data which suggest that genistein aglycone can stimulate tumor cell proliferation and growth in mice having deficient immune systems. In contrast, a recent nested case-control study and meta-analysis of numerous epidemiological studies show an inverse correlation between genistein intake and breast cancer risk."

Green tea (Camellia sinensis) for the prevention of **cancer**. Boehm K, Borrelli F, Ernst E, et al. Cochrane Database Syst Rev. 2009 Jul 8;(3):CD005004. **Key Finding:**"There is insufficient and conflicting evidence to give any firm recommendations regarding green tea consumption for cancer prevention. The results of this review, including its trends of associations, need to be interpreted with caution and their generalisability is questionable, as the majority of included studies were carried out in Asia where the tea drinking culture is pronounced."

Potential of spice-derived phytochemicals for **cancer** *prevention.* Aggarwal BB, Kunnumakkara AB, Harikumar KB, et al. Planta Med. 2008 Oct;74(13):1560-9. **Key Finding:** "The potential of turmeric (curcumin), red chilli (capsaicin), cloves (eugenol), ginger (zerumbone), fennel (anethole), kokum (gambogic acid), fenugreek (diosgenin), and black cumin (thymoquinone) in cancer prevention has been established. Additionally, the mechanism by which these agents mediate anticancer effects is also becoming increasingly evident. The current review describes the active components of some of the major spices, their mechanisms of action and their potential in cancer prevention."

Targeting cancer stem cells with phytochemicals. Kawasaki BT, Hurt EM, Mistree T, Farrar WL. Mol Interv. 2008 Aug;8(4):174-84. **Key Finding:** "Phytochemicals possess anti-cancer properties and represent a promising therapeutic approach for the prevention and treatment of many cancers. This review summarizes the evidence for the **cancer** stem cell hypothesis and discusses the potential mechanisms by which phytochemicals might target cancer stem cells."

Interactive effects of polymethoxy flavones from Citrus on cell growth inhibition in human neuroblastoma SH-SYSY cells. Akao Y, Itoh T, Ohguchi K, Iinuma M, Nozawa Y. Bioorg Med Chem. 2008 Mar 15;16(6):2803-10. **Key Finding:** The interactive effects of polymethoxy flavones from Citrus on cell growth were investigated. "These results indicate the relevance of the combination of phytochemicals for the enhancement of the **anticancer** effect."

Fractionation of polyphenol-enriched apple juice extracts to identify constitutents with **cancer** *chemopreventive potential.* Zessner H, Pan L, Will F, et al. Mol Nutr

Food Res. 2008 Jun;52 Suppl 1:S28-44. **Key Finding:** Apple juice extract was fractionated to determine which constituents contribute to potential chemopreventive activities. "Overall, apple juice constituents belonging to different structural classes have distinct profiles of biological activity in these in vitro test systems. Since carcinogenesis is a complex process, combination of compounds with complementary activities may lead to enhanced preventive effects."

DNA-protective potential of polyphenols in human mucosa cell cultures. Baumeister P, Reiter M, Zieger S, Matthias C, Harreus U. HNO. 2008 Aug;56(8):795-8. **Key Finding:** "By incubating minorgan cultures with the polyphenols (epigallocatechin gallate ECGC, and tannin TA), the DNA damage caused by BPDE was significantly decreased at all concentrations. To our knowledge, this is the first test using cell cultures produced from fresh biopsies that demonstrate ECGC and TA as promising chemopreventive agents and confirms nutritional studies."

Mechanisms of combined action of different chemopreventive dietary compounds: a review. De Kok TM, Van Breda SG, Manson MM. Eur J Nutr. 2008 May;47 Suppl 2:51-9. **Key Finding:** "Evidence is emerging that specific combinations of phytochemicals may be far more effective in protecting against **cancer** than isolated compounds. Our understanding of the molecular mechanisms underlying such synergistic effects is still limited, but it appears that different combinations of complementary modes of actions are involved. In this review, we discuss the molecular mechanisms that are likely to be involved in cancer chemoprevention and summarize the most important findings of those studies that report synergistic chemopreventive effects of dietary compounds."

*The **cancer** chemopreventive actions of phytochemicals derived from glucosinolates.* Hayes JD, Kelleher MO, Eggleston IM. Eur J Nutr. 2008 May;47 Suppl 2:73-88. **Key Finding:** "Isothiocyanates and indoles are capable of affecting cell cycle arrest and stimulating apoptosis. The mechanisms responsible for these anti-proliferative responses are discussed."

Phytochemical composition of nuts. Chen CY, Blumberg JB. Asia Pac J Clin Nutr. 2008; 17 Suppl 1:329-32. **Key Finding:** Tree nuts and peanuts contain numerous phytochemicals that "may contribute to promoting health and reducing the risk of chronic disease," including **cardiovascular disease** and **cancer**. "While many of these bioactive constituents remain to be fully identified and characterized, broad classes include carotenoids, phenols, and phytoesterols." Walnuts are particularly rich in total phenols.

Anticancer activities of cranberry phytochemicals: an update. Neto CC, Amoroso JW, Liberty AM. Mol Nutr Food Res. 2008 Jun;52 Suppl 1:S18-27. **Key Finding:** "Studies employing mainly in vitro tumor models show that extracts and compounds isolated from cranberry fruit inhibit the growth and proliferation of several types of tumor including breast, colon, prostate, and lung. Proanthocyanidin oligomers, flavonol and anthocyanin glycosides and triterpenoids are all likely contributors to the observed anticancer properties and may act in a complementary fashion to limit carcinogenesis."

Inhibition of P-glycoprotein and multidrug resistance protein 1 by dietary phytochemicals. Nabekura T, Yamaki T, Ueno K, Kitagawa S. Cancer Chemother Pharmacol. 2008 Oct;62(5):867-73. **Key Finding:** "These results suggest that dietary phytochemicals, such as glycyrrhetinic acid found in licorice, have dual inhibitory effects on P-glycoprotein and MRP1 and might become useful to enhance the efficacy of **cancer** chemotherapy."

Anticarcinogenesis by dietary phytochemicals: cytoprotection by Nrf2 in normal cells and cytotoxicity by modulation of transcription factors NF-kappa B and Ap-1 in abnormal **cancer** *cells.* Gopalakrishnan A, Tony Kong AN. Food Chem Toxicol. 2008 Apr;46(4):1257-70. **Key Finding:** "This review discusses the most current and up to date understanding of the possible signaling mechanisms by which these natural dietary phytochemicals can differentially modulate signal transduction cascades such that they can bring about apoptosis/cell death in abnormal cancer cells but at the same time induce defensive enzymes to protect against carcinogenesis in normal cells."

Multi-targeted prevention of cancer by sulforaphane. Clarke JD, Dashwood RH, Ho E. Cancer Lett. 2008 Oct 8;269(2):291-304. **Key Finding:** "This review discusses the established **anti-cancer** properties of sulforaphane, an isothiocyanate found especially high in broccoli and broccoli sprouts, with an emphasis on the possible chemoprevention mechanisms. The current status of SFN in human clinical trials also is included, with consideration of the chemistry, metabolism, absorption and factors influencing SFn bioavailability."

*Apple procyanidins induce **tumor cell** apoptosis through mitochondrial pathway activation of caspase-3.* Miura T, Chiba M, Kasai K, et al. Carcinogenesis. 2008 Mar;29(3):585-93. **Key Finding:** "Our results indicate that the oral administration of apple procyanidins inhibits the proliferation of tumor cells by inducing apoptosis through the intrinsic mitochondrial pathway."

*Ins and outs of dietary phytochemicals in **cancer** chemoprevention.* Russo GL. Biochem Pharmacol. 2007 Aug 15;74(4):533-44. **Key Finding:** The bioavailability of phytochemical compounds is discussed, as is whether purified phytochemicals have the same protective effects as whole food mixtures of the compounds; also, the synergistic effects of compounds present in the diet.

***Cancer** control by phytochemicals.* Nishino H, Satomi Y, Tokuda H, Masuda M. Curr Pharm Des. 2007;13(33):3394-9. **Key Finding:** "Chemoprevention is one of the most important strategies in the field of cancer control. Molecular mechanism-based cancer chemoprevention by phytochemicals seems to be a very attractive method. In this review, possible molecular targets for cancer prevention are overviewed, and some examples of cancer prevention phytochemicals, such as carotenoids, are presented."

*Extended treatment with physiologic concentrations of dietary phytochemicals results in altered gene expression, reduced growth, and apoptosis of **cancer** cells.* Moiseeva EP, Almeida GM, Jones GD, Manson MM. Mol Center Ther. 2007 Nov;6(11):3071-9. **Key Finding:** "Curcumin, DIM, EGCG, and genistein reduced cell sensitivity to radiation-induced DNA damage without affecting DNA repair. This model has revealed that apoptosis and not arrest is likely to be responsible for growth inhibition. It also implicated new molecular targets and activities of the agents under conditions relevant to human exposure."

Targeting NOX, INOS and COX-2 inflammatory cells: chemoprevention using food phytochemicals. Murakami A, Ohigashi H. Int J Cancer. 2007 Dec 1;121(11):2357-63. **Key Finding:** "Herein, the **cancer** preventive potentials of several food phytochemicals targeting the induction of NOX, INOS and Cox-2 are described."

*Determining the efficacy of dietary phytochemicals in **cancer** prevention.* Manson MM, Foreman BE, Howells LM, Moiseeva EP. Biochem Soc Trans. 2007 Nov;35(Pt 5):1358-63. **Key Finding:** "Accumulating data suggest that dietary phytochemicals have the potential to moderate deregulated signaling or reinstate checkpoint pathways and apotosis in damaged cells, while having minimal impact on healthy cells. These are ideal characteristics for chemopreventive and combination anticancer strategies."

*Role of nutrition in preventing **cancer**.* Beliveau R, Gingras D. Can Fam Physician. 2007 Nov;53(11):1905-11. **Key Finding:** "Dietary factors play an important role in the high incidence of several types of cancer in Canada. Modification of dietary habits to include daily intake of plant-based food containing anticancer and anti-inflammatory phytochemicals thus represents a promising approach to preventing the development of cancer."

*Phytochemical regulation of UDP-glucuronosyltransferases: implications for **cancer** prevention.* Saracino MR, Lampe JW. Nutr Cancer. 2007;59(2):121-41. **Key Finding:** UGTs are Phase II biotransformation enzymes that metabolize endogenous and exogenous compounds, some of which have been associated with cancer risk. "In this review, we summarize the knowledge of dietary modulation of UGTs, particularly by phytochemicals, and discuss the potential mechanisms by which phytochemicals regulate UGT transcription."

*Cranberry and its phytochemicals: a review of in vitro **anticancer** studies.* Neto CC. J Nutr. 2007 Jan;137(1 Suppl):186S-193S. **Key Finding:** "This article reviews existing research on the anticancer properties of cranberry fruit and key phytochemicals that are likely contributors to chemoprevention. The unique combination of phytochemicals found in cranberry fruit may produce synergistic health benefits."

Molecular basis for chemoprevention by sulforaphane: a comprehensive review. Judge N, Mithen RF, Traka M. Cell Mol Life Sci. 2007 May;64(9):1105-27. **Key Finding:** "It is becoming clear that there are multiple mechanisms activated in response to sulforaphane, including suppression of cytochrome P450 enzymes, induction of apoptotic pathways, suppression of cell cycle progression, inhibition of angiogenesis and anti-inflammatory activity. Moreover, these mechanisms seem to have some degree of interaction to synergistically afford chemoprevention."

*Ins and outs of dietary phytochemicals in **cancer** chemoprevention.* Russo GL. Biochem Pharmacol. 2007 Aug 15;74(4):533-44. **Key Finding:** The bioavailability of phytochemical compounds is discussed, as is whether purified phytochemicals have the same protective effects as whole food mixtures of the compounds; also, the synergistic effects of compounds present in the diet.

*Biomarker and animal models for assessment of retinoid efficacy in **cancer** chemoprevention.* Niles RM. Acta Pharmacol Sin. 2007 Sep;28(9):1383-91. **Key Finding:** "The potential combination of phytochemicals that inhibit DNA methyltransferase activity with retinoids holds promise for more effective chemoprevention of retinoid-unresponsive premalignant lesions."

*Discovery and development of sulforaphane as a **cancer** chemopreventive phytochemical.* Zhang Y, Tang L. Acta Pharmacol Sin. 2007 Sep;28(9):1343-54. **Key Finding:** "We review the discovery of sulforaphane and its development as a cancer chemopreventive agent with the intention of encouraging further research on this important compound and facilitating the identification and development of new phytochemicals for cancer prevention."

*Targeting carcinogen metabolism by dietary **cancer** preventive compounds.* Yu S., Kong AN. Curr Cancer Drug Targets. 2007 Aug;7(5):416-24. **Key Finding:** "In the present review, the specific molecular targets of dietary compounds within carcinogen metabolism, including various enzymes and transporters and their regulatory signaling pathways, are briefly reviewed."

***Cancer** preventive phytochemicals as speed breakers in inflammatory signaling involved in aberrant COX-2 expression.* Surh YJ, Kundu JK. Curr Cancer Drug Targets. 2007 Aug;7(5):447-58. **Key Finding:** "This review highlights the cancer preventive effects of some anti-inflammatory phytochemicals derived from edible plants, and their underlying molecular mechanisms with a focus on representative transcription factors and upstream kinases responsible for COX-2 induction."

Cancer prevention by dietary bioactive components that target the immune response. Ferguson LR, Philpott M. Curr Cancer Drug Targets. 2007 Aug;7(5):459-64. **Key Finding:** "Some of the most potent immunomodulators are phytochemicals such as the polyphenols, EGCG or curcumin, or isothiocyanates such as PEITC."

Interindividual differences in phytochemical metabolism and disposition. Lampe JW, Chang JL. Semin Cancer Biol. 2007 Oct;17(5):347-53. **Key Finding:** "Many phytochemicals possess biologic effects associated with reduced risk of various diseases such as **cancer.** Genetic variation in pathways affecting absorption, metabolism, and distribution of phytochemicals is likely to influence exposure at the tissue level, thus modifying disease risk. Few studies have examined these gene-phytochemical interactions in humans. In this review, we discuss the sources of variation in metabolism and disposition of phytochemicals, and focus on two aspects of phytochemical handling that have received some attention: the impact of intestinal bacteria and genetically polymorphic phase II conjugating enzymes."

Chemopreventive characteristics of avocado fruit. Ding H, Chin YW, Kinghorn AD, D'Ambrosio SM. Semin Cancer Biol. 2007 Oct;17(5):386-94. **Key Finding:** "This review summarizes the reported phytochemicals in avocado fruit and discusses their molecular mechanisms and targets. These studies suggest that individual and combinations of phytochemicals from the avocado fruit may offer an advantageous dietary strategy in **cancer** prevention."

Antigenotoxic effects of the phytoestrogen pelargonidin chloride and the polyphenol chlorogenic acid. Abraham SK, Schupp N, Schmidt U, Stopper H. Mol Nutr Food Res. 2007 Jul;51(7):880-7. **Key Finding:** "Pelargonidin (PEL), a common anthocyanidin with estrogenic activity, was tested in HL-60 cells for its genotoxicity and possible antigenotoxic effects against 4-nitroquinoline 1-oxide, a potent mutagen and carcinogen which induces oxidative stress. The phytoestrogen PEL revealed antioxidative and antigenotoxic properties in HL-60 cells, but no significant additive interaction with the abundant nutritional polyphenol CLA under the tested conditions."

Polyphenols and cancer cell growth. Kampa M, Nifil AP, Notas G, Castanas E. Rev Physiol Biochem Pharmacol. 2007;159:79-113. **Key Finding:** "We briefly review the effects of polyphenols on cancer cell fate, leading towards growth, differentiation and apoptosis. Their action can be attributed not only to their ability to act as antioxidants but also to their ability to interact with basic cellular mechanisms."

Cranberry and blueberry: evidence for protective effects against cancer and vascular diseases. Neto CC. Mol Nutr Food Res. 2007 Jun;51(6):652-64. **Key Finding:** "Growing evidence from tissue culture, animal, and clinical models suggests that the flavonoid-rich fruits of the North American cranberry and blueberry have the potential ability to limit the development and severity of certain cancers and vascular diseases including **atherosclerosis, ischemic stroke**, and neurodegenerative diseases of aging. Cranberry and blueberry constitutents are likely to act by mechanisms that counteract oxidative stress, decrease inflammation, and modulate macromolecular interactions and expression of genes associated with disease processes."

Berry phytochemicals, genomic stability and cancer: evidence for chemoprotection at several stages in the carcinogenic process. Duthie SJ. Mol Nutr Food Res. 2007 Jun;51(6):665-74. **Key Finding:** "There is strong and convincing evidence that berry extracts and berry phytochemicals modulate biomarkers of DNA damage and indicators of malignant transformation in vitro and in vivo. Exactly which berry constituents are cytoprotective remains uncertain and in the majority of in vitro and in vivo studies the concentration of extract or phytochemical employed is non-nutritional. Evidence for an anticarcinogenic effect in human studies is weak."

Phytochemicals and cancer. Johnson IT. Proc Nutr Soc. 2007 May;66(2):207-15. **Key Finding:** "Many phytochemicals present in plant foods are poorly absorbed by human subjects, and this fraction usually undergoes metabolism and rapid excretion. Some compounds that do exert anticarcinogenic effects at realistic doses may contribute to the putative benefits of plant foods such as berries, brassica vegetables and tea, but further research with human subjects is required to fully confirm and quantify such benefits."

Natural dietary anti-cancer chemopreventive compounds: redox-mediated differential signaling mechanisms in cytoprotection of normal cells versus cytotoxicity in tumor cells. Nair S, Li W, Kong AN. Acta Pharmacol Sin. 2007 Apr;28(4):459-72. **Key Finding:** "In the current review, we explore dietary **cancer** chemopreventive phytochemicals, discuss the link between oxidative/electrophilic stresses and the redox circuitry, and consider different redox-sensitive transcription factors."

*Phytosterols as **anticancer** compounds.* Bradford PG, Awad AB. Mol Nutr Food Res. 2007 Feb;51(2):161-70. **Key Finding:** "Phytosterols have effects that directly inhibit tumor growth, including the slowing of cell cycle progression, the induction of apoptosis, and the inhibition of tumor metastasis. This review summarizes the current state of knowledge regarding the anticancer effects of phytosterols."

*Dietary polyphenolic phytochemicals—promising **cancer** chemopreventive agents in humans? A review of their clinical properties.* Thomasset SC, Berry DP, Garcea G, et al. Int J Cancer. 2007 Feb 1;120(3):451-8. **Key Finding:** "We present a review of pilot studies and trials with a cancer chemoprevention-related rationale in which either healthy individuals or patients with premalignant conditions or cancer received polyphenolic phytochemicals. The abundance of flavonoids and related polyphenols in the plant kingdom makes it possible that several hitherto uncharacterized agents with chemopreventive efficacy are still to be identified, which may constitute attractive alternatives to currently used chemopreventive drugs."

*Green tea polyphenols: biology and therapeutic implications in **cancer**.* Shankar S, Ganapathy S, Srivastava RK. Front Biosci. 2007 Sep 1;12:4881-99. **Key Finding:** "Green tea polyphenols inhibit angiogenesis and metastasis, and induce growth arrest and apoptosis through regulation of multiple signaling pathways. This review discusses the molecular mechanisms of green tea polyphenols and their therapeutic implications in cancer."

*Sulforaphane as a promising molecule for fighting **cancer**.* Fimognari C, Hrelia P. Mutat Res. 2007 May-Jun;635(2-3):90-104. **Key Finding:** "Sulforaphane has received a great deal of attention because of its ability to simultaneously modulate multiple cellular targets involved in cancer development. SFN is able to prevent, delay, or reverse preneoplastic lesions, as well as to act on cancer cells as a therapeutic agent."

*Cruciferous vegetables and human **cancer** risk: epidemiologic evidence and mechanistic basis.* Higdon JV, Delage B, Williams DE, Dashwood RH. Pharmacol Res. 2007 Mar;55(3):224-36. **Key Finding:** "Epidemiological studies indicate that human exposure to isothiocyanates and indoles through cruciferous vegetable consumption may decrease cancer risk, but the protective effects may be influenced by individual genetic variation (polymorphisms) in the metabolism and elimination of isothiocyanates from the body. Cooking procedures also affect the bioavailability and intake of glucosinolates and their derivatives."

*Molecular targets of dietary agents for prevention and therapy of **cancer**.* Aggarwal BB, Shishodia S. Biochem Pharmacol. 2006 May 14;71(10):1397-421. **Key Finding:** "In this review, we present evidence that numerous agents identified from fruits and vegetables can interfere with several cell-signaling pathways. The active principle identified in fruit and vegetables and the molecular targets modulated may be the basis for how these dietary agents not only prevent but also treat cancer and other diseases."

*Current trends and perspectives in nutrition and **cancer** prevention.* Barta I, Smerak P, Polivkova Z, et al. Neoplasma. 2006;53(1):19-25. **Key Finding:** "All complete vegetable homogenates and substances of plant origin tested showed a clear antimutagenic and immunomodulatory activities on mutagenicity and immunosuppression induced by reference mutagens."

Pre-exposure to a novel nutritional mixture containing a series of phytochemicals prevents acetaminophen-induced programmed and unprogrammed cell deaths by enhancing BCL-XL expression and minimizing oxidative stress in the liver. Ray SD, Patel N, Shah N, et al. Mol Cell Biochem. 2006 Dec;293(1-2):119-36. **Key Finding:** "We proposed that the additive and synergistic effects of phytochemicals in fruits and vegetables are responsible for these potent **antioxidant** and **anticancer** activities, and that the benefit of a diet rich in fruits and vegetables is attributed to the complex mixture of phytochemicals present in plants. Our investigation suggests that a mixture containing an assortment of phytochemicals/nutraceuticals may serve as a much more powerful blend in preventing drug or chemical-induced organ injuries than a single phytochemical or nutraceutical entity."

Methyl-3-indolylacetate inhibits **cancer** *cell invasion by targeting the MEK1/2-ERK1/2 signaling pathway.* Zhang S, Li Z, Wu X, et al. Mol Cancer Ther. 2006 Dec;5(12):3285-93. **Key Finding:** "Data from this study provided new insight into the anticancer potential of methyl-3-indolylacetate, a cruciferous vegetable-derived indole compound."

Potential synergism of natural products in the treatment of **cancer.** HemaIswarya S, Dobie M. Phytother Res. 2006 Apr;20(4):239-49. **Key Finding:** "This review focuses on a number of reports of herb-drug interactions, their mechanism of action with a special emphasis on dietetic phytochemicals such as quercetin, genistein, curcumin, and catechins. All phytochemicals tend to increase the therapeutic effect by blocking one or more targets of the signal transduction pathway, by increasing the bioavailability of the other drug or, by stabilizing the other drug in the system."

Toxicological aspects of flavonoid interaction with biomacromolecules. Hodek P, Hanustiak P, Krizhova J, et al. Neuro Endocrinol Lett. 2006 Dec;27 Suppl 2:14-7. **Key Finding:** "Some flavonoids show ability of direct interaction with DNA and/or enhance **carcinogen** activation into DNA modifying agents. Induction of CYP1A1 was elicited by the typical citrus flavonoid naringenin in the colon, as well as by flavone in the liver. Moreover, synthetic beta-naphthoflavone and naturally occurring chrysin, quercetin and diosmin induced CYP1A1 in both tissues."

The role of polyphenols in **cancer** *chemoprevention.* Lee KW, Lee HJ. Biofactors. 2006;26(2):105-21. **Key Finding:** "This article reviews the intracellular signaling pathways that respond to oxidative stress and how they are modulated by naturally occurring polyphenols. The possible toxicity and carcinogenicity of polyphenols is also discussed."

Intracellular signaling network as a prime chemopreventive target of (-)-epigallocatechin gallate. Na HK, Surh YJ. Mol Nutr Food Res. 2006 Feb;50(2):152-9. **Key Finding:** "EGCG, a principal antioxidant derived from green tea, has been known to block each stage of **carcinogenesis** by modulating signal transduction pathways involved in cell proliferation, transformation, inflammation, apoptosis, metastasis and invasion. This review addresses the molecular target-based chemoprevention with EGCG."

*Current trends and perspectives in nutrition and **cancer** prevention.* Barta I, Smerak P, Polivkova Z, et al. Neoplasma. 2006;53(1):19-25. **Key Finding:** "We investigated antigenotoxic and immunomodulatory effects of juices and vegetable homogenates (carrot+cauliflower, cauliflower, red cabbage, broccoli, onion, garlic) on the genotoxicity of AFB1 and pyrolysates of amino acids. All complete vegetable homogenates and substances of plant origin tested showed clear antimutagenic and immunomodulatory activities on mutagenicity and immunosuppression induced by reference mutagens."

Purple grape juice inhibits 7,12-dimethylbenz[a]anthracene (DMBA)-induced rat mammary tumorigenesis and in vivo DMBA-DNA adduct formation. Jung KJ, Wallig MA, Singletary KW. Cancer Lett. 2006 Feb 28;233(2):279-88. **Key Finding:** "Grape juice constitutents appear to have benefit in decreasing susceptibility of the rat mammary gland to the **tumor**-initiating action of DMBA."

Apiaceous vegetable constitutents inhibit human cytochrome P-450 1A2 (hCYP1A2) activity and hCYP1A2-mediated mutagenicity of aflatoxin B1. Peterson S, Lampe JW, Bammler TK, Gross-Steinmeyer K, Eaton DL. Food Chem Toxicol. 2006 Sep;44(9):1474-84. **Key Finding:** "In humans, apiaceous vegetables (carrots, parsnips, celery, parsley, etc.) inhibit cytochrome P-450 1A2, a biotranscriptional enzyme known to activate several procarcinogens, including aflatoxin B1. We evaluated eight phytochemicals from apiaceous vegetables for effects on human cytochrome P-450 1A2. These results suggest that in vivo CYP1A2 inhibition by apiaceous vegetables may be due to the phytochemicals present and imply that apiaceous vegetable intake may be chemopreventive by inhibiting CYP1A2-mediated **carcinogent** activation."

Indole-3-carbinol in the maternal diet provides chemoprotection for the fetus against trans-placental carcinogenesis by the polycyclic aromatic hydrocarbon dibenzo[a,l]pyrene. Yu Z, Mahadevan B, Lohr CV, et al. Carcinogenesis. 2006 Oct;27(10):2116-23. **Key Finding:** "The bioavailability of Indole-3-carbinol was determined by dosing a subset of pregnant mice. Addition of chemoprotective agents to the maternal diet during pregnancy and nursing may be an effective new approach in reducing the incidence of **cancers** in children and young adults."

*Natural flavonoids targeting deregulated cell cycle progression in **cancer** cells.* Singh RP, Agarwal R. Curr Drug Targets. 2006 Mar;7(3):345-54. **Key Finding:** "This review is focused on the modulatory effects of natural flavonoids on cell cycle regulators including cyclin-dependent kinases and their inhibitors, cyclins, p53, retinoblastoma family of proteins, E2Fs, check-point kinases, ATM/ATR and surviving controlling G1/S and G2/M check-point transitions in cell cycle progression, and discusses how these molecular changes could contribute to the antineoplastic effects of natural flavonoids."

Neoplastic transformation of BALB/3T3 cells and cell cycle of HL-60 cells are in-hibited by mango (Mangifera indica L.) juice and mango juice extracts. Percival SS, Talcott ST, Chin ST, et al. J Nutr. 2006 May;136(5):1300-4. **Key Finding:** "In this study, whole mango juice and juice extracts were screened for **antioxidant** and **anticancer** activity. Incubation of HL-60 cells with whole mango juice and mango juice fractions resulted in an inhibition of the cell cycle in the G(0)G(1) phase. A fraction of the eluted mango juice with low peroxyl radical scavenging ability was most effective in arresting cells in the G(0)G(1) phase."

Modulation of apoptosis in Na CaT keratinocytes via differential regulation of ERK signaling pathway by flavonoids. Lee ER, Kang YJ, Kim JH, Lee HT, Cho SG. J Biol Chem. 2005 Sep 9;280(36):31498-507. **Key Finding:** "Taken together, our data clearly indicate that a host of phytochemicals, including etoposide and a variety of flavonoids, differentially regulate the apoptosis of human HaCaT keratinocytes via the differential modulation of intracellular ROS production, coupled with the concomitant activation of the ERK signaling pathway."

Modulation of signal transduction by tea catechins and related phytochemicals. Shimizu M, Weinstein IB. Mutat Res. 2005 Dec 11;591(1-2):147-60. **Key Finding:** "The purpose of this paper is to review evidence that these effects (inhibition of growth and induced apoptosis in a variety of **cancer** cell lines) by EGCG, a biologically active component of green tea, are mediated, at least in part, through inhibition of the activity of specific receptor tyrosine kinases and related downstream pathways of signal transduction."

Effects of soy protein and soy phytochemicals on mammary tumor development in female transgenic mice overexpressing human pituitary growth hormone. Hickey J, Bartke A, Winters T, Henry N, Banz W. J Med Food. 2005 Winter;8(4):556-9. **Key Finding:** "These data suggest that a diet rich in soy protein may provide protective benefits regarding tumor development in female **cancer**-prone mice."

Redox-sensitive transcription factors as prime targets for chemoprevention with anti-inflammatory and antioxidative phytochemicals. Surh YJ, Kundu JK, Na HK, Lee JS. J Nutr. 2005 Dec;135(12 Suppl):2993S-3001S. **Key Finding:** "The modulation of cellular signaling by anti-inflammatory phytochemicals hence provides a rational and pragmatic strategy for molecular target-based chemoprevention."

***Cancer** prevention by phytochemicals.* Nishino H, Murakoshi M, Mou XY, et al. Oncology. 2005;69 Suppl 1:38-40. **Key Finding:** "A mixture of natural carotenoids has been studied extensively and proven to show beneficial effects on human cancer prevention."

Chinese cabbage extracts and sulforaphane can protect H2O2-induced inhibition of gap junctional intercellular communication through the inactivation of ERK1/2 and p38 MAP kinases. Hwang JW, Park JS, Jo EH, et al. J Agric Food Chem. 2005 Oct 19;53(21):8205-10. **Key Finding:** "The results suggest that cruciferous vegetables and their components, sulforaphane glucosinolate, may exert the **anticancer** effect by targeting the GJIC (gap junctional intercellular communication) as a functional dietary chemopreventive agent."

*Antioxidant intervention as a route to **cancer** prevention.* Collins AR. Eur J Cancer. 2005 Sep;41(13):1923-30. **Key Finding:** "It is certainly true that we do not yet fully understand the role of phytochemicals as antioxidants, or as modulators of other processes related to carcinogenesis and its prevention."

Breaking the relay in deregulated cellular signal transduction as a rationale for chemoprevention with anti-inflammatory phytochemicals. Kundu JK, Surh YJ. Mutat Res. 2005 Dec 11;591(1-2):123-46. **Key Finding:** "Center to the **cancer** biology is disrupted intracellular signaling network, which transmits improper signals resulting in abnormal cellular functioning. Modulation of cellular signaling involved in chronic inflammatory response by anti-inflammatory phytochemicals may comprise a rational and pragmatic strategy in molecular target-based chemoprevention."

*The **antitumor** activities of flavonoids.* Kandaswami C, Lee LT, Lee PP, et al. In Vivo. 2005 Sep-Oct;19(5):895-909. **Key Finding:** "Experimental animal studies indicate that certain dietary flavonoids possess antitumor activity. The hydroxylation pattern of the B ring of the flavones and flavonols, such as luteolin and quercetin, seems to critically influence their activities, especially the inhibition of protein kinase activity and antiproliferation. "

*Induction of **cancer** cell apoptosis by flavonoids is associated with their ability to inhibit fatty acid synthase ctivity.* Brusselmans K, Vrolix R, Verhoeven G, Swinnen JV. J Biol Chem. 2005 Feb 18;280(7):5636-45. **Key Finding:** "These findings indicate that the potential of flavonoids to induce apoptosis in cancer cells is strongly associated with their fatty acid synthase inhibitory properties, thereby providing a new mechanism by which polyphenolic compounds may exert their cancer-preventive and antineoplastic effects."

Does an apple a day keep the oncologist away? Gallus S, Talamini R, Giacosa A, et al. Ann Oncol. 2005 Nov;16(11):1841-4. **Key Finding:** "We analyzed data from multicenter case-control studies conducted between 1991 and 2002 in Italy. This investigation found a consistent inverse association between apples and risk of various **cancers**."

Targets for indole-3-carbinol in **cancer** *prevention.* Kim YS, Milner JA. J Nutr Biochem. 2005 Feb;16(2):65-73. **Key Finding:** "Modification of nuclear transcription factors including Sp1, estrogen receptor, nuclear factor kappaB and aryl hydrocarbon receptor may represent a common site of action to help explain downstream cellular responses to dietary I3C and ultimately, to its anticancer properties."

Total cranberry extract versus its phytochemical constitutents: antiproliferative and synergistic effects against human **tumor cell** *lines.* Seeram NP, Adams LS, Hardy ML, Heber D. J Agric Food Chem. 2004 May 5;52(9):2512-7. **Key Finding:** "The enhanced antiproliferative activity of total polyphenols compared to total cranberry extract and its individual phytochemicals suggests synergistic or additive antiproliferative interactions of the anthocyanins, proanthocyanidins, and flavonoid glycosides within the cranberry extract."

Antimicrobial *and chemopreventive properties of herbs and spices.* Lai PK, Roy J. Curr Med Chem. 2004 Jun;11(11):1451-60. **Key Finding:** "A growing body of research has demonstrated that the commonly used herbs and spices such as garlic, black cumin, cloves, cinnamon, thyme, allspices, bay leaves, mustard and rosemary possess antimicrobial properties that, in some cases, can be used therapeutically. Other spices, such as saffron, turmeric, green or black tea, and flaxseed do contain potent phytochemicals, including carotenoids, curcumins, catechins, lignin, which provide significant protection against **cancer.**"

Chemopreventive *potential of epigallocatechin gallate and genistein: evidence from epidemiological and laboratory studies.* Park OJ, Surh YJ. Toxicol Lett. 2004 Apr 15;150(1):43-56. **Key Finding:** "The purpose of this review is to provide perspectives on the molecular basis of chemopreventive activities of EGCG and genistein as representative functional food phytochemicals with emphasis on their ability to control intracellular signaling cascades responsible for regulating cell growth and differentiation."

Vitamins, phytochemicals, diets, and their implementation in **cancer** *chemoprevention.* Lee KW, Lee HJ, Lee CY. Crit Rev Food Sci Nutr. 2004;44(6):437-52. **Key Finding:** "These results suggest that a metabolomics approach might demonstrate that antioxidant rich whole diets play a more important role, rather than individual antioxidants in cancer prevention. On the other hand, the chemopreventive mechanisms of dietary vitamins and phenolic phytochemicals may be associated with the inhibition of other carcinogenic processes, particularly tumor promotion, rather than that of tumor initiation."

Cancer-preventive isothiocyanates: dichotomous modulators of oxidative stress. Zhang Y, Li J, Tang L. Free Radic Biol Med. 2005 Jan 1;38(1):70-7. **Key Finding:** "Although ITC (isothiocyanaes) induced stress may lead to oxidative damage, it has become increasingly clear that much of the chemopreventive activity of ITCs stems from the response of cells to the stress induced by these compounds."

Health benefits of soy isoflavonoids and strategies for enhancement: a review. McCue P, Shetty K. Crit Rev. Food Sci Nutr. 2004;44(5):361-7. **Key Finding:** "We discuss the current state of knowledge concerning soybean isoflavonoids, their chemopreventive actions against postmenopausal health problems, **cancer**, and **cardiovascular disease**."

Dietary antioxidants and human cancer. Borek C. Integr Cancer Ther. 2004 Dec;3(4):333-41. **Key Finding:** "While clinical studies on the effect of anti-oxidants in modulating cancer treatment are limited in number and size, experimental studies show that antioxidant vitamins and some phytochemicals selectively induce apoptosis in cancer cells but not in normal cells and prevent angiogenesis and metastatic spread."

Luteolin inhibitis vascular endothelial growth factor-induced angiogenesis; inhibition of endothelial cell survival and proliferation by targeting phosphatidylinositol 3'-kinase activity. Bagli E, Stefaniotou M, Morbidelli L, et al. Cancer Res. 2004 Nov 1;64(21):7936-46. **Key Finding:** "In an attempt to identify phytochemicals contributing to the well-documented preventive effect of plant-based diets on **cancer** incidence and mortality, we have previously shown that certain flavonoids inhibit in vitro angiogenesis. Here, we show that the flavonoid luteolin inhibited tumor growth and angiogenesis in a murine xenograft model."

Dietary isothiocyanates inhibit Caco-2 cell proliferation and induce G2/M phase cell cycle arrest, DNA damage, and G2/M checkpoint activation. Visanji JM, Duthie SJ, Pirie L, Thompson DG, Padfield PJ. J Nutr. 2004 Nov;134(11):3121-6. **Key Finding:** "Benzyl isothiocyanate and phenethyl isothiocyanate, two aromatic phytochemicals present in substantial concentrations in edible vegetables of the genus brassica, were investigated for their effects on Caco-2 cell proliferation. This study indicates they may exert an antiproliferative effect through activation of the G(2)/M DNA damage checkpoint."

Cancer *prevention by natural compounds.* Tsuda H, Ohshima Y, Nomoto H, et al. Drug Metab Pharmakinet. 2004 Aug;19(4):245-63. **Key Finding:** "Natural agents are advantageous for application to humans because of their combined mild mechanism. Here we review naturally occurring compounds useful for cancer chemoprevention based on in vivo studies with reference to their structures, sources and mechanisms of action."

Molecular basis of chemoprevention by resveratrol: NF-kappaB and AP-1 as potential targets. Kundu JK, Surh YJ. Mutat Res. 2004 Nov 2;555(1-2):65-80. **Key Finding:** "This review aims to update the molecular mechanisms underlying chemoprevention by resveratrol with special focus on its effect on cellular signaling cascades mediated by NF-kappaB and Ap-1."

Role of chemopreventive agents in **cancer** *therapy.* Dorai T, Aggarwal BB. Cancer Lett. 2004 Nov 25;215(2):129-40. **Key Finding:** "Chemopreventive agents include genistein, resveratrol, diallyl sulfide, S-allyl cysteine, allicin, lycopene, capsaicin, curcumin, 6-gingerol, ellagic acid, ursolic acid, silymarin, anethol, catechins and eugenol. Because these agents have been shown to suppress cancer cell proliferation, inhibit growth factor signaling pathways, induce apoptosis, inhibit NF-kappaB, AP-1 and JAK-STAT activation pathways, inhibit angiogenesis, suppress the expression of anti-apoptotic proteins, inhibit cyclooxygenase-2, they may have untapped therapeutic value. These chemopreventive agents also have very recently been found to reverse chemoresistance and radioresistance in patients undergoing cancer treatment."

The effect of cruciferous and leguminous sprouts on genotoxicity in vitro and in vivo. Gill CI, Haldar S, Porter S, et al. Cancer Epidemiol Biomarkers Prev.

2004 Jul;13(7):1199-205. **Key Finding:** "Some putative protective phytochemicals are found in higher amounts in young sprouts than in mature plants. The effect of an extract of mixed cruciferous and legume sprouts on DNA damage induced by H(2)O(2) was measured in HT29 cells using single cell microgelelectrophoresis. A significant antigenotoxic effect against H(2)O(2)-induced DNA damage was shown in peripheral blood lymphocytes of volunteers who consumed the supplemented diet when compared with the control diet. No significant induction of detoxifying enzymes was observed during the study, neither were plasma antioxidant levels or activity altered. The results support the theory that consumption of cruciferous vegetables is linked to a reduced risk of **cancer** via decreased damage to DNA."

Phytochemical-induced changes in gene expression of carcinogen-metabolizing enzymes in cultured human primary hepatocytes. Gross-Steinmeyer K, Stapleton PL, Liu F, et al. Xenobiotica 2004 Jul;34(7):619-32. **Key Finding:** "The present study investigated the effects of these phytochemicals (curcumin, 3,3'-diindolymethane, isoxanthohumol, 8-prenylnaringenin, phenethyl isothiocyanate, and sulforaphane) on the expression of four carcinogenesis-relevant enzymes in primary cultures of freshly isolated human hepatocytes. The findings show novel and unexpected effects of these phytochemicals on the expression of human hepatic biotransformation enzymes that play key roles in chemical-induced **carcinogenesis.**"

*Polyphenolic phytochemicals versus non-steroidal anti-inflammatory drugs: which are better **cancer** chemopreventive agents?* Gescher A. J Chemother. 2004 Nov;16 Suppl 4:3-6. **Key Finding:** "As non-steroidal anti-inflammatory drugs possess unwanted side effects, polyphenolic phytochemicals such as curcumin and resveratrol are promising alternatives. They suppress carcinogenesis in the ApcMin+ mouse model. Clinical pilot studies of curcumin show that it is safe at doses of up to 3.6g daily, and that the levels of curcumin which can be achieved in the gastrointestinal tract exert pharmacological activity."

Antimutagenic activity of berry extracts. Hope Smith S, Tate PL, Huang G, et al. J Med Food. 2004 Winter;7(4):450-5. **Key Finding:** "Fresh juices and organic solvent extracts from the fruits of strawberry, blueberry, and raspberry were evaluated for their ability to inhibit the production of mutations by the direct-acting mutagen methyl methanesulfonate and the metabolically activated carcinogen benzo[a]pyrene. Juice from strawberry, blueberry and raspberry fruit significantly inhibited mutagenesis caused by both carcinogens."

Allyl-isothiocyanate causes mitotic block, loss of cell adhesion and disrupted cytoskeletal structure in HT29 cells. Smith TK, Lund EK, Parker ML, Clarke RG, Johnson IT. Carcinogenesis. 2004;25(8):1409-1415. **Key Finding:** "We have examined the effects of allyl-isothiocyanate (AITC), a major breakdown product of the glucosinolate sinigrin, on proliferation and death of colorectal cancer cells. AITC inhibits proliferation of **cancer** cells by causing mitotic block associated with disruption of a-tubulin in a manner analogous to a number of chemotherapeutic agents."

Protection against ionizing radiation by antioxidant nutrients and phytochemicals. Weiss JF, Landauer MR. Toxicology. 2003 Jul 15;189(1-2):1-20. **Key Finding:** "Many antioxidant nutrients and phytochemicals have antimutagenic properties, and their modulation of long-term radiation effects, such as **cancer**, needs further examination. In addition, further studies are required to determine the potential value of specific antioxidant nutrients and phytochemicals during radiotherapy for cancer."

Synergistic suppression of superoxide and nitric-oxide generation from inflammatory cells by combined food factors. Murakami A, Takahashi D, Koshimizu K, Ohigashi H. Mutat Res. 2003 Feb-Mar;523-524:151-61. **Key Finding:** "The present findings suggest that individual food phytochemicals have complex interactions that can be antagonistic, additive, and/or synergistic in biological systems, depending upon certain environmental factors including concentrations. Further, these results support and emphasize the concept that combinations of different types of chemicals at low concentrations are one of the essential areas of study for **chemopreventive** strategies."

Why whole grains are protective: biological mechanisms. Slavin J. Proc Nutr Soc. 2003 Feb;62(1):129-34. **Key Finding:** "Epidemiological studies find that whole-grain intake is protective against **cancer, cardiovascular disease, diabetes and obesity**. As a consequence of the traditional models of conducting nutrition studies on isolated nutrients, few studies exist on the biological effects of increased whole-grain intake. The few whole-grain feeding studies that are available show improvements in bio-markers with whole-grain consumption, such as weight loss, blood lipid improvement and antioxidant protection."

Plant-derived triterpenoids as potential antineoplastic agents. Setzer WN, Setzer MC. Mini Rev Med Chem. 2003 Sep;3(6):540-56. **Key Finding:** "A number of triterpenoids have shown promise as antineoplastic agents. Members of the cycloartane, lupine, ursane, oleanane, friedelane (especially quinine methides), dammarane, cucurbitacin, and limonoid triterpenoids, have demonstrated anti-proliferative activity on various **cancer** cell lines. This review covers the recent developments regarding antienoplastic/cytotoxic triterpenoids, excluding saponins."

Redox-sensitive mechanisms of phytochemical-mediated inhibition of **cancer** *cell proliferation (review).* Loo G. J Nurt Biochem. 2003 Feb;14(2):64-73. **Key Finding:** "Cancer cells, particularly those that are highly invasive or metastatic, may require a certain level of oxidative stress to maintain a balance between undergoing either proliferation or apoptosis. They constitutively generate large but tolerable amounts of H_2O_2 that apparently function as signaling molecules in the mitogen-activated protein kinase pathway to constantly activate redox-sensitive transcription factors and responsive genes that are involved in the survival of cancer cells as well as their proliferation. Phytochemicals can either scavenge the constitutive H_2O_2 or paradoxically generate additional amounts of H_2O_2 to inhibit the proliferation of cancer cells."

Spicing up a vegetarian diet: chemopreventive effects of phytochemicals. Lampe JW. Am J Clin Nutr. 2003 Sep;78(3 Suppl):579S-583S. **Key Finding:** "Embracing a cuisine rich in spice, as well as in fruit and vegetables, may further enhance the **chemopreventive** capacity of one's diet."

Sulforaphane and quercetin modulate PhIP-DNA adduct formation in human HepG2 cells and heptocytes. Bacon JR, Williamson G, Garner RC, et al. Carcinogenesis. 2003 Dec;24(12):1903-11. **Key Finding:** "This study indicates that dietary isothiocyanates and flavonoids modulate phase I and phase

II enzyme expression, hence increasing the rate of detoxification of the dietary **carcinogen** PhIP in human HepG2 cells but do not affect the rate of PhIP-DNA adduct repair."

*Tumor angiogenesis: a potential target in **cancer** control by phytochemicals.* Singh RP, Agarwal R. Curr Cancer Drug Targets. 2003 Jun;3(3):205-17. **Key Finding:** "This review is focused on recent developments and comprehensive mechanistic aspects of phytochemicals related to an interplay of angiogenic promoters and inhibitors, and associated signaling in both tumor as well as endothelial cells. Since vascular endothelial cells constitute the first line exposure to the blood-borne agents, it is plausible that anti-angiogenic activity of phytochemicals could be associated with lowering the risk of cancer by preventing the growth and metastasis of tumor."

*Reduction of **cancer** risk by consumption of selenium-enriched plants: enrichment of broccoli with selenium increases the anticarcinogenic properties of broccoli.* Finley JW. J Med Food. 2003 Spring;6(1):19-26. **Key Finding:** "Selenium from high-selenium broccoli decreased the incidence of aberrant crypts in rats with chemically induced colon cancer by more than 50%, compared with controls. Selenium from high-selenium broccoli also decreased the incidence of mammary tumors in rats treated with DMBA and tumor number and volume in APC(min) mice. These results suggest that development of methods to increase the natural accumulation of selenium in broccoli may greatly enhance its health-promoting properties."

Mechanisms of vanilloid-induced apoptosis. Hail N Jr. Apoptosis. 2003 Jun;8(3):251-62. **Key Finding:** "Vanilloids have demonstrated the ability to induce apotosis in various cell types. This review will examine the cellular targets, cytotoxic effects, and the downstream effector mechanisms associated with vanilloid phytochemical-induced apoptosis."

The anticarcinogenic potential of soybean lectin and lunasin. De Mejia EG, Bradford T, Hasler C. Nutr Rev. 2003 Jul;61(7):239-46. **Key Finding:** "Soybean contains a variety of anticarcinogenic phytochemicals. Lunasin is a polypeptide that arrests cell division and induces apoptosis in malignant cells. Lectins are glycoproteins that selectively bind carbohydrates. Additional research, including clinical trials, should continue to examine and elucidate the therapeutic effects."

The antioxidant responsibe element (ARE) may explain the protective effects of crucifer-ous vegetables on **cancer**. Finley JW. Nutr Rev. 2003 Jul;61(7):250-4. **Key Finding:** "Most studies show that phytochemicals in crucifers up-regulate many detoxification enzyme systems in the animal that consumes them. Recent reports of the molecular events involved in the activation of a gene promoter called the antioxidant responsive element have begun to provide clues as to how a single substance may induce a battery of many genes."

Chemoprevention *of 2-amino-3-methyllimidazo[4,5-f]quinoline (IQ)-induced colonic and hepatic preneoplastic lesions in the F344 rat by cruciferous vegetables ad-ministered simultaneously with the carcinogen.* Kassie F, Uhi M, Rabot Sd, et al. Carcinogenesis. 2003 Feb;24(2):255-61. **Key Finding:** "The induction effect of brussels sprouts on the activity of UDPGT-2 was more marked than that of the red cabbage cultivars, suggesting that increased gluc-uronidation of IQ may account for the reduction of the preneoplastic lesions. Our findings support the assumption that brassica vegetables pro-tect against the carcinogenic effects of heterocyclic amines."

Flavonoids: promising anticancer agents. Ren W, Qiao Z, Wang H, Zhu L, Zhang L. Med Res Rev. 2003 Jul;23(4):519-34. **Key Finding:** "Compel-ling data from laboratory studies, epidemiological investigations, and hu-man clinical trials indicate that flavonoids have important effects on **can-cer** chemoprevention and chemotherapy. Many mechanisms of action have been identified, including carcinogen inactivation, antiproliferation, cell cycle arrest, induction of apoptosis and differentiation, inhibition of angiogenesis, antioxidation and reversal of multidrug resistance or a combination of these mechanisms."

Phytochemicals as cell cycle modulators—a less toxic approach in halting human **can-cers**. Singh RP, Dhanalakshmi S, Agarwal R. Cell Cycle. 2002 May-Jun;1(3):156-61. **Key Finding:** "A number of phytochemicals inhibit cell cycle progression in cancer cells, yet their clinical applications are still in infancy. The present review is focused on the modulatory effects of phy-tochemicals on critical cell cycle molecules, and discusses how they inhibit proliferation and/or induce apoptotic death in cancer cells."

*Anti-**tumor** promoting potential of selected spice ingredients with antioxidative and anti-inflammatory activities: a short review.* Surh YJ. Food Chem Toxicol. 2002 Aug;40(8):1091-7. **Key Finding:** "This review summarizes the molecular mechanisms underlying chemopreventive effects of the spice ingredients curcumin, [6]-gingerol, and capsaicin, in terms of their effects on intracellular signaling cascades, particularly those involving NF-kappaB and mitogen-activated protein kinases."

Soy isoflavone genistein modulates cell cycle progression and induces apoptosis in HER-2/neu oncogene expressing human breast epithelial cells. Katdare M, Osborne M, Telang NT. Int J Oncol. 2002 Oct;21(4):809-15. **Key Finding:** "These data provide evidence that natural soy isoflavone genistein may be a potential chemopreventive lead compound for human comedo DCIS, carcinoma in situ."

***Cancer** preventive effects of flavonoids—a review.* Le Marchand L. Biomed Pharmacother. 2002 Aug;56(6):296-301. **Key Finding:** "This review focuses on the biological effects of the main flavonoids, as well as the epidemiological evidence that support their potential cancer protective properties."

Inhibition of estrogenic stimulation of gene expression by genistein. Ratna WN. Life Sci. 2002 Jul 12;71(8):865-77. **Key Finding:** "Two principle soy-derived isoflavones, genistein and daidzein, are believed to play a key role in inhibiting **tumor growth**. The molecular basis of the anti-tumor activity of these two isoflavones has not yet been fully established. To determine the mechanism of action of the above phytochemicals on estrogen-responsive genes, we tested the effect of the same on the expression of Estrogen-Regulation mRNA Stabilizing Factor, which is expressed in the liver in response to estrogen. Genistein generally appears to behave as a partial agonist. An agonist creates cell binding by itself. However, daidzein did not display any estrogenic or antiestrogenic activity at the concentrations tested."

*Botanicals in **cancer** chemoprevention.* Park EJ, Pezzuto JM. Cancer Metastasis Rev. 2002;21(3-4):231-55. **Key Finding:** "In this review, we discuss the cancer chemopreventive activity of cruciferous vegetables such as cabbage and broccoli, Allium vegetables such as garlic and onion, green tea, citrus fruits, tomatoes, berries, ginger and ginseng. Phytochemicals of these types have great potential in the fight against human cancer, and a variety of delivery methods are available as a result of their occurrence in nature."

Food and **cancer:** *state of the art about the protective effect of fruits and vegetables.* Gerber M, Boutron-Ruault MC, Hercberg S, et al. Bull Cancer. 2002 Mar;89(3):293-312. **Key Finding:** "To date, a high intake of fruits and vegetables (at least 400 g per day) is appropriate to lower the risk of cancer. Fruits and vegetables provide numerous phytochemicals which, in part, may explain their beneficial effect."

Phytochemicals as cell cycle modulators —a less toxic approach in halting human cancers. Singh RP, Dhanalakshmi S, Agarwal R. Cell Cycle. 2002 May-Jun;1(3):156-61. **Key Finding:** "A number of phytochemicals inhibit cell cycle progression in cancer cells, yet their clinical applications are still in infancy. The present review is focused on the modulatory effects of phytochemicals on critical cell cycle molecules, and discusses how they inhibit proliferation and/or induce apoptotic death in **cancer** cells."

17beta-Estradiol and the phytoestrogen genistein attenuate neuronal apoptosis induced by the endoplasmic reticulum calcium-ATPase inhibitor thapsigargin. Linford NJ, Dorsa DM. Steroids. 2002 Dec;67(13-14):1029-40. **Key Finding:** "Our results demonstrate that genistein and 17beta-estradiol have comparable anti-apoptotic properties in primary cortical neurons and that these properties are mediated through estrogen receptors."

Epigallocatechin gallate protects U937 cells against nitric oxide-induced cell cycle arrest and apoptosis. Kelly MR, Geigerman CM, Loo G. J Cell Biochem. 2001;81(4):647-58. **Key Finding:** "These data suggest that nitric oxide or downstream products induced cell cycle arrest and apoptosis that was not due to single-strand breaks in DNA, and that EGCG (the tea phenolic) scavenged cytotoxic nitric oxide or downstream products, thus reducing the number of cells in a state of cell cycle arrest or apoptosis."

Molecular mechanisms underlying chemopreventive activities of anti-inflammatory phytochemicals: down-regulation of COX-2 and iNOS through suppression of NF-

kappa B activation. Surh YJ, Chun KS, Cha HH, et al. Mutat Res. 2001 Sep 1;480-481:243-68. **Key Finding:** "Curcumin, EGCG and reservatrol have been shown to suppress activation of NF-kappa B. One of the plausible mechanisms underlying inhibition of NF-kappa B activation by aforementioned phytochemicals involves repression of degradation of the inhibitory unit I kappa B alpha, which hampers subsequent nuclear translocation of the functionally active subunit of NF-kappa B."

Phytochemical glyceollins, isolated from soy, mediate antihormonal effects through estrogen receptor alpha and beta. Burow ME, Boue SM, Collins-Burow BM, et al. J Clin Endorcrinol Metab. 2001 Apr;86(4):1750-8. **Key Finding:** "We describe the phytoalexin compounds known as glyceollins, which exhibit unique antagonistic effects on ER signaling in both HEK 293 and MCF-7 cells. The glyceollins as well as other phytoalexin compounds may represent an important component of the health effects of soy-based foods."

*Current prospects for controlling **cancer** growth with non-cytotoxic agents—nutrients, phytochemicals, herbal extracts, and available drugs.* McCarty MF. Med Hypotheses. 2001 Feb;56(2):137-54. **Key Finding:** "In animal or cell culture studies, the growth and spread of cancer can be slowed by many nutrients, food factors, herbal extracts, and well-tolerated available drugs that are still rarely used in the clinical management of cancer, in part because they seem unlikely to constitute definitive therapies in themselves. However, it is reasonable to expect that mechanistically complementary combinations of these measures could have a worthwhile impact on survival times and, when used as adjuvants, could improve the cure rates achievable with standard therapies."

*Phytochemicals from cruciferous plants protect against **cancer** by modulating carcinogen metabolism.* Talalay P, Fahey JW. J Nutr. 2001 Nov;131(11 Suppl):30275-335. **Key Finding:** "Many isothiocyanates are also potent inducers of phase 2 proteins. Substantial evidence supports the view that phase 2 enzyme induction is a highly effective strategy for reducing susceptibility to carcinogens."

*Cruciferous vegetables and **cancer** prevention.* Murillo G, Mehta RG. Nutr Cancer. 2001;41(1-2):17-28. **Key Finding:** "Results clearly point toward a positive correlation between cancer prevention of many target organs and consumption of cruciferous vegetable or their active constitutents. Yet we are still far from complete understanding of the effects of combinations of chemopreventive phytochemicals present in these cruciferous vegetables and their overall mechanisms of action in providing protective effects."

Dietary indoles and isothiocyanates that are generated from cruciferous vegetables can both stimulate apoptosis and confer protection against DNA damage in human colon cell lines. Bonnesen C, Eggleston IM, Hayes JD. Cancer Res. 2001 Aug 15;61(16):6120-30. **Key Finding:** "These phytochemicals together may prevent **colon tumorigenesis** by both stimulating apoptosis and enhancing intracellular defenses against genotoxic agents."

*Role of diet modification in **cancer** prevention.* Abdulla M, Gruber P. Biofactors. 2000;12(1-4):45-51. **Key Finding:** "A number of epidemiological and experimental studies have shown that vitamin C and E, Beta-carotene and the essential trace element selenium can reduce the risk of cancer. Consistent observations during the last few decades that cancer risk is reduced by a diet rich in vegetables, fruits, legumes, grains and green tea have encouraged research to identify several plant components, especially phytochemicals, that protect against DNA damage. This paper reviews current knowledge."

Natural killer cells from aging mice treated with extracts from Echinacea purpurea are quantitatively and functionally rejuvenated. Currier NL, Miller SC. Exp Gerontol. 2000 Aug;35(5):627-39. **Key Finding:** "Our results revealed that E. purpurea, but not thyroxin, had the capacity to increase NK cell numbers in aging mice, reflecting increased new NK cell production in their bone marrow generation site, leading to an increase in absolute numbers in NK cells in the spleen, their primary destiny. The E. purpurea-mediated increase in NK cell numbers was indeed paralleled by an increase in their **anti-tumor**, lytic functional capacity."

***Cancer** Chemoprevention by Phytochemicals and their Related Compounds.* Nishino H, Tokuda H, Satomi Y, et al. Asian Pac J Cancer Prev. 2000;1(1):49-55. **Key Finding:** "Cancer chemoprevention by phytochemicals may be one of the most feasible approaches for cancer control. For example, phyotchemicals obtained from vegetables, fruits, spices, teas, herbs and medicinal plants, such as carotenoids, phenolic compounds and terpenoids, have been proven to suppress experimental carcinogenesis in various organs."

Role of **antioxidant** *lycopene in* **cancer** *and* **heart disease**. Rao AV, Agarwal S. J Am Coll Nutr. 2000 Oct;19(5):563-9. **Key Finding:** "Serum and tissue lycopene levels have been inversely related with chronic disease risk, such as cancer and cardiovascular disease. Although the antioxidant properties of lycopene are thought to be primarily responsible for its beneficial properties, evidence is accumulating to suggest other mechanisms such as modulation of intercellular gap junction communication, hormonal and immune system and metabolic pathways may also be involved."

Isoprenoid-mediated inhibition of mevalonate synthesis: potential application to **cancer**. Elson CE, Peffley DM, Hentosh P, Mo H. Proc Soc Exp Biol Med. 1999 Sep;221(4):294-311. **Key Finding:** "Isoprenoid-mediated activities are additive, and, sometimes synergistic. Therefore, the combined actions of the estimated 23,000 isoprenoid constitutents of plant materials, acting in concert with other chemopreventive phytochemicals, may explain the lowered cancer risk associated with a diet rich in plant products."

Apoptosis and cell-cycle arrest in human and **murine tumor** *cells are initiated by isoprenoids.* Mo H, Elson CE. J Nutr. 1999 Apr;129(4):804-13. **Key Finding:** "The additive and potentially synergistic actions of isoprenoids in the suppression of tumor cell proliferation and initiation of apoptosis coupled with the mass action of the diverse isoprenoid constitutents of plant products may explain, in part, the impact of fruit, vegetable and grain consumption on cancer risk."

Antimutagens in food plants eaten by Polynesians: micronutrients, phytochemicals and protection against bacterial mutagenicity of the heterocyclic amine 2-amino-3-methyylimidazo (4,5-flquinoline. Botting KJ, Young MM, Pearson AE, Harris PJ, Ferguson LR. Food Chem Toxicol. 1999 Feb-Mar;37(2-3):95-103. **Key Finding:** "We have previously suggested that differences in **cancer** incidence between Polynesians (including Maoris and people from several Pacific islands) and Europeans in New Zealand may at least partially relate to differences in the species of food plants preferentially eaten by these groups. Twenty-five food plants that are typically eaten in different amounts by these two population groups were selected for detailed study. The data revealed strong antimutagenic properties in several of the food plants commonly eaten by Polynesians, especially rice, watercress, pawpaw, taro leaves, green banana and mango."

Phytochemicals as modulators of **cancer** *risk.* Bradlow HL, Telang NT, Sepkovic DW, Osborne MP. Adv Exp Med Biol. 1999;472:207-21. **Key Finding:** "Dietary changes could play a role in decreasing the incidence of a variety of tumors. 13C and the other compounds discussed may well be only prototypes for other as yet unexplored phytochemicals present in the diet. There have been no attempts to explore the possibilities of synergistic action among the various phytochemicals, 13C, limonene, curcumin, epigallocatechin gallate, sulforaphene, or genistein. Mixtures of these compounds might well show potency at lower doses for each of the compounds and show even greater promise than that already demonstrated."

*Anti-***tumor*** promoting activites of selected pungent phenolic substances present in ginger.* Surh YJ, Park KK, Chun KS, et al. J Environ Pathol Toxicol Oncol. 1999;18(2):131-9. **Key Finding:** "In our study, we found anti-tumor promoting properties of [6]-gingerol and [6]-paradol. These substances also significantly inhibited the tumor-promoter-stimulated inflammation, TNF-alpha production, and activation of epidermal ornithine descarboxylase in mice. In another study, [6]-gingerol and [6]-pardol suppressed the superoxide production stimulated by TPA in differentiated HL-60 cells. Taken together, these findings suggest that pungent vanilloids found in ginger possess potential chemopreventive activities."

Alkylperoxyl radical-scavenging activity of various flavonoids and other phenolic compounds: implications for the **anti-tumor*****-promoter effect of vegetables.* Sawa T, Nakao M, Akaike T, Ono K, Maeda H. J Agric Food Chem. 1999 Feb;47(2):397-402. **Key Finding:** "Here we describe the ROO(*)-scavenging activity of flavonoids and nonflavonoid phenolics and their role in anti-tumor promoter effects. Of 17 authentic plant phenolics tested, 9 compounds (including rutin, cholorgenic acid, vanillin, vanillic acid, neohesperidin, gallic acid, shikimic acid, rhamnetin, and kaempferol) showed remarkably high Roo(*)-scavenging activity. Some of them were detected and quantified in hot-water extracts of mung bean sprouts, used as the model vegetable, and their contents increased after germination. Thus, a diet rich in these radical scavengers would reduce the cancer-promoting action of ROO(*)."

Effect of dietary phytochemicals on **cancer** *development (review).* Waladkhani AR, Clemens MR. Int J Mol Med. 1998 Apr;1(4):747-53. **Key Finding:** "Phytochemicals can inhibit carcinogenesis by inhibiting phase I enzymes, and induction of phase II DNA reactive enzymes. Scavenge DNA reactive agents suppress the abnormal proliferation of early, prenoeplastic lesions, and inhibit certain properties of the cancer cell. There are many biologically plausible reasons why consumption of plant foods might slow or prevent the appearance of cancer. These include the presence in plant foods of such potentially anticarcinogenic substances as carotenoids, chlorophyll, flavonoids, indole, isothiocyanate, polyphenolic compounds, protease inhibitors, sulfides, and terpens. The specific mechanisms of action of most phytochemicals in cancer prevention are not yet clear but appear to be varied."

Antimutagenicity of flavones and flavonols to heterocyclic amines by specific and strong inhibition of the cytochrome P450 1A family. Kanazawa K, Yamashita T, Ashida H, Danno G. Biosci Biotechnol Biochem. 1998 May;62(5):970-7. **Key Finding:** "The antimutagenicity of the flavones and flavonols was thus concluded to be due to inhibition of the activation process of Trp-P-2 by P450 1A1 to be the ultimate carcinogenic form. They were also able to act as antimutagens toward other indirect mutagens that were activated by P450 1A1."

Plant anticarcinogens. Johnson IT. Eur J Cancer Prev. 1997 Dec;6(6):515-7. **Key Findings:** "There is strong epidemiological evidence to suggest that the consumption of diets rich in plant materials is associated with a reduced risk of **cancer**. Human beings are probably adapted to consume relatively large quantities of biologically active phytochemicals derived from as many as 300 different plant genera. Plant foods contain a variety of potentially anticarcinogenic secondary metabolites, and these can conveniently be classified as blocking agents and suppressing agents. Blocking agents modulate the activation and detoxification of carcinogens, whereas suppressing agents are thought to modify post-initiation events including cellular differentiation, proliferation and apoptosis."

Experimental evidence for **cancer** *preventive elements in foods.* Wargovich MJ. Cancer Lett. 1997 Mar 19;114(1-2):11-7. **Key Finding:** "Food components can modify carcinogenesis in one of five different ways. They may: (1) modify carcinogen activation by inhibiting Phase 1 enzymes; (2) modify how carcinogens are detoxified through Phase 2 pathways; (3) scavenge DNA reactive agents; (4) suppress the abnormal proliferation of early, preneoplastic lesions; and (5) inhibit certain properties of the cancer cell."

Dietary flavonoids, quercetin, luteolin and genistein, reduce oxidative DNA damage and lipid peroxidation and quench free radicals. Cai Q, Rahn RO, Zhang R. Cancer Lett. 1997 Oct 28;119(1):99-107. **Key Finding:** "The effects of quercetin, luteolin and genistein as antioxidants were investigated. Of the test compounds, luteolin exhibited the most potent quenching effect on Fenton-induced 8-OHdG formation. The scavenging of oxygen free radicals, the inhibitory effect on lipid peroxidation and the quenching effect on 8-OHdG formation by quercetin, luteolin and genistein, may, at least in part, be responsible for their **anticarcinogenic** effects."

Dietary levels of plant phenols and other non-nutritive components: could they prevent **cancer***?* Dragsted LO, Strube M, Leth T. Eur J Cancer Prev. 1997 Dec;6(6):522-8. **Key Finding:** "Meta-analyses of cohort studies on specific food items rich in specific non-nutritive components, indicate that carotenoid or glucosinolate-rich foods protect against some cancers, while flavonoid rich food items do not uniformly show protective effects."

A review of mechanisms underlying **anticarcinogenicity** *by brassica vegetables.* Verhoeven DT, Verhagen H, Goldbohm RA, Van den Brandt PA, van Poppel G. Chem Biol Interact. 1997 Feb 28;103(2):79-129. **Key Finding:** "Most evidence concerning anticarcinogenic effects of glucosinolate hydrolysis products and brassica vegetables has come from studies in animals. Animal studies are invaluable in identifying and testing potential anticarcinogens. In addition, studies carried out in human using high but still realistic human consumption levels of indoles and brassica vegetables have shown putative positive effects on health."

*Anti-**tumor** promotion with food phytochemicals: a strategy for cancer chemoprevention.* Murakami A, Ohigashi H, Koshimizu K. Biosci Biotechnol. Biochem. 1996 Jan;60(1):1-8. **Key Finding:** In this review, the anti-tumor promoting properties of vegetables, fruits, and edible marine algae are described. "Anti-tumor promotion with food phytochemicals may be characterized as an efficient and reliable strategy for cancer chemoprevention."

Vegetables, fruit and phytoestrogens as preventive agents. Potter JD, Steinmetz K. IARC Sci Publ. 1996; (139):61-90. **Key Finding:** "In the presence of a diet and lifestyle high in potential carcinogens (whether derived from fungai contamination, cooking or tobacco) or high in promoters (such as salt and alcohol), overall risk of **cancer** at many epithelial sites is elevated. Plant foods appear to exert a general risk-lowering effect."

Bioactive organosulfur phytochemicals in Brassic oleracea vegetables—a review. Stoewsand GS. Food Chem Toxicol. 1995 Jun;33(6):537-43. **Key Finding:** "The **cancer** chemopreventive effects of brassica vegetables that have been shown in human and animal studies may be due to the presence of both types of sulfur-containing phytochemicals (i.e. certain glucosinolates and S-methyl cysteine sulfoxide)."

*Flavonoid intake and long-term risk of **coronary heart disease** and **cancer** in the seven countries study.* Hertog MG, Kromhout D, Aravanis C, et al. Arch Intern Med. 1995 Feb;155(4):381-386. **Key Finding:** "Average flavonoid intake may partly contribute to differences in coronary heart disease mortality across populations, but it does not seem to be an important determinant of cancer mortality."

*Chemoprotection against **cancer** by Phase 2 enzyme induction.* Talalay P, Fahey JW, Holtzclaw WD, Prestera T, Zhang Y. 1995 Dec;82-83:173-179. **Key Finding:** "Inducers are widely, but unequally, distributed among edible plants. Search for such inducer activity in broccoli led to the isolation of sulforaphane, an isothiocyanate that is a very potent Phase 2 enzyme inducer and blocks mammary tumor formation in rats."

*Dietary flavonoids and **cancer** risk in the Zutphen Elderly Study.* Hertog MG, Feskens EJ, Hollman PC, Katan MB, Krombout D. Nutr Cancer. 1994;22(2):175-84. **Key Finding:** "A high intake of flavonoids from vegetables and fruits only was inversely associated with risk of cancer of the alimentary and respiratory tract. These results suggest the presence of other nonvitamin components with anticarcinogenic potential in these foods. We conclude that intake of flavonoids, mainly from tea, apples and onions, does not predict a reduced risk of all-cause cancer or of cancer of the alimentary and respiratory tract in elderly men. The effect of flavonoids on risk of cancer at specific sites needs further investigation in prospective cohort studies."

Actions of carotenoids in biological systems. Krinsky NI. Annual Review of Nutrition. 1993 Jul;13:561-587. **Key Finding:** This review discusses the evidence to date for carotenoid actions in vitro and in vivo **antioxidant,** antimutagenesis, protection against genotoxicity and malignant transformation, and its **anticarcinogenic** role.

Oxidants, antioxidants, and the degenerative diseases of **aging**. Ames BN, Shigenaga MK, Hagen TM. Proc Natl Acad Sci. 1993 Sep 1;90(17):7915-22. **Key Finding:** "Metabolism, like other aspects of life, involves tradeoffs. Oxidant by-products of normal metabolism cause extensive damage to DNA, protein, and lipid. We argue that this damage (the same as that produced by radiation) is a major contributor to aging and to degenerative diseases of aging such as cancer, cardiovascular disease, immune-system decline, brain dysfunction, and cataracts. Antioxidant defenses against this damage include ascorbate, tocopherol, and carotenoids. Dietary fruits and vegetables are the principal source. Low dietary intake of fruits and vegetables doubles the risk of most types of **cancer** and also markedly increase the risk of **heart disease** and **cataracts**."

Fruit, vegetables, and **cancer** *prevention: a review of the epidemiological evidence.* Block G, Patterson B, Subar A. Nutr Cancer. 1992;18(1):1-29. **Key Finding:** "Approximately 200 studies that examined the relationship between fruit and vegetable intake and cancers of the lung, colon, breast, cervix, esophagus, oral cavity, stomach, bladder, pancreas and ovary are reviewed. A statistically significant protective effect of fruit and vegetable consumption was found in 128 of 156 dietary studies in which results were expressed in terms of relative risk. For most cancer sites, persons with low fruit and vegetable intake experience about twice the risk of cancer compared with those with high intake. For lung cancer, significant protection was found in 24 of 25 studies after control for smoking. Fruits, in particular, were significantly protective in cancers of the esophagus, oral cavity, and larynx, for which 28 of 29 studies were significant. Strong evidence of a protective effect of fruit and vegetable consumption was seen in cancers of the pancreas and stomach (26 of 30 studies) as well as in colorectal and bladder cancer (23 of 38 studies.) For cancers of the cervix, ovary, and endometrium, a significant protective effect was shown in 11 of 13 studies, and for breast cancer a protective effect was found to be strong and consistent in a meta analysis."

Vegetables, fruits, and carotenoids and the risk of **cancer***.* Ziegler RG. Am J Clin Nutr. 1991 Jan;53(1 Suppl):251S-259S. **Key Finding:** "Both prospective and retrospective studies suggest that vegetable and fruit intake may reduce the risk of cancers of the mouth, pharynx, larynx, esophagus, stomach, colon, rectum, bladder, and cervix. But because of fewer studies and less consistency among studies, the epidemiologic evidence is at present less persuasive than for lung cancer."

Carotenoids enhance gap junctional communication and inhibit lipid peroxidation in C3H/10T1/2 cells: relationship to their **cancer** *chemopreventive action.* Zhang LX, Cooney RV, Bertram JS. Carcinogenesis. 1991 Nov;12(11):2109-14. **Key Finding:** "We have previously demonstrated that diverse carotenoids inhibit chemically induced neoplastic transformation in 10T1/2 cells. To address their mechanism of action, the effects of six diverse carotenoids, with or without provitamin A activity, on gap junctional communication and lipid peroxidation have been investigated. Beta-carotene, canthaxanthin, lutein, lycopene and alpha-carotene increased gap junctional intercellular communication in a dose-dependent manner in the above order of potency."

Vegetables, fruit, and **cancer***. I. Epidemiology.* Steinmetz KA, Potter JD. Cancer Causes Control. 1991 Sep;2(5):325-57. **Key Finding:** "It is concluded that consumption of higher levels of vegetables and fruit is associated consistently, although not universally, with a reduced risk of cancer at most sites."

*Vegetable and fruit consumption and **cancer** risk.* Negri E, La Vecchia C, Franceschi S, D'Avanzo B, Parazzini F. Int J Cancer. 1991 May 30;48(3):350-4. **Key Finding:** "The relationship between cancer risk and frequency of consumption of green vegetables and fruit has been analyzed using data from an integrated series of case-controlled studies conducted in northern Italy. For vegetables, there was a consistent pattern of protection from all epithelial cancers, with relative risks in the upper tertile ranging from 0.2 for oesophagus, liver and larynx to 0.7 for breast. All the trends in risk were in the same direction and significant for all carcinomas except gall-bladder. In contrast, no protection was afforded by high vegetable consumption against non-epithelial lymphoid neoplasms. The lower the location of the tumour in the digestive tract, the weaker appeared to be the protection afforded. Significant inverse relationships were observed for liver, pancreas, prostate and urinary sites, but not for rectum, breast and female genital cancers or thyroid."

*A review of epidemiologic evidence that carotenoids reduce the risk of **cancer**.* Ziegler RG. J Nutr. 1989 Jan;119(1):116-22. **Key Finding:** "Low intake of vegetables and fruits and carotenoids is consistently associated with an increased risk of lung cancer in both prospective and retrospective studies. In addition, low levels of serum or plasma beta-carotene are consistently associated with the subsequent development of lung cancer. The simplest explanation is that beta-carotene is indeed protective."

*Can dietary beta-carotene materially reduce human **cancer** rates?* Peto R, Doll R, Buckley JD, Sporn MB. Nature. 1981 Mar 19;290(5803):201-8. **Key Finding:** "Human cancer risks are inversely correlated with (a) blood retinol and (b) dietary beta-carotene. Although retinol in the blood might well be truly protective, this would be of little immediate value without discovery of the important external determinants of blood retinol which (in developed countries) do not include dietary retinol or beta-carotene. If dietary beta-carotene is truly protective—which could be tested by controlled trials—there are a number of theoretical mechanisms whereby it might act, some of which do not directly involve its 'provitamin A' activity."

Alimentary

New approaches to the role of diet in the prevention of **cancers of the alimentary tract.** Johnson IT. Mutat Res. 2004 Jul 13;551(1-2):9-28. **Key Finding:** "Plant foods contain a variety of components including micronutrients, polyunsaturated fatty acids, and secondary metabolites such as glucosinolates and flavonoids, many of which can inhibit cell proliferation and induce apoptosis, and which may well act synergistically when combined in the human diet. The future challenge is to fully characterize and evaluate these effects at the cellular and molecular level, so as to exploit their full potential as protective mechanisms for the population as a whole."

Tomatoes, tomato-rich foods, lycopene and cancer of the upper aerodigestive tract: a case-control in Uruguay. De Stefani E, Oreggia F, Boffetta P, Deneo-Pellegrini H, Ronco A, Mendilaharsu M. Oral Oncol. 2000 Jan;36(1):47-53. **Key Finding:** " In order to study the relationship between tomatoes, tomato products, lycopene and **cancers** of the upper aerodigestive tract; **oral cavity, pharynx, larynx, esophagus**, a case-control study was carried out in Uruguay involving 238 cases and 491 hospitalized controls. We found that the joint effect of lycopene and total phytosterols was associated with a significant reduction in risk for these cancers."

Bladder

Consumption of vegetables and fruit and the risk of **bladder cancer** *in the European Prospective Investigation Into Cancer and Nutrition.* Buchner FL, Bueno-de-Mesquite HB, Ros MM, et al. Int J Cancer. 2009 Dec 1;125(11):2643-51. **Key Finding:** "Data on food consumption and complete follow-up for cancer occurrence was available for a total of 478,533 participants who were recruited in 10 European countries. Increments of 100 g/day in fruit and vegetable consumption combined did not affect **bladder cancer** risk. Borderline statistically significant lower bladder cancer risks were found among never smokers with increased consumption of fruit and vegetables combined with increments of 100 g/day and increased consumption of apples and pears with increments of 25 g/day. For none of the associations a statistically significant interaction with smoking status was found. Our findings do not support an effect of fruit and vegetable consumption, combined or separately, on bladder cancer risk."

Soy phytochemicals prevent orthotopic growth and metastasis of **bladder cancer** *in mice by alterations of cancer cell proliferation and apoptosis and tumor angiogenesis.* Singh AV, Franke AA, Blackburn GL, Zhou JR. Cancer Res. 2006 Feb 1;66(3):1851-8. **Key Finding:** "The results from our studies suggest that further clinical investigation should be warranted to apply soy phytochemicals, such as isoflavone-rich soy phytochemical concentrate, as a potent prevention regimen for bladder cancer progression."

The principal urinary metabolite of dietary isothiocyanates, N-acetylcystein conjugates, elicit the same anti-proliferative response as their parent compounds in human **bladder cancer** *cells.* Tang L, Li G, Song L, Zhang Y. Anticancer Drugs. 2006 Mar;17(3):297-305. **Key Finding:** "Isothiocyanates (ITCs) are a class of well-known cancerpreventive phytochemicals, but are primarily disposed of and concentrated in the urine as N-acetylcysteine (NAC-ITC) conjugates in vivo. Because human urinary bladder cancers occur almost exclusively in the bladder epithelium, which is directly exposed to the urine stored in the bladder, we undertook to examine the anti-cancer activity of NAC-ITCs in cultured human bladder cancer cells. In this paper we report that the NAC conjugates of four naturally occurring ITCS, including allyl ITC, benzyl ITC, phenethyl ITC and sulforaphane, potently inhibited the growth of cells derived from both low-grade superficial and high-grade invasive human bladder cancers and drug-resistant bladder cancer cells."

Silibinin causes cell cycle arrest and apoptosis in human bladder transitional cell carcinoma cells by regulating CDKI-CDK-cyclin cascade, and caspase 3 and PARP cleavages. Tyagi A, Agarwal C, Harrison G, Glode LM, Agarwal R. Carcinogenesis. 2004 Sep;25(9):1711-20. **Key Finding:** "These results suggest that silibinin modulates CDKI-CDK-cyclin cascade and activates caspase 3 causing growth inhibition and apoptotic death of human TCC cells, providing a strong rationale for future studies evaluating preventive and/or intervention strategies for silibinin in **bladder cancer** pre-clinical models."

Silibinin down-regulates survivin protein and mRNA expression and causes caspases activation and apoptosis in human bladder transitional-cell papilloma RT4 cells. Tyagi AK, Agarwal C, Singh RP, Shrover KR, Glode LM, Agarwal R. Biochem Biophys Res Commun. 2003 Dec 26;312(4):1178-84. **Key Finding:** "Silibinin treatment of cells for 24 hours at 100 microM dose resulted in approximately 50% decrease in surviving protein levels; however, treatment at 200 microM for 24 and 48 hours showed a complete loss in surviving protein. Together, these findings suggest that more studies are needed to investigate in vivo effect of silibinin on survivin expression and associated biological effects in **bladder cancer.**"

*High intake of specific carotenoids and flavonoids does not reduce the risk of **bladder cancer.*** Garcia R, Gonzalez CA, Agudo A, Riboli E. Nutr Cancer. 1999;35(2):212-4. **Key Finding:** "The study included 497 cases first diagnosed with bladder cancer, 547 neighborhood controls, and 566 hospital controls. The results of this study do not support the hypothesis that intake of specific carotenoids and flavonoids is protective against bladder cancer risk."

Breast

*Blueberry phytochemicals inhibit growth and metastatic potential of MDA-MB-231 **breast cancer** cells through modulation of the phosphatidylinositol 3-kinase pathway.* Adams LS, Phung S, Yee N, Seeram NP, Li L, Chen S. Cancer Res. 2010 May 1;70(9):3594-605. **Key Finding**: Blueberry phytochemicals have an inhibitory effect on the growth and metastatic potential of MDA-MB-231 breast cancer cell line in blueberry fed mice.

Pomegranate extract inhibits the proliferation and viability of MMTV-Wnt-1 mouse mammary cancer stem cells in vitro. Dai Z, Nair V, Khan M, Ciolino HP, Oncol Rep. 2010 Oct;24(4):1087-91. **Key Finding**: "These data suggest that pomegranate extract, which is a proven and safe dietary supplement, has promise as a treatment against **breast cancer** by preventing proliferation of cancer stem cells."

*Dietary consumption of phytochemicals and **breast cancer** risk in Mexican women.* Torres-Sanchez L, Galvan-Portillo M, Wolff MS, Lopez-Carrillo L. Public Health Nutr. 2009 Jun;12(6):825-31. **Key Finding:** "Among postmenopausal women, high dietary intake of **flavonoids and flavones** was associated with a significant reduction of breast cancer risk. Our results support a protective role of specific dietary phytochemicals in breast cancer risk by menopausal status, independent of other reproductive factors."

*Phytochemicals for **breast cancer** prevention by targeting aromatase.* Adams LS, Chen S. Front Biosci. 2009 Jan 1;14:3846-63. **Key Finding:** Aromatase is a cytochrome P450 enzyme (CYP19) and is the rate-limiting enzyme in the conversion of androgens to estrogens, which can be a trigger for breast cancer. This review discusses whole food extracts and the phytochemicals which have been investigated for potential aromatase inhibitory activity.

Genistein protects against polycyclic aromatic hydrocarbon-induced oxidative DNA damage in non-cancerous breast cells MCF-10A. Leung HY, Yung LH, Poon CH, Shi G, Lu AL, Leung LK. Br J Nutr. 2009 Jan;101(2):257-62. **Key Finding:** "The soya isoflavone genistein has been shown previously in our laboratory to be an inhibitor of PAH metabolite binding to DNA. In the present study, we investigated the effect of genistein on oxidative DNA damage induced by PAH in the **non-tumorigenic breast cell** line MCF-10A." **Genistein** was found to "significantly suppress" the expressions of enzymes which metabolize the PAH into their ultimate carcinogenic forms.

*Dietary carotenoids and the risk of invasive **breast cancer**.* Mignone LI, Giovannucci E, Newcomb PA, et al. Int J Cancer. 2009 Jun 15;124(12):2909-37. **Key Finding:** "Results from this study are comparable to previous prospective studies, and suggest that a high consumption of carotenoids may reduce the risk of premenopausal but not postmenopausal breast cancer, particularly among smokers."

Dietary carotenoids and certain cancers, heart disease, and age-related macular degeneration: a review of recent research. Cooper DA, Eldrigde

AL, Peters JC. Nutr Rev. 2009 Apr 27;57(7):201-214. **Key Finding:** "Key epidemiologic studies show associations between high dietary intakes of certain carotenoid-containing fruits and vegetables and reduced risk of **prostate cancer, breast cancer, head and neck cancers, cardiovascular disease** and age-related **macular degeneration**, although overall the evidence is inconsistent. Little is known about the potential biochemical mechanisms whereby carotenoids might protect against disease, and human intervention trials are limited to high dose B-carotene, which is not protective against lung cancer or cardiovascular disease."

Longitudinal study of serum carotenoid, retinol, and tocopherol concentrations in relation to breast cancer risk among postmenopausal women. Kabat GC, Kim M, Adams-Campbell LL, et al. Am J Clin Nutr. 2009;90(1):162-169. **Key Finding:** "The present study, which was the first to assess repeated measurements of serum carotenoids and micronutrients in relation to breast cancer, adds to the evidence of an inverse association of specific carotenoids with breast cancer."

Adolescent and adult soy food intake and breast cancer risk: results from the Shanghai Women's Health Study. Lee SA, Shu XO, Li H, et al. Am J Clin Nutr. 2009 Jun;89(6):1920-6. **Key Finding:** "This large, population-based, prospective cohort study provides strong evidence of a protective effect of soy food intake against premenopausal breast cancer."

Plasma isoflavone level and subsequent risk of breast cancer among Japanese women: a nested case-control study from the Japan Public Health Center-based prospective study group. Iwasaki M, Inoue M, Otani T, et al. J Clin Oncol. 2008 Apr 1;26(10):1677-83. **Key Finding:** "We found a statistically significant inverse association between plasma genistein and risk of breast cancer, but no association for plasma daidzein."

Extended treatment with physiologic concentrations of dietary phytochemicals results in altered gene expression, reduced growth, and apoptosis of cancer cells. Moiseeva EP, Almedia GM, Jones GD, Manson MM. Mol Cancer Ther. 2007 Nov;6(11):3071-9. **Key Finding:** "We investigated antitumor activity of curcumin, 3,3'-dindolylmethane (DIM), epigallocatechin gallate (EGCG), denistein, or indole-3-carbinol (I3C) in

breast cancer MDA-MB-231 cells. Curcumin and EGCG increased cell doubling time. Curcumin, EGCG, and I3C inhibited clonogenic growth by 55% to 60% and induced 1.5- to 2-fold higher levels of the basal caspase-3/7 activity. No changes in expression of cell cycle-related proteins or survivin were found; however, I3C reduced epidermal growth factor receptor expression, contributing to apoptosis. Curcumin, DIM, EGCG, and genistein reduced cell sensitivity to radiation-induced DNA damage without affecting DNA repair."

*Phytochemicals induce **breast cancer** resistance protein in Caco-2 cells and enhance the transport of benzo[a]pyrene-3-sulfate.* Ebert B, Seidel A, Lampen A. Toxicol Sci. 2007 Apr;96(2):227-36. **Key Finding:** "We have previously reported that breast cancer resistance protein (BCRP) is involved in the transport of phase II metabolites of the food carcinogen benzo[a]pyrene (BP) in the human intestinal cell line Caco-2. In this study, we found that apart from the modulation of detoxifying enzymes in the intestine, induction of BCRP by dietary constitutents (such as quercetin and green tea component (-)-epicatechin) may contribute to the detoxification of food-derived procarcinogens such as BP."

Cancer chemoprevention by phytochemicals: potential molecular targets, biomarkers and animal models. Kwon KH, Barve A, Yu S, Huang MT, Kong AN. Acta Pharmacol Sin. 2007 Sep;28(9):1409-21. **Key Finding:** "In this review, we summarize the potential mechanisms that certain daily-consumed dietary phytochemicals could have as **cancer** protective effects."

*Interactions among GSTM1, GSTT1 and GSTP1 polymorphisms, cruciferous vegetable intake and **breast cancer risk**.* Steck SE, Gaudet MM, Britton JA, et al. Carcinogenesis. 2007 Sep;28(9):1954-9. **Key Finding:** "Isothiocyanates are anticarcinogenic phytochemicals found in cruciferous vegetables that both induce and are substrates for the gluthatione S-transferases (GSTs). The GSTs are phase II metabolizing enzymes involved in metabolism of various bioactive compounds. We found no joint effects among GST polymorphisms and cruciferous vegetable intake and breast cancer risk. In conclusion, we found associations between specific combinations of three GST gene polymorphisms and breast cancer risk but these did not modify the association between cruciferous vegetable intake and breast cancer."

Antiestrogenic effects of phytochemicals on human primary mammary fibroblasts MCF-7 cells and their co-culture. Van Meeuwen JA, Korthagen N, de Jong PC, Piersma AH, Van den Berg M. Toxicol Appl Pharmacol. 2007 Jun 15;221(3):372-83. **Key Finding:** "In the present study, biochanin A. chrysin, naringenin, apigenin, genistein and quercetin were studied for their estrogenic properties (cell proliferation, p52 mRNA) and aromatase inhibition in MCF-7 **breast tumor cells**, healthy mammary fibroblasts and their co-culture. The results of these studies show that these phytochemicals can induce cell proliferation or inhibit aromatase in the same concentration range (1-10 microM). Results from co-cultures did not elucidate the dominant effect of these compounds. MCF-7 cell proliferation occurs at concentrations that are not uncommon in blood of individuals using food supplements. It is suggested that perhaps a more cautionary approach should be taken for these phytochemicals before taken as food supplements."

Inhibition of **cancer** *cell proliferation and suppression of TNF-induced activation of NFkappaB by edible berry juice.* Boivin D, Blanchette M, Barrette S, Moghrabi A, Beliveau R. Anticancer Res. 2007 Mar-Apr;27(2):937-48. **Key Finding:** "The growth of various cancer cell lines, including those of **stomach, prostate, intestine and breast,** was strongly inhibited by raspberry, black currant, white currant, gooseberry, velvet leaf blueberry, low-bush blueberry, sea buckhorn and cranberry juice, but not (or only slightly) by strawberry, high-bush blueberry, serviceberry, red currant, or blackberry juice."

Effect of selected phytochemicals and apple extracts on NF-kappaB activation in human **breast cancer** *MCF-7 cells.* Yoon H, Liu RH. J Agric Food Chem. 2007 Apr 18;55(8):3167-73. **Key Finding:** "These results suggest that apple extracts and curcumin have the capabilities of inhibiting TNF-alpha-induced NF-kappaB activation of MCF-7 cells by inhibiting the proteasomal activities instead of IkappaB kinase activation."

*Soy phytochemicals synergistically enhance the preventive effect of tamoxifen on the growth of estrogen-dependent **human breast carcinoma** in mice.* Mai Z, Blackburn GL, Zhou JR. Carcinogenesis. 2007 Jun;28(6):1217-23. **Key Finding:** "Genistein and tamoxifen combination synergistically delayed the growth of breast tumor via decreased estrogen level and activity, and down-regulation of EGFR expressions. The results from our studies suggest that further investigations may be warranted to determine if the combination of tamoxifen and bioactive soy components may be used for prevention and/or treatment of estrogen-dependent **breast cancer**."

Anthocyanin-rich grape extract blocks breast cell DNA damage. Singletary KW, Jung KJ, Giusti M. J Med Food. 2007 Jun;10(2):244-51. **Key Finding:** "These data suggest that Concord grape extract and a component grape anthocyanin have **breast cancer** chemopreventive potential due in part to their capacity to block carcinogen-DNA adduct formation, modulate activities of carcinogen-metabolizing enzymes, and suppress ROS in these noncancerous human breast cells."

*Genistein and quercetin increase connexin43 and suppress growth of **breast cancer** cells.* Conklin CM, Bechberger JF, MacFabe D, et al. Carcinogenesis. 2007 Jan;28(1):93-100. **Key Finding:** "Genistein and quercetin increase Cx43 and suppress MDA-MB-231 cell proliferation at physiologically relevant concentrations. These results demonstrate that genistein and quercetin are potential anti-breast cancer agents."

*Dietary flavonoid intake and **breast cancer** survival among women on Long Island.* Fink BN, Steck SE, Wolff MS, et al. Cancer Epidemiol Biomarkers Prev. 2007 Nov;16(11):2295-92. **Key Finding:** "Mortality may be reduced in association with high levels of dietary flavones and isoflavones among postmenopausal U.S. breast cancer patients."

*Cranberry phytochemical extracts induce cell cycle arrest and apoptosis in human MCF-7 **breast cancer cells**.* Sun J, Hai Liu R. Cancer Lett. 2006 Sep 8;241(1):124-34. **Key Finding:** "Epidemiological studies have consistently suggested the inverse association between cancer risk and intake of fruits and vegetables. These health benefits have been linked to the additive and synergistic combination of phytochemicals in fruits and vegetables. Our results suggest that cranberry phytochemical extracts possess the ability to suppress the proliferation of human breast cancer MCF-7 cells and this suppression is at least partly attributed to both the initiation of apoptosis and the G1 phase arrest."

Gene expression profiling revealed surviving as a target of 3,3'-diindolyl-methane-induced cell growth inhibition and apoptosis in **breast cancer** *cells.* Rahman KW, Li Y, Wang Z, Sarkar SH, Sarkar FH. Cancer Res. 2006 May 1;66(9):4952-60. **Key Finding:** "These results suggest that targeting suivivin by 3,3'-diindolylmethane could be a new and novel approach for the prevention and/or treatment of breast cancer."

3,3'-Diindolylmethane is a novel mitochondrial H(+)-ATP synthase inhibitor that can induce p21(Cip1/Waf1) expression by induction of oxidative stress in human **breast cancer** *cells.* Gong Y, Sohn H, Xue L, Firestone GL, Bidldanes LF. Cancer Res. 2006 May 1;66(9):4880-7. **Key Finding:** "We have established the critical role of enhanced mitochondrial ROS release in 3,3'-diindolylmethane-induced p21 up-regulation in human breast cancer cells."

Influence of phytoestrogens on the proliferation and expression of adhesion receptors in human mammary epithelial cells in vitro. Nebe B, Peters A, Duske K, Richter DU, Briese V. Eur J Cancer Prev. 2006 Oct;15(5):405-15. **Key Finding:** "Accumulating evidence suggests that phytoestrogens could inhibit tumorigenesis during the development of breast cancer. As the phytoestrogens do not up-regulate adhesion receptors in **human breast cells** and, regarding proliferation, are able to abolish the stimulatory effect of 17beta-estradiol, we suggest that phytoestrogens could have beneficial effects for the prevention or inhibition of carcinogenesis in hormone-dependent malignancies."

Polymethoxylated flavones induce Ca(2+)-mediated apoptosis in **breast cancer** *cells.* Sergeev IN, Li S, Colby J, Ho CT, Dushenkov S. Life Sci. 2006 Dec 23;80(3):245-53. **Key Finding:** "Here we report that polymethoxyflavones derived from sweet orange inhibit growth of human **breast cancer** cells. Our results strongly suggest that the cellular Ca(2+) modulating activity of flavonoids underlies their apoptotic mechanism and that hydroxylation of PMFs is critical for their ability to induce an increase in [Ca(2+)](i) and, thus, activate Ca(2+)-dependent apoptotic proteases."

Flavonoids and vitamin E reduce the release of the angiogenic peptide vascular endothelial growth factor from human tumor cells. Schindler R, Mentlein R, J Nutr. 2006 Jun;136:1477-1482. **Key Finding:** "The rank order of inhibitory potency on MDA human breast cancer cells was naringin>rutin>a-tocopheryl su ccinate>lovastatin>apigenin>genistein>a-tocopherol>kaempferol. Chrysin and curcumin were inactive except at a concentration of 100 umol/L. Overall, the glycosylated flavonoids (i.e. naringin, a constitutent of citrus fruits, and rutin, a constitutent of cranberries) induced the greatest response to treatment at the lowest concentration in MDA human **breast cancer** cells. Inhibition of VEGF release by flavonoids, tocopherols, and lovastatin suggests a novel mechanism for mammary cancer prevention."

*Dietary factors modifying **breast cancer** risk and relation to time of intake.* Tsubura A, Uehara N, Kiyozuka Y, Shikata N. J Mammary Gland Biol Neoplasia. 2005 Jan;10(1):87-100. **Key Finding:** "Some phytochemicals present in fruits and vegetables are protective. Time of intake appears to be important: lifetime protection may be achieved if one is exposed to a dietary factor that lowers breast cancer risk early in life. Synergistic and antisynergistic interactions between dietary factors can modify breast cancer risk. The available evidence suggests that breast cancer risk can be reduced by early dietary intervention."

Apples prevent mammary tumors in rats. Liu RH, Liu J, Chen B. J Agric Food Chem. 2005 Mar 23;53(6):2341-3. **Key Finding:** "This study demonstrated that whole apple extracts effectively inhibited **mammary cancer** growth in the rat model; thus, consumption of apples may be an effective therapy for cancer protection."

Sulforaphane, erucin, and iberin up-regulate thioredoxin reductase 1 expression in human MCF-7 cells. Wang W, Wang S, Howie AF, et al. J Agric Food Chem. 2005 Mar 9;53(5):1417-21. **Key Finding:** "In this study, we have shown that three isothiocyanates, sulforaphane, erucin and iberin, are potent inducers of thioredoxin reductase in human **breast cancer** MCF-7 cells."

3,3'-Diindolylmethane inhibits angiogenesis and the growth of transplantable human **breast carcinoma** *in athymic mice.* Chang X, Tou JC, Hong C, et al. Carcinogenesis. 2005;26(4):771-778. **Key Finding:** "This is the first study to show that 3,3'-Diindolylmethane can strongly inhibit the development of human breast tumor in a xenograft model and to provide evidence for the antiangiogenic properties of this dietary indole."

Inhibition of nuclear translocation of nuclear factor-kB contributes to 3,3'-Diindolylmethane-induced apoptosis in **breast cancer** *cells.* Rahman KMW, Sarkar FH. Cancer Res. 2005 Jan 1;65:364-371. **Key Finding:** "These results showed for the first time that the inactivation of Akt and NF-nB activity also plays important roles in Diindolylmethane-induced apoptosis in breast cancer cells, which seems to be more relevant to in vivo situations."

Flavonoids and **breast cancer** *risk in Italy.* Bosetti C, Spertini L, Parpinei M, et al. Cancer Epidemiol Biomarkers Prev. 2005 Apr;14(4):805-8. **Key Finding:** "After allowance for major confounding factors and energy intake, a reduced risk of breast cancer was found for increasing intake of flavones. No significant association was found for other flavonoids, including flavanones, anthocyanidins, as well as for isoflavones. The findings of this large study of an inverse association between flavones and breast cancer risk confirm the results of a Greek study."

The role of nutrition in the prevention of **breast cancer.** Duncan AM. AACN Clin Issues. 2004 Jan-Mar;15(1):119-35. **Key Finding:** "Results of epidemiological studies relating consumption of these dietary factors (such as phytochemicals) to breast cancer have increased the knowledge base that provides rationale for various nutritional strategies to contribute to breast cancer prevention."

Phytochemicals inhibit catechol-O-methyltransferase activity in cytosolic fractions from healthy human **mammary** *tissues: implications for catechol estrogen-induced DNA damage.* Van Duursen MB, Sanderson JT, De Jong PC, Kraaij M, van den Berg M. Toxicol Sci. 2004 Oct;81(2):316-24. **Key Finding:** "We investigated the effects of several phytochemicals on COMT activity in cytosolic fractions of seven healthy human mammary tissues from reduction mammoplasty. Both Ro 41-0960 and quercetin caused a decrease of methoxy estradiol formation and an increase of catechol estrogen-induced DNA damage in MCF-7 cells. This suggests that phytochemicals with a catechol structure have the potential to reduce COMT activity in mammary tissues and may consequently reduce the inactivation of potentially mutagenic estradiol metabolites and increase the chance of DNA damage."

Biphasic modulation of cell proliferation by quercetin at concentrations physiologically relevant in humans. Van der Woude H, Gliszczynska-Swigio A, Struijs K. Smeets A, Alink GM, Rietjens IM. Cancer Lett. 2003 Oct 8;200(1):41-7. **Key Finding:** "Optimal in vitro conditions regarding quercetin solubility and stability were defined. Using these conditions, the effect of quercetin on proliferation of the **colon carcinoma** cell lines HCT-116 and HT29 and the **mammary adenocarcinoma** cell line MCF-7 was investigated. For the colon carcinoma cell lines, at relatively high concentrations, a significant decrease in cell proliferation was observed, providing a basis for claims on the anti-carcinogenic activity of quercetin. However, at lower concentrations, a subtle but significant stimulation of cell proliferation was observed for all cell lines tested. These results point at a dualistic influence of quercetin on cell proliferation that may affect present views on its supposed beneficial anti-proliferative effect."

Potential risks and benefits of phytoestrogen-rich diets. Cassidy A. Int J Vitam Nutr Res. 2003 Mar;73(2):120-6. **Key Finding:** "The limited studies conducted so far in humans clearly confirm that soya isoflavones can exert hormonal effects. These effects may be of benefit in the prevention of many of the common diseases observed in Western populations (such as **breast cancer, prostate cancer, menopausal symptoms, osteoporosis**) where the diet is typically devoid of these biologically active naturally occurring compounds."

Intake of fruits, vegetables and selected micronutrients in relation to the risk of **breast cancer**. Malin AS, Qi D, Shu XO, et al. Int J Cancer. 2003 Jun 20;105(3):413-8. **Key Finding:** "Intake of fruits, except watermelons and apples, was inversely associated with breast cancer risk. Our study suggests that high intake of certain vegetables and fruits may be associated with a reduced risk of breast cancer."

*Dietary carotenoids and risk of **breast cancer**.* Terry P, Jain M, Miller AB, Howe GR, Rohan TE. Am J Clin Nutr. 2002 Oct;76(4):883-8. **Key Finding:** "Our data do not support any association between dietary intakes of the studied carotenoids (beta-carotene, alpha-carotene, beta-cryptoxanthin, lycopene, and lutein) and breast cancer risk. However, prospective cohort studies of carotenoids in relation to breast cancer are scarce and further studies are warranted."

The action of dietary phytochemicals quercetin, catechin, resveratrol and naringenin on estrogen-mediated gene expression. Ratna WN, Simonelli JA. Life Sci. 2002 Feb 15;70(13):1577-89. **Key Finding:** "To determine whether dietary phytochemicals purported to prevent hormone-dependent **breast and prostate cancers, and atherosclerosis**, acted via the estrogen-cell-signaling pathway, roosters were administered increasing doses up to 1 mmole/kg of resveratrol, quercetin, catechin, or naringenin parenterally and tested for hepatic expression of E-RmRNASF. Besides estrogen, the expression of E-RmRNASF in the liver was stimulated by resveratrol and catechin, indicating these agents to be estrogenic. A lack of E-Rm-RNASF expression was seen with the roosters treated with the naringenin or quercetin."

*White button mushroom phytochemicals inhibit aromatase activity and **breast cancer** cell proliferation.* Grube BJ, Eng ET, Kao YC, Kwon A, Chen S. J Nutr. 2001 Dec;131(12):3288-93. **Key Finding:** "Phytochemicals in the mushroom aqueous extract inhibited aromatase activity and proliferation of MCF-7aro cells. These results suggest that diets high in mushrooms may modulate the aromatase activity and function in chemoprevention in postmenopausal women by reducing the in situ production of estrogen."

Estrogenic and antiestrogenic activities of flavonoid phytochemicals through estrogen receptor binding-dependent and –independent mechanisms. Collins-Burow BM, Burow ME, Duong BN, McLachlan JA. Nutr Cancer. 2000;38(2):229-44. **Key Finding:** "We conclude that antiestrogenic activities of flavonoid phytochemicals may occur through ER binding-dependent and –independent mechanisms and that the binding-independent antiestrogen activity of certain flavonoids is biologically significant in regulation of **breast cancer** cell proliferation."

Phytoestrogens and human health effects: weighing up the current evidence. Humfrey CD. Nat Toxins. 1998;6(2):51-9. **Key Finding:** "Epidemiological studies suggest that foodstuffs containing phytoestrogens may have a beneficial role in protecting against a number of chronic diseases and conditions. For cancer of the **prostate, colon, rectum, stomach and lung,** the evidence is most consistent for a protective effect resulting from a high intake of grains, legumes, fruits and vegetables. Dietary intervention studies indicate that in women soya and linseed may have beneficial effects on the risk of **breast cancer** and may help to alleviate **postmenopausal symptoms.** For **osteoporosis,** tentative evidence suggests phytoestrogens may have similar effects in maintaining **bone density.** Soya also appears to have beneficial effects on blood lipids which may help to reduce the risk of **cardiosvascular disease** and **atherosclerosis.** Generally, however, little evidence exists to link these effects directly to phytoestrogens; many other components of soy and linseed are biologically active in various experimental systems and may be responsible for the observed effects in humans."

Phyto-oestrogens: where are we now? Bingham SA, Atkinson C, Liggins J, Bluck L, Coward A. Br J Nutr. 1998 May;79(5):393-406. **Key Finding:** "Evidence is beginning to accrue that they may begin to offer protection against a wide range of human conditions, including **breast, bowel, prostate** and other cancers, **cardiovascular disease,** brain function, alcohol abuse, **osteoporosis** and **menopausal symptoms.** There are few indications of harmful effects at present, although possible proliferative effects have been reported."

Urinary excretion of isoflavonoids and the risk of **breast cancer.** Zheng W, Dai Q, Custer LJ, et al. Cancer Epidemiol Biomarkers Prev. 1999 Jan;8(1):35-40. **Key Finding:** Overnight urine samples from 60 incident breast cancer cases and their individually matched controls were assayed for urinary excretion rates of five major isoflavonoids (daidzein, genistein, glycitein, equci, and O-desmethylangolensin.) "Individuals in the highest textile of daidzein, glycitein, and total isolflavonoids had about half the cancer risk of those in the lowest textile. The adjusted odds ratio for breast cancer was 0.14 (95% confidence interval, 0.02-0.88) for women whose urinary excretion of both phenol and total isoflavonoids was in the upper 50%

compared with those in the lower 50%. The results from this study support the hypothesis that a high intake of soy foods may reduce the risk of breast cancer."

*Vegetables, fruits, and related nutrients and risk of **breast cancer**: a case-control study in Uruguay.* Ronco A, De Stefani E, Boffetta P, et al. Nutr Cancer. 1999;35(2):111-9. **Key Finding:** "We carried out a case-control study in Uruguay including 400 cases and 405 controls. The results related to vegetable and nutrient intakes are consistent with antioxidant and antiestrogenic effects. This could be mediated, among other nutrients, by dietary fiber and lycopene intake. The role of other unmeasured phytochemicals, correlated with dietary fiber and lycopene intakes, cannot be ruled out."

*Inhibition of aberrant proliferation and induction of apoptosis in pre-neoplastic human **mammary epithelial cells** by natural phytochemicals.* Katdare M, Osborne MP, Telang NT. Oncol Rep. 1998 Mar-Apr;5(2):311-5. **Key Finding:** "Aberrant proliferation and modulated apoptosis leading to impaired cellular homeostatis represent crucial early events in the multistep carcinogenic process. Regulation of these perturbed biomarkers may predict efficacious prevention of cancer development. In long-term (21 day) experiments, BP (pyrene) treatment induced a 145.3% increase in anchorage-dependent colony formation. This aberrant proliferation was inhibited by 44.2% to 65.3% in the presence of three phytochemicals (cruciferous glucosinolate indole-3-carbinol, tea polyphenol epigallo catechin gallate, and soy isoflavone genistein.)"

*Modulation of androgen and progesterone receptors by phytochemicals in **breast cancer** cell lines.* Rosenberg RS, Grass L, Jenkins DJ, Kendall CW, Diamandis EP. Biochem Biophys Res Commun. 1998 Jul 30;248(3):935-9. **Key Finding:** "Our study indicates that a significant number of natural compounds have the ability to bind to steroid hormone receptors and act as weak blockers. A fewer number of compounds not only bind to the receptors but they also mediate transcriptional activity, acting as agonists."

*Micronutrients and **breast cancer**.* Franceschi S. Eur J Cancer Prev. 1997 Dec;6(6):535-9. **Key Finding:** "A large case-control study of 2,569 breast cancer and 2,588 hospital controls conducted in six Italian areas suggested that a diet rich in several micronutrients was associated with significantly lowered risk of breast cancer. Beta-carotene, vitamin E and calcium were associated with odds ratios in the highest intake quintile. Among agents that have only recently been investigated, isoflavones, which are weak oestrogens, are of particular interest."

Dose-ranging study of indole-3-carbinol for **breast cancer** *prevention.* Wong GY, Bradlow L, Sepkovic D, et al. J Cell Biochem Suppl. 1997;28-29:111-6. **Key Finding:** "The results of this study suggest that I3C at a minimum effective dose schedule of 300 mg per day is a promising chemopreventive agent for breast cancer prevention."

Cervical

The flavonoid quercetin induces cell cycle arrest and mitochondria-mediated apoptosis in human **cervical cancer** *(HeLa) cells through p53 induction and NF-KB inhibition.* Vidya Priyadarsini R, Senthil Murugan R, et al. Eur J Pharmacol. 2010 Dec 15;649(1-3):84-91. **Key Finding**: "The results demonstrate that quercetin suppressed the viability of HeLa cells in a dose-dependent manner. Quercetin that exerts opposing effects on different signaling networks to inhibit cancer progression is a classic candidate for anticancer drug design."

Multiple, disparate roles for calcium signaling in apoptosis of **human prostate and cervical cancer** *cells exposed to diindolylmethane.* Savino JA, Evans JF, Rabinowitz D, Auborn KJ, Carter TH. Mol Cancer Therap. 2006 Mar 1;5:556. **Key Finding:** "Diindolylmethane (DIM) derived from indole-3-carbinol in cruciferous vegetables causes growth arrest and apoptosis of cancer cells in vitro. We asked whether elevated cytosolic free calcium [Ca2+] is required for cytotoxicity of DIM and thapsigargin in two cancer cell lines from cervix and prostate was measured. Our results suggest that DIM induces apoptosis by different mechanisms in these two cell lines and/or that calcium mobilization also activates different survival pathways."

Anti-estrogenic activities of indole-3-carbinol in cervical cells: implication for prevention of **cervical cancer**. Yuan F, Chen DZ, Liu K, et al. Anticancer Res.

1999 May-Jun;19(3A):1673-80. **Key Finding:** "I3C has anti-estrogenic activities which should prevent cancer in cervical cells."

Colon

Curcumin therapeutic promises and bioavailability in **colorectal cancer.** Shehzad A, Khan S, Shehzad O, Lee YS. Drugs Today. 2010 Jul;46(7):523-32. **Key Finding:** "Curcumin, a polyphenol and derivative of turmeric is one of the most commonly used and highly researched phytochemicals. Although curcumin's poor absorption and low systemic bioavailability limit its translation into clinics, some of the methods for its use can be approached to enhance the absorption and achieve a therapeutic level of curcumin. Recent clinical trials suggest a potential role for curcumin in regards to colorectal cancer therapy."

Dietary intake of pterostilbene, a constitutent of blueberries, inhibits the beta-catenin/ p65 downstream signaling pathway and **colon carcinogenesis** *in rats.* Paul S, DeCastro AJ, Lee HJ, et al. Carcinogenesis. 2010 Jul;31(7):1272-8. **Key Finding:** "Our data with pterostilbene in suppressing colon tumorigenesis, cell proliferation as well as key inflammatory markers in vivo and in vitro suggest the potential use of peterostilbene for colon cancer prevention."

Colorectal cancer *prevention by flavonoids.* Hoensch H, Richling E, Kruis W, Krich W. Med Klin (Munich). 2010 Aug;105(8):554-9. **Key Finding:** "Selected flavonoids possess antimutagenic and anticarcinogenic properties and could reduce the incidence of colorectal neoplasias as shown in epidemiologic trials. Randomized controlled clinical studies with flavonoid intervention are necessary to provide evidence for their role in colorectal cancer prevention."

Urinary isothiocyanates; glutathione S-transferase M1, T1, and P1 polymorphisms; and risk of **colorectal cancer:** *the Multiethnic Cohort Study.* Epplein M, Wilkens LR, Tiirikainen M, et al. Cancer Epidemiol Biomarkers Prev. 2009 Jan;18(1):314-20. **Key Finding:** "A detectable amount of urinary isothiocyanates was associated with a 41% decrease in colorectal cancer risk. This is only the second study published on the association between urinary isothiocyanates and colorectal cancer risk. The results suggest that further studies, with larger numbers, examining a possible interaction with the GSTP1-polymorphisms are warranted."

The effect of strict adherence to a high-fiber, high-fruit and vegetable, and low-fat eating pattern on **adenoma** *recurrence.* Sansburn LB, Wanke K, Albert PS, et al. Am J Epidemiol. 2009 Sep 1;170(5):576-84. **Key Finding:** "The authors examined the effect of strict adherence to a low-fat, high-fiber, high-fruit and vegetable intervention over 4 years among participants in the US Polyp Prevention Trial on **colorectal adenoma** recurrence. The authors observed a 35% reduced odds of adenoma recurrence among super compliers compared with controls. Findings suggest that high compliance with a low-fat, high-fiber diet is associated with reduced risk of adenoma recurrence."

Fruit and vegetable intakes are associated with lower risk of **colorectal adenomas**. Wu H, Dai Q, Shrubsole MJ, et al. J Nutr. 2009 Feb;139(2):340-4. **Key Finding:** "This study provides additional evidence that high total fruit intake and certain fruit and vegetable intakes may be associated with a reduced risk of colorectal adenomas (cancerous polyps of the colon.)"

Phytochemical induction of cell cycle arrest by glutathione oxidation and reversal by N-acetylcysteine in **human colon carcinoma** *cells.* Odom RY, Dansby MY, Rollins-Hairston AM, Jackson KM, Kirlin WG. Nutr Cancer. 2009;61(3):332-9. **Key Finding: Cancer** prevention by dietary phytochemicals has been shown to involve decreased cell proliferation and cell cycle arrest. "One potential mechanism for cancer prevention by dietary phytochemicals is inhibition of the growth of cancer cells through modulation of their intracellular redox environment."

Fruit and vegetable intakes are associated with lower risk of **colorectal adenomas**. Wu H, Dai Q, Shrubsole MJ, et al. J Nutr. 2009 Feb;139(2):340-4. **Key Finding:** "This study provides additional evidence that high total fruit intake and certain fruit and vegetable intakes may be associated with a reduced risk of colorectal adenomas."

3,3'-diindolylmethane enhances the efficacy of butyrate in **colon cancer** *prevention through down-regulation of survivin.* Bhatnagar N, Li X, Chen Y, et al. Cancer

Prev Res. 2009 Jun;2(6):581-9. **Key Finding:** "Butyrate is an inhibitor of histone deacetylase and has been extensively evaluated as a chemoprevention agent for colon cancer. We showed that 3,3'-diindolylmethane (DIM) was able to down-regulate survivin and enhance the effects of butyrate in apoptosis induction and prevention of familiar adenomatous polypsis in APC mice. Thus, the combination of DIM and butyrate is potentially an effective strategy for the prevention of colon cancer."

Induction of p53 contributes to apoptosis of HCT-116 human **colon cancer** *cells induced by the dietary compound fisetin.* Lim DY, Park JH. Am J Physiol Gastrointest Liver Physiol. 2009 May;296(5):G1060-8. **Key Finding:** "These results show that fisetin induces apoptosis in HCT-116 cells via the activation of the death receptor and mitochondrial-dependent pathways and subsequent activation of the caspase cascade."

A plant flavonoid fisetin induces apoptosis in **colon cancer** *cells by inhibition of COX2 and Wnt/EGFR/NF-kappaB-signaling pathways.* Suh Y, Afaq F, Johnson JJ, Mukhtar H. Carcinogenesis. 2009 Feb;30(2):300-7. **Key Finding:** 'We provide evidence that the plant flavonoid fisetin can induce apoptosis and suppress the growth of colon cancer cells. We suggest that fisetin could be a useful agent for prevention and treatment of colon cancer."

Dietary flavonoid intake and **colorectal cancer***: a case control study.* Kyle JA, Sharp L, Little J, Duthie GG, McNeill G. Br J Nutr. 2009 Sep 7:1-8. **Key Finding:** "Non-tea flavonol intake was inversely associated with colorectal cancer risk. We conclude that flavonols, specifically quercetin, obtained from non-tea components of the diet may be linked with reduced risk of developing colon cancer."

Dietary flavonol, flavone and catechin intake and risk of **colorectal cancer** *in the Netherlands Cohort Study.* Simons CC, Hughes LA, Arts IC, et al. Int J Cancer. 2009 Dec 15;125(12):2945-52. **Key Finding:** "Our findings generally do not support an association of dietary flavonol, flavone and catechin intake with colorectal cancer endpoints. Dietary catechin intake may be associated with a decreased risk in overweight men. Dietary flavonol and catechin intake may also be associated with a decreased colorectal cancer risk in overweight women."

Growth inhibition of human **colon cancer** *cells by plant compounds.* Duessel S, Heuertz RM, Ezekiel UR. Clin Lab Sci. 2008 Summer;21(3):151-7. **Key Finding:** "Cinnamaldehyde, piperine, and resveratrol offer significant in vitro anti-proliferative effects on cultured human colon cancer cells. While each phytochemical exhibited significant anti-proliferative effects, resveratrol results were most impressive in that lower concentrations administered at regular intervals were significantly effective. These results taken together with everyday dietary availability of concentrations used in this study strongly suggest that regular intake of low doses of these phytochemicals offer preventive effects against colon cancer."

Flavonoids and **intestinal cancers.** Pierini R, Gee JM, Belshaw NJ, Johnson IT. Br J Nutr. 2008 May;99 E Suppl 1:ES53-9. **Key Finding:** "Many flavonoids exert anticarcinogenic effects in vitro and in animals, and many of these effects occur via signaling pathways known to be important in the pathogenesis of colorectal, gastric and oesophageal cancers. However, dietary flavonoid intakes are generally low and their metabolism in humans is extremely complex."

Mechanisms of **colorectal** *and* **lung cancer** *prevention by vegetables: a genomic approach.* Van Breda SG, De Kok TM, Van Delft JH. J Nutr Biochem. 2008 Mar;19(3):139-57. **Key Finding:** "This review evaluates current knowledge on the mechanisms of colorectal cancer and lung cancer prevention by vegetables, thereby focusing on the modulation of gene and protein expressions."

Dietary chemoprevention of **colorectal cancer.** Forte A, De Sanctis R, Leonetti G, et al. Ann Ital Chir. 2008 Jul-Aug;79(4):261-7. **Key Finding:** "The authors analyze the possible mechanisms by which certain nutritive factors may interfere with the complex process of carcinogenesis. At present, the data suggest that vegetables are associated with lower risk for colorectal cancer and that their fibre content alone does not account for this association. Several micronutrients of the diet may be associated with reduced risk, including folate, methionine, calcium and vitamin D. Short chain fatty acids also contribute to colonic health. Meat consumption is associated with an increased risk. Mutagenic compounds, particularly heterocyclic amines, produced when protein is cooked, plausibly explain the meat association."

*Lack of prospective associations between plasma and urinary phytoestrogens and risk of **prostate** or **colorectal cancer** in the European Prospective Into Cancer Norfolk study.* Ward H, Chapelais G, Kuhnie GG, et al. Cancer Epidemiol Biomarkers Prev. 2008 Oct;17(10):2891-4. **Key Finding:** "Serum and urine samples were analyzed for seven phytoestrogens (daidzein, enterodiol, enterolactone, genistein, glycitein, O-desmethylangolensin, and equci) among 193 cases of prostate cancer and 828 controls, and 221 cases of colorectal cancer with 889 controls. There was no significant association between prostate cancer risk and total serum isoflavones, or between colorectal cancer risk and total serum isoflavones. Similarly, null associations were observed for individual serum phytoestrogens and for all urinary phytoestrogen biomarkers. In conclusion, we have found no evidence to support an inverse association between phytoestrogen exposure and prostate or colorectal cancer risk."

*Structure-function relationships of anthocyanins from various anthocyanin-rich extracts on the inhibition of **colon cancer** cell growth.* Jing P, Bomser JA, Schwartz SJ, et al. J Agric Food Chem. 2008 Oct 22;56(20):9391-8. **Key Finding:** "Anthocyanins played a major role in anthocyanin-rich extracts chemoprotection and exerted an additive interaction with the other phenolics present." Anthocyanins color red, purple and blue fruits. Purplecorn and bilberry were more potent than the radish. Anthocyanin pigments obtained from black carrots and radishes slowed the growth of cancer cells by 50% to 80%.

*Dietary soy and isoflavone intake and risk of **colorectal cancer** in the Japan public health cancer-based prospective study.* Akhter M, Inoue M, Kurahashi N, et al. Cancer Epidemiol Biomarkers Prev. 2008 Aug;17(8):2128-35. **Key Finding:** "These findings suggest that the intake of isoflavones, miso soup, and soy food has no substantial effect on the risk of colorectal cancer in Japanese men and women."

*Dietary flavonoids and **colorectal adenoma** recurrence in the Polyp Prevention Trial.* Bobe G, Sansbury LB, Albert PS, et al. Cancer Epidemiol Biomarkers

Prev. 2008 Jun;17(6):1344-53. **Key Finding:** "Our data suggest that a flavonol-rich diet may decrease the risk of advanced adenoma recurrence."

Green tea polyphenols in the prevention of **colon cancer.** Kumar N, Shibata D, Helm J, Coppola D, Malafa M. Front Biosci. 2007 Jan 1;12:2309-15. **Key Finding:** "The goal of this review is to provide the rationale and discuss the use of EGCG in green tea polyphenols as a chemopreventive agent for prevention of colon carcinogenesis and present evidence for the efficacy and safety of these agents based on epidemiological, animal, in vitro studies and Phase I clinical trials."

Inhibition of **cancer** *cell proliferation and suppression of TNF-induced activation of NFkappaB by edible berry juice.* Boivin D, Blanchette M, Barrette S, Moghrabi A, Beliveau R. Anticancer Res. 2007 Mar-Apr;27(2):937-48. **Key Finding:** "The growth of various cancer cell lines, including those of **stomach, prostate, intestine and breast,** was strongly inhibited by raspberry, black currant, white currant, gooseberry, velvet leaf blueberry, low-bush blueberry, sea buckhorn and cranberry juice, but not (or only slightly) by strawberry, high-bush blueberry, serviceberry, red currant, or blackberry juice."

Colon-available raspberry polyphenols exhibit anti-cancer effects on in vitro models of **colon cancer.** Coates EM, Popa G, Gill CI, et al. J Carcinog. 2007 Apr 18;6:4. **Key Finding:** "A 'colon available' raspberry extract was prepared that contained phytochemicals surviving a digestion procedure that mimicked the physiochemical conditions of the upper gastrointestinal tract. The results indicate that raspberry phytochemicals likely to reach the colon are capable of inhibiting several important stages in **colon carcinogenesis** in vitro."

Berry phenolic extracts modulate the expression of p21(WAF1) and Bax but not Bcl-2 in HT-29 **colon cancer** *cells.* Wu QK, Koponen JM, Mykkanen HM, Torronen AR. J Agric Food Chem. 2007 Feb 21;55(4):1156-63. **Key Finding:** "the objective of this study was to compare the effects of berry extracts containing different phenolic profiles on cell viability and expression of markers of cell proliferation and apoptosis in human colon cancer HT-29 cells. A 14-fold increase in the expression of p21WAF1, an inhibitor of cell proliferation and a member of the cyclin kinase inhibitors, was seen in cells exposed to cloudberry extract compared to other berry treatments. Cloudberry, despite its very low anthocyanin content, was a potent inhibitor of cell proliferation. Therefore, it is concluded that, in addition to anthocyanins, also other phenolic or nonphenolic phytochemicals are responsible for the antiproliferative activity of berries."

Chemoprevention of aberrant crypt foci in the colon of rats by dietary onion. Tache S, Ladam A, Corpet DE. Eur J Cancer. 2007 Jan;43(2):454-8. **Key Finding:** "Onion intake might reduce the risk of **colorectal cancer**, according to epidemiology. However, Femia showed in 2003 that diets with a 20% onion intake increase carcinogenesis in rats. We speculated this dose was too high. Prevention of initiation was thus tested in 60 rats given a 5% dried onion diet. Phytochemicals diet and pluronic diet reduced aberrant crypt foci growth similarly. Data show that a 5% onion diet reduced carcinogenesis during initiation and promotion stages, and suggest this chemoprevention is due to known phytochemicals."

Green tea polyphenols in the prevention of **colon cancer**. Kumar N, Shibata D, Helm J, Coppola D, Malafa M. Front Biosci. 2007 Jan 1;12:2309-15. **Key Finding:** "The goal of this review is to provide the rationale, and discuss the use of EGCG in green tea polyphenols as a chemopreventive agent for prevention of colon carcinogenesis and present evidence for the efficacy and safety of these agents based on epidemiological, animal, in vitro studies and Phase I clinical trials."

Dietary flavonoids and the risk of **colorectal cancer**. Theodoratou E, Kyle J, Catnarsky FL, et al. Cancer Epidemiol Biomarkers Prev. 2007 Apr;16(4):684-93. **Key Finding:** "The significant dose dependent reductions in colorectal cancer risk that were associated with consumption of flavonols, quercetin, catechin, and epicatechin remained robust after controlling for other vegetable consumption. The risk reductions were greater among nonsmokers."

Dietary anthocyanin-rich tart cherry extract inhibits intestinal tumorigenesis in APC(Min) mice fed suboptimal levels of sulindac. Bobe G, Wang B, Seeram NP, Nair MG, Bourquin LD. J Agric Food Chem. 2006 Dec 13;54(25):9322-8. **Key Finding:** "These results suggest that a dietary combination of tart cherry anthocyanins and sulindac (a nonsteroidal anti-inflammatory drug) is more protective against **colon cancer** than sulindac alone."

*Blackberry, black raspberry, blueberry, cranberry, red raspberry, and strawberry extracts inhibit growth and stimulate apoptosis of human **cancer** cells in vitro.* Seeram NP, Adams LS, Zhang Y, et al. J Agric Food Chem. 2006 Dec 13;54(25):9329-39. **Key Finding:** "With increasing concentration of berry extract, increasing inhibition of cell proliferation in all of the cell lines were observed, with different degrees of potency between cell lines. The berry extracts were also evaluated for their ability to stimulate apoptosis of the COX-2 expressing **colon cancer** cell line, HT-29. Black raspberry and strawberry extracts showed the most significant pro-apoptotic effects against this cell line."

*Anthocyanin-rich extracts inhibit multiple biomarkers of **colon cancer** in rats.* Lala G, Malik M, Zhao C, et al. Nutr Cancer. 2006;54(1):84-93. **Key Finding:** "Extracts from bilberry, chokeberry and grape were assessed by multiple biomarkers of colon cancer in male rats treated with a colon carcinogen. These results support our previous in vitro studies suggesting a protective role of anthocyanin-rich extracts in colon carcinogenesis and indicate multiple mechanisms of action."

Tumors from rats given 1,2-dimethylhydrazine plus chlorophyllin or indole-3-carbinol contain transcriptional changes in beta-catenin that are independent of beta-catenin mutation status. Wang R, Dashwood WM, Bailey GS, Williams DE, Dashwood RH. Mutat Res. 2006 Oct 10;601(1-2):11-8. **Key Finding:** "Tumors induced in the rat by 1,2-dimethylhydrazine contain mutations in beta-catenin, but the spectrum of such mutations can be influenced by phytochemicals such as chlorophyllin and indole-3-carbinol. In the present study, we determined the mutation status of beta-catenin in more than 50 DMH-induced **colon tumors** and small intestine tumors. Similar findings have been reported in primary human colon cancers and their liver metastases."

*Pomegranate juice, total pomegranate ellagitannins, and punicalagin suppress inflammatory cell signaling in **colon cancer** cells.* Adams LS, Seeram NP, Aggarwal BB, et al. J Agric Food Chem. 2006 Feb 8;54(3):980-5. **Key Find-**

ing: "The polyphenolic phytochemicals in the pomegranate can play an important role in the modulation of inflammatory cell signaling in colon cancer cell."

High dry bean intake and reduced risk of advanced **colorectal adenoma** *recurrence among participants in the polyp prevention trial.* Lanza E, Hartman TJ, Albert PS, et al. J Nutr. 2006 Jul;136(7):1896-903. **Key Finding:** "There were no significant associations between nonadvanced adenoma recurrence and overall change in fruit and vegetable consumption; however, those in the highest quartile of change in dry bean intake (greatest increase) compared with those in the lowest had a significantly reduced odds ratio for advanced adenoma recurrence."

Heme and chlorophyll intake and risk of **colorectal cancer** *in the Netherlands cohort study.* Balder HF, Vogel J, Jansen MC, et al. Cancer Epidemiol Biomarkers Prev. 2006 Apr;15(4):717-25. **Key Finding:** "Our data suggest an elevated risk of colon cancer in men with increasing intake of heme iron and decreasing intake of chlorophyll. Further research is needed to confirm these results."

Flavonoids and **colorectal cancer** *in Italy.* Rossi M, Negri E, Talamini R, et al. Cancer Epidemiol Biomarkers Prev. 2006 Aug;15(8):1555-8. **Key Finding:** "The findings of this large study provide support for an inverse association of selected classes of flavonoids with colorectal cancer risk."

Flavonoid intake and **colorectal cancer** *risk in men and women.* Lin J, Zhang SM, Wu K, et al. Am J Epidemiol. 2006 Oct 1;164(7):644-51. **Key Finding:** "The authors prospectively evaluated the association between intake of flavonoids and colorectal cancer incidence in 71,976 women from the Nurses' Health Study and 35,425 men from the Health Professionals Follow-Up Study by means of a food frequency questionnaire. These data provide little support for the hypothesis of an association between flavonoid intake and colorectal cancer risk, at least within the ranges of intakes consumed in the populations studied."

In vitro antiproliferative, apoptotic and antioxidant activities of punicalagin, ellagic acid and a total pomegranate tannin extract are enhanced in combination with other polyphenols as found in pomegranate juice. Seeram NP, Adams LS, Henning SM, et al. J Nutr Biochem. 2005 Jun;16(6):360-7. **Key Finding:** "Pomegranate juice showed greatest antiproliferative activity against all **colon cancer** cell lines by inhibiting proliferation from 30% to 100%. The superior bioactivity of pomegranate juice compared to its purified polyphenols illustrated the multifactorial effects and chemical synergy of the action of multiple compounds compared to single purified active ingredients."

Inhibition of cytokine-induced prostanoid biogenesis by phytochemicals in human **colonic fibroblasts**. Russell WR, Drew JE, Scobbie L, Duthie GG. Biochem Biophys Acta. 2006 Jan;1762(1):124-30. **Key Finding:** "Many of the inflammatory pathways regulating the production of prostanoids are implicated in the development of **colon cancer**. Diets rich in fruits and vegetables are associated with decreased rates of colon cancer and this may reflect anti-inflammatory properties of some phytochemicals. In order to ascertain which of the many dietary compounds may be protective, a cell-based screening method was established to determine their effects on the production of prostanoids. Several of the compounds signficiantly inhibited prostanoid biogenesis by up to 81% and others enhanced prostanoid production. All of the compounds that enhanced prostanoid production belonged to the hydroxylated benzoic acid family. Common structure features of the inhibitors were the presence of 4-hydroxyl and 3-methoxyl substituents on the aromatic ring and/or the presence of a three-carbon side-chain on C1."

Primary prevention of **colorectal cancer**: *lifestyle, nutrition, exercise.* Martinez ME. Recent Results Cancer Res. 2005;166:177-211. **Key Finding:** "Diets high in red and processed meat increase risk for colorectal cancer. Excess alcohol consumption, probably in combination with a diet low in some micronutrients such as folate and methionine, appear to increase risk. There is also recent evidence supporting a protective effect of calcium and vitamin D in the etiology of colorectal neoplasia. The relationship between intake of dietary fiber and risk of colon cancer has been studied for three decades but the results are still inconclusive. However, some micronutrients or phytochemicals in fiber-rich foods may be important; folic acid is one such micronutrient that has been shown to protect against the development of colorectal neoplasma."

Modulation of aberrant crypt foci and apoptosis by dietary herbal supplements quercetin, curcumin, silymarin, ginseng and rutin. Volate SR, Davenport DM, Muga SJ, Wargovich MJ. Carcinogenesis. 2005 Aug;26(8):1450-6. **Key Finding:** "The results of this study suggest that these herbal supplements may exert significant and potentially beneficial effects on decreasing the amount of **precancerous lesions** and inducing apoptosis in the **large intestine**."

The effects of quercetin on SW480 human **colon carcinoma** *cells: a proteomic study.* Mouat MF, Kolli K, Orlando R, Hargrove JL, Grider A. Nutr J. 2005 Mar 4;4:11. **Key Finding:** "Several proteins were determined to have altered expression following treatment with quercetin. Such changes in the levels of these particular proteins could underlie the chemo-protective action of quercetin towards colon cancer."

Green vegetables, red meat and **colon cancer***: chlorophyll prevents the cytotoxic and hyperproliferative effects of haem in rat colon.* De Vogel J, Jonker-Termon DS, Van Lieshout EM, Katan MB, Van der Meer R. Carcinogenesis. 2005 Feb;26(2):387-93. **Key Finding:** "We studied whether green vegetables inhibit the unfavourable colonic effects of haem (from red meat) in rat colons. We conclude that green vegetables may decrease colon cancer risk because chlorophyll prevents the detrimental, cytotoxic and hyperproliferative colonic effects of dietary haem."

Fisetin inhibits the activities of cyclin-dependent kinases leading to cell cycle arrest in HT-29 human **colon cancer** *cells.* Lu X, Jung J, Cho HJ, et al. J Nutr. 2005 Dec;135(12):2884-90. **Key Finding:** "Fisetin dose dependently inhibited both cell growth and DNA synthesis with a 79+/- 1% decrease in cell number observed 72 h after the addition of 60 micromol/L fisetin. These results indicate that inhibition of cell cycle progression in HT-29 cells after treatment with fisetin can be explained, at least in part, by modification of CDK activities."

Indian food ingredients and cancer prevention – an experimental evaluation of anticarcinogenic effects of garlic in rat colon. Sengupta A, Ghosh S, Bhattacharjee S, Das S. Asian Pac J Cancer Prev. 2004 Apr-Jun;5(2):126-32. **Key Finding:** "Following treatment, significant inhibition of cell proliferation and induction of apoptosis, as well as suppression of cyclooxygenase-2 activity were observed, associated with significant reduction in the incidence of aberrant crypt foci. The study points to combined protective effects of garlic components on **colon carcinogenesis**."

Modulatory properties of various natural chemopreventive agents on the activation of NF-kappaB signaling pathway. Jeong WS, Kim IW, Hu R, Kong AN. Pharm Res. 2004 Apr;21(4):661-70. **Key Finding:** "To study and compare effects of selected natural chemopreventive agents on the transcription activation of nuclear factor-kappa B in human HT-29 colon cancer cells, isothiocyanates found in cruciferous vegetables, flavonoids found in green tea, resveratrol and curcumin were examined. We found that ITCs such as phenethyl isothiocyanate (PEITC), sulforaphane (SUL), allyl isothiocyanate (AITC) and curcumin strongly inhibited LPS-induced NF-kappaB-luciferase activations, whereas resveratrol increased activation at lower dose, but inhibited at higher doses, and tea flavonoids and procyanidin dimmers had little or no effects. PEITC, SUL, and curcumin also potently inhibited cell growth. These results suggest that natural chemopreventive agents have differential biological functions on the signal transduction pathways in the colon and/or **colon cancer**."

*Effects of commercial anthocyanin-rich extracts on **colonic cancer** and nontumorigenic colonic cell growth.* Zhao C, Giusti MM, Malik M, Moyer MP, Magnuson BA. J Agric Food Chem. 2004 Oct 6;52(20):6122-8. **Key Finding:** "Commercially prepared grape, bilberry, and chokeberry anthocyanin-rich extracts were investigated for their potential chemopreventive activity against colon cancer. All extracts inhibited the growth of HT-29 colon cancer cells with chokeberry being the most potent inhibitor. The varying compositions and degrees of growth inhibition suggest that the antocyanin chemical structure may play an important role in the growth inhibitory activity."

*Tart cherry anthocyanins inhibit tumor development in Apc(Min) mice and reduce proliferation of human **colon cancer** cells.* Kang SY, Seeram NP, Nair MG, Bourquin LD. Cancer Lett. 2003 May 8;194(1):13-9. **Key Finding:** "Mice consuming the cherry diet, anthocyanins, or cyaniding, had significantly fewer and smaller cecal adenomas than mice consuming the control diet or sulindac. Anthocyanins and cyanidin also reduced cell growth of human colon cancer cell lines HT29 and HCT 116."

Biphasic modulation of cell proliferation by quercetin at concentrations physiologically relevant in humans. Van der Woude H, Gliszczynska-Swigio A, Struijs K, et al.Cancer Lett. 2003 Oct 8;200(1):41-7. **Key Finding:** "Optimal in vitro conditions regarding quercetin solubility and stability were defined. Using these conditions, the effect of quercetin on proliferation of the **colon carcinoma** cell lines HCT-116 and HT29 and the **mammary adenocarcinoma** cell line MCF-7 was investigated. For the colon carcinoma cell lines, at relatively high concentrations, a significant decrease in cell proliferation was observed, providing a basis for claims on the anti-carcinogenic activity of quercetin. However, at lower concentrations, a subtle but significant stimulation of cell proliferation was observed for all cell lines tested. These results point at a dualistic influence of quercetin on cell proliferation that may affect present views on its supposed beneficial anti-proliferative effect."

Dietary factors and risk of **colon cancer** *in Shanghai, China.* Chiu BC, Ji BT, Dai Q, et al. Cancer Epidemiol Biomarkers Prev. 2003 Mar;12(3):201-8. **Key Finding:** "For dietary nutrients, risk generally declined with greater consumption of fiber and micronutrients common in fruit and vegetables, including vitamin C, carotene, and vitamin E. Our findings suggest that diets high in fruit and antioxidant vitamins that are common in plant foods reduce the risk of colon cancer, whereas diets high in red meat, eggs, and preserved foods increase the risk."

Promotion versus suppression of rat **colon carcinogenesis** *by chlorophyllin and chlorophyll: modulation of apoptosis, cell proliferation, and beta-carenin/ Tcf signaling.* Blum CA, Xu M, Orner GA, et al. Mutat Res. 2003 Feb-Mar;523-524:217-23. **Key Finding:** "The results suggest that further investigation of the dose-response for suppression versus promotion by chlorophyll and chlorophyllin is warranted, including studies of the beta-catenin/Tcf signaling pathway and its influence on cell proliferation and apoptosis in the colonic crypt."

Novel approaches for **colon cancer** *prevention by cyclooxygenase-2 inhibitors.* Reddy BS, Rao CV. J Environ Pathol Toxicol Oncol. 2002;21(2):155-64. **Key Finding:** "Naturally occurring COX-2 inhibitors such as curcumin and certain phytosterols have been proven to be effective as chemopreventive agents against colon carcinogenesis with minimal gastrointestinal toxicity."

Nutritional chemoprevention of **colon cancer**. Mason JB. Semin Gastrointest Dis. 2002 Jul;13(3):143-53. **Key Finding:** "Overall, a diet habitually high in fresh fruits and vegetables, modest in calories and alcohol, and low in red meat and animal fat, is cancer protective. There is little question that diet has a major impact on colorectal cancer risk."

Primary prevention: phytoprevention and chemoprevention of **colorectal cancer**. Turini ME, DuBois RN. Hematol Oncol Clin North Am. 2002 Aug;16(4):811-40. **Key Finding:** "Phytochemicals have been identified as strong candidates for use as agents to prevent colorectal cancer in cell culture and in rodent models of carcinogenesis. Their potential as chemoprevention agents must be demonstrated in clinical trials."

Dietary carotenoid intake and **colorectal cancer** *risk*. Terry P, Jain M, Miller AB, Howe GR, Rohan TE. Nutr Cancer. 2002;42(2):167-72. **Key Finding:** "In this study we examined the relationships between dietary intakes of beta-carotene, alpha-carotene, lycopene, lutein, and beta-crypotoxanthin and colorectal cancer risk in a large cohort study of 56,837 Canadian women. Our data do not support any association between dietary intakes of the studied carotenoids and colorectal cancer risk. However, given that this is the first prospective cohort study of carotenoids in relation to colorectal cancer, further studies are warranted."

Chemopreventive effect of farnesol and lanosterol on **colon carcinogenesis**. Rao CV, Newmark HL, Reddy BS. Cancer Detect Prev. 2002;26(6):419-25. **Key Finding:** "In this study we have assessed the chemopreventive efficacy of farnesol and lanosterol on azoxymethane (AOM)-induced colonical aberrant crypt foci in rats. Farnesol and lanosterol significantly suppress colonic ACF formation and crypt multiplicity strengthens the hypothesis that these agents possess cheompreventive activity against colon carcinogenesis."

Modifiable risk factors for **colon cancer**. Giovannucci E. Gastroenterol Clin North Am. 2002 Dec;31(4):925-43. **Key Finding:** "Recent epidemiologic studies have tended not to support a strong influence of fiber; instead, some micronutrients or phytochemicals in fiber-rich foods may be important in decreasing the risk of colon cancer. The overwhelming evidence indicates that primary prevention of colon cancer is feasible. At least 70% of colon cancers may be preventable by moderate changes to diet and lifestyle."

Fruits, vegetables, and **adenomatous polyps***: the Minnesota Cancer Prevention Research Unit case-control study.* Smith-Warner SA, Elmer PJ, Fosdick L, et al. Am J Epidemiol. 2002 Jun 15;155(12):1104-13. **Key Finding:** "The results for fruits, vegetables, total fruits and vegetables, green leafy vegetables, and several botanically and phytochemically defined subgroups generally were not statistically significant. Because elevated vegetable consumption has been associated with a lower risk of **colorectal cancer**, vegetables may have a stronger role in preventing the progression of adenomas to carcinomas rather than in preventing the initial appearance of adenomas."

Beta-Catenin mutation in rat colon tumors initiated by 1,2-dimethylhydrazine and 2-amino-3-methylimidazo (4,5-quinoline, and the effect of post-initiation treatment with chlorophyllin and indole-3-carbinol. Blum CA, Xu M, Orner GA, et al. Carcinogenesis. 2001 Feb;22(2):315-20. **Key Finding:** "Two dietary phytochemicals, chlorophyllin and indole-3-carbinol, given post-initiation, shifted the pattern of beta-catenin mutations in rat **colon tumors**. The results indicate that the mechanism might involve the altered expression of beta-catenin/Tcf/Lef target genes."

Dietary indoles and isothiocyanates that are generated from cruciferous vegetables can both stimulate apoptosis and confer protection against DNA damage in human **colon cell** *lines.* Bonnesen C, Eggleston IM, Hayes JD. Cancer Res. 2001 Aug 15;61(16):6120-30. **Key Finding:** "Evidence is presented that the ability of indoles and isothiocyanates to stimulate either xenobiotic response element- or antioxidant response element-driven gene expression accounts for the two groups of phytochemicals inducing different gene batteries. These phytochemicals together may prevent colon tumorigenesis by both stimulating apoptosis and enhancing intracellular defenses against genotoxic agents."

Chemoprevention of **colon carcinogenesis** *by dietary non-nutritive compounds.* Tanaka T, Kohno H, Mori H. Asian Pac J Cancer Prev. 2001;2(3):165-177. **Key Finding:** "Previous studies in our laboratory demonstrated protective effects of several naturally occurring products against rat colon tumorgenesis. This article will introduce our recent studies in our search for chemopreventive effects of flavonoids (diosmin and hesperidin) and other phytochemicals in edible plants on rat colon carcinogenesis."

(+)-Catechin inhibits intestinal tumor formation and suppresses focal adhesion kinase activation in the min/+ mouse. Weyant MJ, Carothers AM, Dannenberg AJ, Bertagnolli MM. Cancer Res. 2001 Jan 1;61(1):118-25. **Key Finding:** "The natural abundance and favorable bioavailability of (+)-catechin make it a promising addition to the list of potential **colorectal cancer** chemopreventive agents."

Carotenoids and **colon cancer.** Slattery ML, Benson J, Curtin K, et al. Am J Clin Nutr. 2000 Feb;71(2):575-82. **Key Finding:** "Lutein was inversely associated with colon cancer in both men and women studied. The major dietary sources of lutein in subjects with colon cancer and in control subjects were spinach, broccoli, lettuce, tomatoes, oranges and orange juice, carrots, celery, and greens. These data suggest that incorporating these foods into the diet may help reduce the risk of developing colon cancer."

Dietary flavones is a potent apoptosis inducer in human **colon carcinoma** *cells.* Wenzel U, Kuntz S, Brendel MD, Daniel H. Cancer Res. 2000 Jul 15;60(14):3823-31. **Key Finding:** "Flavone was found to reduce cell proliferation in HT-29 cells and to potential induce differentiation as well as apoptosis. The flavonoid proved to be a stronger apoptosis inducer than the clinically established antitumor agent camptothecin."

Prevention of precancerous **colonic lesions** *in rats by soy flakes, soy flour, genistein, and calcium.* Thiagarajan DG, Bennink MR, Bourquin LD, Kavas FA. Am J Clin Nutr. 1998 Dec;68 (6Suppl):1394S-1399S. **Key Finding:** "Eating soybeans and soy flour may reduce the early stages of colon cancer."

Soyfoods, isoflavones and risk of **colonic cancer:** *a review of the in vitro and in vivo data.* Messina M, Bennink M, Baillieres Clin Endocrinol. Metab. 1998 Dec;12(4):707-28. **Key Finding:** "Although the relationship between soy intake and colonic cancer risk is certainly worthy of further investigation, there is, at the moment, very limited support for soy exerting a protective effect against this type of cancer."

Phytoestrogens and human health effects: weighing up the current evidence. Humfrey CD. Nat Toxins. 1998;6(2):51-9. **Key Finding:** "Epidemiological studies suggest that foodstuffs containing phytoestrogens may have a beneficial role in protecting against a number of chronic diseases and conditions. For cancer of the **prostate, colon, rectum, stomach and lung,** the evidence is most consistent for a protective effect resulting from a high intake of grains, legumes, fruits and vegetables. Dietary intervention studies indicate that in women soya and linseed may have beneficial effects on the risk of **breast cancer** and may help to alleviate **postmenopausal symptoms**. For **osteoporosis**, tentative evidence suggests phytoestrogens may have similar effects in maintaining **bone density**. Soya also appears to have beneficial effects on blood lipids which may help to reduce the risk of **cardiosvascular disease** and **atherosclerosis**. Generally, however, little evidence exists to link these effects directly to phytoestrogens; many other components of soy and linseed are biologically active in various experimental systems and may be responsible for the observed effects in humans."

Phyto-oestrogens: where are we now? Bingham SA, Atkinson C, Liggins J, Bluck L, Coward A. Br J Nutr. 1998 May;79(5):393-406. **Key Finding:** "Evidence is beginning to accrue that they may begin to offer protection against a wide range of human conditions, including **breast, bowel, prostate** and other cancers, **cardiovascular disease**, brain function, alcohol absue, **osteoporosis** and **menopausal symptoms.** There are few indications of harmful effects at present, although possible proliferative effects have been reported."

*Enhancement of experimental **colon cancer** by genistein.* Rao CV, Wang CX, Simi B, et al. Cancer Res. 1997 Sept 1;57(17):3717-22. **Key Finding:** "The present study was designed to investigate the effect of genistein on azoxymethane-induced colon carcinogenesis. Administration of genistein significantly increased noninvasive and total adenocarcinoma multiplicity in the colon, compared to the control diet, but it had no effect on the colon adenocarcinoma incidence nor on the multiplicity of invasive adenocarcinoma."

Dietary factors and risk of **colon cancer.** Giovannucci E, Willett WC. Ann Med. 1994 Dec;26(6):443-52. **Key Finding:** "Intake of red meat appears to increase the risk of colon cancer. High consumption of vegetables and fruits and the avoidance of highly refined sugar containing foods are likely to reduce risk of colon cancer, although the responsible constituents remain unclear."

Dietary Fiber, Vegetables, and **Colon Cancer:** *Critical Review and Meta-analysis of the Epidemiologic Evidence.* Trock B, Lanza E, Greenwald P. J Natl Cancer Inst.1990;82(8):650-661. **Key Finding:** "This review consisted of an aggregate assessment of the strength of evidence from 37 observational epidemiologic studies as well as meta-analyses of data from 16 of the 23 case-control studies. Both types of analyses revealed that the majority of studies gave support for a protective effect associated with fiber-rich diets. But the data do not permit discrimination between effects due to fiber and nonfiber effects due to vegetables."

Gastric

Eugenol induces apoptosis and inhibits invasion and angiogenesis in a rat model of **gastric carcinogenesis** *induced by MNNG.* Mankiandan P, Murugan RS, Priyadarsini RV, Vinothini G, Nagini S.Life Sci. 2010 Jun 19;86(25-26):936-41. **Key Finding**: "Phytochemicals such as eugenol that are capable of manipulating the equilibrium between pro- and anti-apoptotic proteins as well as the delicate balance between stimulators and inhibitors of invasion and angiogenesis are attract candidates for preventing tumour progression."

Isothiocyanates, glutathione S-transferase M1 and T1 polymorphisms and gastric cancer risk: a prospective study of men in Shanghai, China. Moy KA, Yuan JM, Chung FL, et al. Int J Cancer. 2009 Dec 1;125(11):2652-9. **Key Finding:** "In this cohort of Chinese men at high risk for gastric cancer, isothiocyanates may protect against the development of **gastric cancer**. The protection may be stronger for individuals genetically deficient in enzymes that metabolize these chemopreventive compounds."

Suppressive effects of selected food phytochemicals on CD74 expression in NCI-N87 **gastric carcinoma cells**. Sekiguchi H, Washida K, Murakami A. J Clin Biochem Nutr. 2008 Sep;43(2):109-17. **Key Finding:** Human gastric carcinoma cells were treated with 25 different food phytochemicals. A citrus coumarin, bergamottin, was found to be the most promising compound for suppression, followed by luteolin, nobiletin, and quercetin.

Hepatocellular carcinoma

Phytochemicals as potential chemopreventive and chemotherapeutic agents in hepatocarcinogenesis. Mann CD, Neal CP, Garcea G, et al. Eur J Cancer Prev. 2009 Feb;18(1):13-25. **Key Finding: Hepatocellular carcinoma** is the fifth commonest malignancy worldwide. Both in-vitro and animal studies show several phytochemicals, including curcumin, resveratrol, green tea catechins, oltipraz and silibinin, possess promising chemopreventive and chemotherapeutic properties.

Green tea polyphenol epigallocatechin-3-gallate inhibits thrombin-induced hepatocellular **carcinoma** *cell invasion and p42/p44-MAPKinase activation.* Kaufmann R, Henklein P, Henklein P, Settmacher U. Oncol Rep. 2009 May;21(5):1261-7. **Key Finding:** "In this study, we investigated the effect of EGCG on thrombin-PAR1/PAR4-mediated hepatocellular carcinoma cell invasion and p42/p44 MAPKinase activation. The results suggest that EGCG might have therapeutic potential for hepatocellular carcinoma."

Laryngeal

Flavonoids and **laryngeal cancer** *risk in Italy.* Garavello W, Rossi M, McLaughlin JK, et al. Ann Oncol. 2007 Jun;18(6):1104-9. **Key Finding:** "This study provides support for a beneficial effect of selected flavonoids on laryngeal cancer risk. Significant inverse relations were found for flavan-3-ols, flavones, flavonols and total flavonoids, although the overall trends in risk were significant only for flavones and flavonols. No consistent associations were observed for isoflavones, anthocyanidins and flavones."

Tomatoes, tomato-rich foods, lycopene and cancer of the upper aerodigestive tract: a case-control in Uruguay. De Stefani E, Oreggia F, Boffetta P, et al. Oral Oncol. 2000 Jan;36(1):47-53. **Key Finding:** " In order to study the relationship between tomatoes, tomato products, lycopene and **cancers** of the upper aerodigestive tract; **oral cavity, pharynx, larynx, esophagus;** a case-control study was carried out in Uruguay involving 238 cases and 491 hospitalized controls. We found that the joint effect of lycopene and total phytosterols was associated with a significant reduction in risk for these cancers."

Leukemia

*Quercetin induced apoptosis in association with death receptors and fludarabine in cells isolated from chronic lymphocytic **leukaemia** patients.* Russo M, Spagnuolo C, Volpe S, et al. Br J Cancer. 2010 Aug 24;103(5):642-8. **Key Finding**: "Quercetin significantly enhanced anti-CD95- and rTRAIL-induced cell death as shown by decreased cell viability."

Involvement of glutathione in the cytotoxicity of 9-isothiocyanatoacridine. Paulikova H, Bajdichova M, Sovcikova A, Sabolova D. Biomed Pap Med Fac Unive Palacky Olomouc Czech Repub. 2005 Dec;149(2):413-7. **Key Finding:** "Our results indicated that apoptosis of **leukemia cells** induced by isothiocyanates is possible only if intracellular glutathione is not entirely depleted."

*Flavonoids induce apoptosis in human **leukemia** U937 cells through caspase- and caspase-calpain-dependent pathways.* Monasterio A, Urdaci MC, Pinchuk IV, Lopez-Moratalla N, Martinze-Irujo JJ. Nutr Cancer. 2004;50(1):90-100. **Key Finding:** "In this study we tested the apoptotic activity of 22 flavonoids and related compounds in leukemic U937 cells. Several flavones but none of the isoflavones or flavonoids tested induced apoptotic cell death. Galangin, luteolin, chrysin and quercetin induced apoptosis in a way that required the activation of caspases 3 and 8, but not caspase 9. In contrast, an active role calpains in addition to caspases was demonstrated in apoptosis induced by fisetin, apigenin, and 3,7-dihydroxyflavone."

*Volatile isoprenoid constitutents of fruits, vegetables and herbs cumulatively suppress the proliferation of murine B16 melanoma and human HL-60 **leukemia** cells.* Tatman D, Mo H. Cancer Lett. 2002 Jan 25;175(2):129-39. **Key Finding:** "A search for volatile isoprenoid constituents of food products spanning seven plant families identified 179 isoprenoids. Of these, 41 were screened for efficacy in suppressing the proliferation of murine B16 melanoma cells. Individual isoprenoids suppressed the proliferation of B16 and HL-60 promyelocytic leukemia cells with varying degrees of potency. Blends of isoprenoids suppressed B16 and HL-60 cells proliferation with efficacies equal to the sum of the individual impacts. These findings suggest that the cancer-protective property of fruits, vegetables and related products is partly conferred by the cumulative impact of volatile isoprenoid constitutents."

Piceatannol, a hydroxylated analog of the chemopreventive agent resveratrol, is a potent inducer of apoptosis in the lymphoma cell line BJAB and in primary, leukemic lymphoblasts. Wieder T, Prokop A, Bagci B, et al. Leukemia. 2001 Nov;15(11):1735-42. **Key Finding:** "In the present study, we show that resveratrol, as well as the hydrooxylated analog piceatannol, are potent inducers of apoptotic cell death in BJAB Burkitt-like lymphoma cells. To explore the antileukemic properties of both compounds in more detail, we extended our study to primary leukemic lymphblasts. Interestingly, piceatannol but not resveratrol is a very efficient inducer of apoptosis in this ex vivo assay with leukemic lymphoblasts of 21 patients suffering from childhood lymphoblastic **leukemia.**"

Antiproliferative effects of compounds derived from plants of Northeast Brazil. Pessoa C, Silveira ER, Lemos TL, et al. Phytother Res. 2000 May;14(3):187-91. **Key Finding:** "This study demonstrated the antiproliferative activity (on **leukemia, lung tumor, and normal skin fibroblast** cells) of four novel phytochemicals, three of which are DNA-reactive and inhibit DNA synthesis. Further studies are warranted to evaluate these compounds for antitumour potential."

Liver

Resveratrol in the chemoprevention and treatment of **hepatocellular carcinoma**. Bishayee A, Politis T, Darvesh AS. Cancer Treat Rev. 2010 Feb;36(1):43-53. **Key Finding**: "Using naturally occurring phytochemicals and dietary compounds endowed with potent antioxidant and anti-inflammatory properties is a novel approach to prevent and control hepatocellular carcinoma. One such compound, resveratrol, present in grapes, berries, peanuts, has emerged as a promising molecule that inhibits carcinogenesis with a pleiotropic mode of action."

Studies of structure-activity relationship on plant polyphenol-induced suppression of human **liver cancer** *cells.* Loa J, Chow P, Zhang K. Cancer Chemother Pharmacol. 2009 May;63(6):1007-16. **Key Finding:** "To study anticancer activities of 68 plant polyphenols on human liver cancer cells, the polyphenols were sub-classed to flavonoids (chalcones, flavanones, flavones and isoflavones), chromones and courmarins. The order of their potency to suppress the human liver cancer cells is chalcones>flavones>chromones>isoflavones>flavanones>courmarins. Top nine most potent chalcones in the group have hydroxylation at 2'-carbon position in B-ring. The most potent chalcone, 2,2'-dihydroxychalcone could induce G2/M arrest and then apoptosis of the cancer cells."

Inhibitory effects of polyphenolic compounds on human arylamine N-acetyltransferase 1 and 2. Kukongvirivapan V, Phromsopha N, Tassaneevakul W, et al. Xenobiotica. 2006 Jan;36(1):15-28. **Key Finding:** "Arylamine N-acetyltransferases are important enzymes involved in the metabolic activation of aromatic and heterocyclic amines and inhibitors of NAT enzymes and may be valuable as chemopreventive agents. Phytochemicals including cinnamic acid derivatives, various classes of flavonoids and coumarins were tested for the inhibitory activity on NAT1 and NAT2 from human **liver** and the human cholangiocarcinoma cell lines. Quercetin inhibited both enzymes and was the most potent inhibitor of all compounds tested."

Lung

*Candidate dietary phytochemicals modulate expression of phase II enzymes GSTP1 and NQO1 in human **lung cells**.* Tan XL, Shi M, Tang H, et al. J Nutr. 2010 Aug;140(8):1404-10. **Key Finding**: Many phytochemicals possess cancer-preventive properties. We applied human lung cells in vitro to investigate the effects of several candidate phytopreventive agents, including broccoli sprout extracts, epigallocatechin gallate and sulforaphane. We conclude that modulation of lung cell phase II metabolism by chemopreventive agents requires cell and agent specific discovery and testing.

*Cruciferous vegetable intake is inversely associated with **lung cancer** risk among smokers: a case-control study.* Tang L, Zirpoli GR, Jayaprakash V, et al. BMC Cancer. 2010 Apr 27;10:162. **Key Finding**: "Our findings are consistent with the smoking-related carcinogen-modulating effect of isothiocyanates, a group of phytochemicals uniquely present in cruciferous vegetables. Our data support consumption of a diet rich in cruciferous vegetables may reduce the risk of lung cancer among smokers."

*Flavonoids intake and risk of **lung cancer**: a meta-analysis.* Tang NP, Zhou B, Wang B, Yu RB, Ma J. Jpn J Clin Oncol. 2009 Jun;39(6):352-9. **Key Finding:** "Eight prospective studies and four case-control studies involving 5,073 lung cancer cases and 237,981 non-cases were included in the meta-analysis. The combined results indicated a statistically significant association between highest flavonoid intake and reduced risk of developing lung cancer."

*Cruciferous vegetable consumption and **lung cancer** risk: a systematic review.* Lam TK, Gallicchio L, Lindsley K, et al. Can Epidemio Biomarkers Prev. 2009 Jan;18(1):184-95. **Key Finding:** "Epidemiologic evidence suggest that cruciferous vegetable intake may be weakly and inversely associated with lung cancer risk. Because of a gene-diet interaction, the strongest inverse association was among those with homozygous deletion for GSTM1 and GSTT1."

Soy photochemicals decrease nonsmall cell lung cancer growth in female athymic mice. Gallo D, Zannoni GF, De Stefano I, et al. J Nutr. 2008 Jul;138(7):1360-4.

Key Finding: "Our research provides further support for the concept that consumption of phytoestrogens may be effective in delaying **lung cancer** progression."

Mechanisms of **colorectal** *and* **lung cancer** *prevention by vegetables: a genomic approach.* Van Breda SG, De Kok TM, Van Delft JH. J Nutr Biochem. 2008 Mar;19(3):139-57. **Key Finding:** "This review evaluates current knowledge on the mechanisms of colorectal cancer and lung cancer prevention by vegetables, thereby focusing on the modulation of gene and protein expressions."

Silibinin inhibits cytokine-induced signaling cascades and down-regulates inducible nitric oxide synthase in human **lung carcinoma** *A549 cells.* Chittezhath M, Deep G, Singh RP, Agarwal C, Agarwal R. Mol Cancer Ther. 2008 Jul;7(7):1817-26. **Key Finding:** "These results suggest that silibinin could target multiple cytokine-induced signaling pathways to down-regulate INOS expression in lung cancer cells and that could contribute to its overall cancer preventive efficacy against lung tumoringenesis."

A review of the epidemiological evidence on tea, flavonoids, and **lung cancer.** Arts IC. J Nutr. 2008 Aug;138(8):1561S-1566S. **Key Finding:** "In general, the studies on tea, flavonoids, and lung cancer risk indicate a small beneficial association, particularly among never-smokers. More well-designed cohort studies, in particular for catechins, are needed to strengthen the evidence on effects of long-term exposure to physiological doses of dietary flavonoids."

Dietary quercetin inhibits proliferation of lung carcinoma cells. Hung H. Forum Nutr. 2007;60:146-57. **Key Finding:** "In this study, we report that quercetin-inhibited A549 **lung carcinoma** cell proliferation was associated with activation of the extracellcular signal-regulated kinase (ERK). Inhibition of MEK1/2 but not PI3 kinase, p38 kinase or JNK abolished quercetin-induced apoptosis suggesting MEK-ERK activation was required to trigger apoptosis."

Clove (Syzygium aromaticum L.), a potential chemopreventive agent for **lung cancer.** Banerjee S, Panda CK, Das S. Carcinogenesis. 2006 Aug;27(8):1645-

54. **Key Finding:** "In the present work we assess the chemopreventive potential of aqueous infusion of clove during benzo[a]pyrene (BP)-induced lung carcinogenesis in strain A mice. The observations signifiy the chemopreventive potential of clove in view of its apoptogenic and anti-proliferative properties."

Role of mitochondria in quercetin-enhanced chemotherapeutic response in human non-small cell lung carcinoma H-520 cells. Kuhar M, Sen S, Singh N. Anticancer Res. 2006 Mar-Apr;26(2A):1297-303. **Key Finding:** "Based on these findings, it can be concluded that quercetin might act as an effective chemosensitizer in the chemotherapy of **lung cancer** by regulating the expression of various apoptosis-related genes."

*Apigenin inhibits expression of vascular endothelial growth factor and angiogenesis in human **lung cancer** cells: implication of chemoprevention of lung cancer.* Liu LZ, Fang J, Zhou Q, et al. Mol Pharmacol. 2005 Sep;68(3):635-43. **Key Finding:** "Our data suggested that apigenin may inhibit human lung cancer angiogenesis by inhibiting HIF-1alpha and VEGF expression, thus providing a novel explanation for the anticancer action of apigenin."

*Dietary flavonoids and **cancer** risk: evidence from human population studies.* Neuhouser ML. Nutr Cancer. 2004;50(1):1-7. **Key Finding:** "This article reviews data from four cohort studies and six case-control studies, which have examined associations of flavonoid intake with cancer risk. There is consistent evidence from these studies that flavonoids, especially quercetin, may reduce the risk of **lung cancer**. Further research using new dietary databases for food flavonoid content is needed to confirm these findings before specific public health recommendations about flavonoids can be formulated."

*The role of activated MEK-ERK pathway in quercetin-induced growth inhibition and apoptosis in A549 **lung cancer** cells.* Nguyen TT, Tran E, Nguyen TH, et al. Carcinogenesis. 2004 May;25(5):647-59. **Key Finding:** "Dietary phytochemicals have been shown to be protective against various types of cancers. However, the precise underlying protective mechanisms are poorly understood. In the present study, we report that treatment of A549 lung carcinoma cells with quercetin resulted in a dose-dependent reduction in cell viability and DNA synthesis."

Silibinin induces growth inhibition and apoptotic cell death in human lung carcinoma cells. Sharma G, Singh RP, Chan DC, Agarwal R. Anticancer Res. 2003 May-Jun;23(3B):2649-55. **Key Finding:** "Silibinin significantly induces growth inhibition, a moderate cell cycle arrest and a strong apoptotic death in both small cell and non-small cell human **lung carcinoma** cells, which warrants further studies to assess the efficacy of this non-toxic agent in animal lung tumor models."

*Fruits and vegetables are associated with lower **lung cancer** risk only in the placebo arm of the beta-carotene and retinol efficacy trial (CARET).* Neuhouser ML, Patterson RE, Thornquist MD, et al. Cancer Epidemiol Biomarkers Prev. 2003 Apr;12(4):350-8. **Key Finding:** "We did not observe any statistically significant associations of fruit and vegetable intake with lung cancer risk among participants randomized to receive the CARET supplements (30 mg of beta-carotene and 25,000 IU of retinyl palmitate. This report provides evidence that plant foods have an important preventive influence in a population at high risk for lung cancer. However, persons who use beta-carotene supplements do not benefit from the protective compounds in plant foods."

Flavonoid intake and risk of chronic diseases. Knekt P, Kumpulainen J, Jarvinen R, et al. Am J Clin Nutr. 2002 Sep;76(3):560-68. **Key Finding:** "The total dietary intakes of 10,054 men and women were determined with a dietary history method. Persons with higher quercetin intakes had lower mortality from ischemic **heart disease**. The incidence of **cerebrovascular disease** was lower at higher kaempferol, naringenin, and hesperetin intakes. Men with higher quercetin intakes had a lower **lung cancer** incidence and men with higher myricetin intakes had a lower **prostate cancer** risk. **Asthma** incidence was lower at higher quercetin, naringenin, and hesperetin. A trend toward a reduction in risk of **type 2 diabetes** was associated with higher quercetin and myricetin intakes."

Antiproliferative effects of compounds derived from plants of Northeast Brazil. Pessoa C, Silveira ER, Lemos TL, et al. Phytother Res. 2000 May;14(3):187-91. **Key Finding:** "This study demonstrated the antiproliferative activity (on **leukemia, lung tumor, and normal skin fibroblast** cells) of four novel phytochemicals, three of which are DNA-reactive and inhibit DNA synthesis. Further studies are warranted to evaluate these compounds for antitumour potential."

*Isothiocyanates, glutathione S-transferase M1 and T1 polymorphisms, and **lung-cancer** risk: a prospective study of men in Shanghai, China.* London S, Yuan J, Chung F, et al.The Lancet. 2000;356(9231):724-729. **Key Finding:** "Isothiocyanates appeared to reduce lung cancer risk in this cohort of Chinese men. Reduction in risk was strongest among persons genetically deficient in enzymes that rapidly eliminate these chemopreventive compounds."

*Intake of flavonoids and **lung cancer**.* Marchand LL, Murphy SP, Hankin JH, Wilkens LR, Kolonel LN. J Natl Cancer Inst. 2000 Jan 19;92(2):154-60. **Key Finding:** "After adjusting for smoking and intakes of saturated fat and B-carotene, we found statistically significant inverse associations between lung cancer risk and the main food sources of the flavonoids quercetin (onions and apples) and naringin (white grapefruit.)"

*Intake of specific carotenoids and flavonoids and the risk of **lung cancer** in women in Barcelona, Spain.* Garcia-Closas R, Agudo A, Gonzalez CA, Riboli E. Nutr Cancer. 1998;32(3):154-8. **Key Finding:** "With adjustment for smoking habit and vitamin E, vitamin C, and total flavonoid intake, no association was found for the intake of alpha-carotene, beta-carotene, or lutein. No protective effect was observed for quercetin or luteolin or for total flavonoid intake."

Beta-carotene, carotenoids, and disease prevention in humans. Mayne ST. FASEB J. 1996 May;10(7):690-701. **Key Finding:** "Researchers should now seek explanations for the apparently discordant findings of observational studies vs. intervention trials. The most pressing research issues include studies of interactions of carotenoids with themselves and with other phytochemicals and mechanistic studies of the actions of beta-carotene in **lung carcinogenesis** and **cardiovascular disease**."

*Dietary flavonoids and the risk of **lung cancer** and other malignant neoplasms.* Knekt P, Jaryinen R, Seppanen R, et al. Am J Epidemiol. 1997 Aug 1;146(3):223-30. **Key Finding:** "Of the major dietary flavonoid sources, the consumption of apples showed an inverse association with lung cancer incidence. The results are in line with the hypothesis that flavonoid intake in some circumstances may be involved in the cancer process, resulting in lowered risks."

Importance of a-carotene, B-carotene, and other phytochemicals in the etiology of **lung cancer**. Ziegler RG, Colavito EA, Harge P, et al. JNatl Cancer Inst. 1996 May 1; vol 88, no. 9: 612-615. **Key Finding:** Analysis of white male smokers with lung and related cancers found that "B-carotene is not the dominant protective factor in vegetables and fruit. Intakes of a-carotene, yellow-orange vegetables, and dark-green vegetables were each more predictive of reduced lung cancer risk. The most rational way to reduce lung cancer risk is to eat a variety of vegetables and fruits and, most important, not to smoke."

Dietary antioxidants and the risk of **lung cancer**. Knekt P, Jaryinen R, Seppanen R, et al. Am J Epidemiol. 1991 Sep 1;134(5):471-9. **Key Finding:** "The relation between the intake of retinoids, carotenoids, vitamin E, vitamin C, and selenium and the subsequent risk of lung cancer was studied among 4,538 initially cancer-free Finnish men aged 20-69 years. The results suggest that carotenoids, vitamin E, and vitamin C may be protective against lung cancer among nonsmokers. Food sources rich in these micronutrients may also have other constitutents with independent protective effects against lung cancer."

Protective dietary factors and **lung cancer**. Fontham ET. Int J Epidemiol. 1990;19 Suppl 1:532-42. **Key Finding:** "Since the first report of a protective effect of dietary vitamin A on lung cancer risk was issued in 1975, a succession of retrospective (case-control) and prospective (cohort) epidemiological studies have examined the association. The dietary studies have been notably consistent, finding an approximate 50% reduction in risk associated with high compared to low consumption of carotene-containing fruits and vegetables."

Carotenoid intake, vegetables, and the risk of **lung cancer** *among white men in New Jersey.* Ziegler RG, Mason TJ, Stemhagen A, et al. Am J Epidemiol. 1986 Jun:123(6):1080-93. **Key Finding:** "Consumption of dark yellow-orange vegetables was consistently more predictive of reduced risk than consumption of any other food group or the total carotenois index, possibly because of the high content of beta-carotene relative to other carotenoids in this particular food group."

Non-Hodgkin's lymphoma

Intakes of fruits, vegetables, and related nutrients and the risk of **non-Hodgkin's lymphoma** *among women.* Zhang SM, Hunter DJ, Rosner BA, et al. Cancer Epidemiology Biomarkers & Prevention. 2000 May; vol 9:477-485. **Key Finding:** "Higher intake of vegetables, particularly cruciferous vegetables, may reduce the risk of non-Hodgkin's lymphoma among women."

Neck

Dietary carotenoids and certain cancers, heart disease, and age-related macular degeneration: a review of recent research. Cooper DA, Eldrigde AL, Peters JC. Nutr Rev. 2009 Apr 27;57(7):201-214. **Key Finding:** "Key epidemiologic studies show associations between high dietary intakes of certain carotenoid-containing fruits and vegetables and reduced risk of **prostate cancer**, **breast cancer**, **head and neck cancers**, **cardiovascular disease** and age-related **macular degeneration**, although overall the evidence is inconsistent. Little is known about the potential biochemical mechanisms whereby carotenoids might protect against disease, and human intervention trials are limited to high dose B-carotene, which is not protective against lung cancer or cardiovascular disease."

Oral

Association between fruit and vegetable consumption and **oral cancer**: *a meta-analysis of observational studies.* Pavia M, Pileggi C, Nobile CG, Angelillo IF. Am J Clin Nutr. 2006 May;83(5):1126-34. **Key Finding:** "Sixteen studies met the inclusion criteria and were included in the meta-analysis. For vegetable consumption, the meta-analysis showed a significant reduction in the overall risk of oral cancer of 50%. The multivariate meta-regression showed that the lower risk of oral cancer associated with fruit consumption was significantly influenced by the type of fruit consumed and by the time interval of dietary recall."

Inhibition of the growth of premalignant and malignant human oral cell lines by extracts and components of black raspberries. Han C, Ding H, Casto B, Stoner GD, D'Ambrosio SM. Nutr Cancer. 2005;51(2):207-17. **Key Finding:** "These results show for the first time that the growth inhibitory effects of black raspberries on premalignant and **malignant human oral cells** may reside in specific components (ferulic acid and beta-sitosterol) that target aberrant signaling pathways regulating cell cycle progression."

*Effect of yerba mate (Ilex paraguariensis) tea on topoisomerase inhibition and **oral carcinoma** cell proliferation.* Gonzalez de Mejia E, Song YS, Ramirez-Mares MV, Kobayashi H. J Agric Food Chem. 2005 Mar 23;53(6):1966-73. **Key Finding:** "Tea flavonoids have antitopoisomerase activity and can inhibit cell proliferation. The objectives of this study were to determine the phenolic content of yerba mate tea products and evaluate their capacity to inhibit topoisomerase activities and oral carcinoma cell proliferation. It is concluded that yerba mate tea is rich in phenolic constitutents and can also inhibit oral cancer proliferation. The lack of correlation between polyphenol content and the inhibition of topoisomerases suggests that the effect of yerba mate tea on topoisomerase inhibition may be due to other still unidentified biologically active phytochemicals constitutents."

Tomatoes, tomato-rich foods, lycopene and cancer of the upper aerodigestive tract: a case-control in Uruguay. De Stefani E, Oreggia F, Boffetta P, et al. Oral Oncol. 2000 Jan;36(1):47-53. **Key Finding:** " In order to study the relationship between tomatoes, tomato products, lycopene and **cancers** of the upper aerodigestive tract; **oral cavity, pharynx, larynx, esophagus;** a case-control study was carried out in Uruguay involving 238 cases and 491 hospitalized controls. We found that the joint effect of lycopene and total phytosterols was associated with a significant reduction in risk for these cancers."

Ovarian

*A prospective study of dietary flavonoid intake and incidence of epithelial **ovarian cancer.*** Gates MA, Tworoger SS, Hecht JL, et al. Int J Cancer. 2007;121(10):2225-2232. **Key Finding:** "These data suggest that dietary intake of certain flavonoids in the flavonol and flavones subclasses may reduce ovarian cancer risk."

*Risk of human **ovarian cancer** is related to dietary intake of selected nutrients, phytochemicals and food groups.* McCann SE, Freudenheim JL, Marshall JR, Graham S. J Nutr. 2003 Jun;133(6):1937-42. **Key Finding:** "We conducted a case-control study of diet and ovarian cancer in western New York involving 124 primary, histologically confirmed ovarian cancer cases and 696 population-based controls. These results support a protective effect on ovarian cancer of phytoestrogen intakes, and our results support the hypothesis that a plant-based diet may be important in reducing risk of hormone-related neoplasms."

Pancreatic

*Flavonoid intake and risk of **pancreatic cancer** in male smokers (Finland).* Bobe G, Weinstein SJ. Albanes D, et al. Cancer Epidemiol Biomarkers Prev. 2008 Mar;17(3):553-62. **Key Finding:** "Our data suggest that a flavonoid-rich diet may decrease pancreatic cancer risk in male smokers not consuming supplemental alpha-tocopherol and/or beta-carotene."

*A food pattern that is predictive of flavonol intake and risk of **pancreatic cancer.*** Nothlings U, Murphy SP, Wilkens LR, et al. Am J Clin Nutr. 2008 Dec;88(6):1653-62. **Key Finding:** "A food pattern associated with the intake of quercetin, kaempferol, and myricetin was associated with lower pancreatic cancer risk in smokers in a US-based population. However, failure to replicate the associations in an independent study weakens the conclusions and raises questions about the utility of food patterns for flavonols across populations."

*Flavonols and **pancreatic cancer** risk: the multiethnic cohort study.* Nothlings U, Murphy SP, Wilkens LR, Henderson BE, Kolonel LN. Am J Epidemiol. 2007 Oct 15;166(8):924-31. **Key Finding:** "Total flavonols, quercetin, kaempferol, and myricetin were all associated with a significant inverse trend among current smokers, former smokers, or those who have never smoked. This study provides evidence for a preventive effect of flavonols on pancreatic cancer, particularly for current smokers."

*3,3'-diindolylmethane (DIM) and its derivatives induce apoptosis **in pancreatic cancer** cells through endoplasmic reticulum stress-dependent upregulation of DR5.* Abdelrahim M, Newman K, Vanderlaag K, Samudio I, Safe S. Carcinogenesis. 2006 Apr;27(4):717-28. **Key Finding:** "DIM, ring-substituted DIMs and 1,1-bis(3'indolyl)-1-(p-substituted phenylmethanes (D-DIMs) inhibit growth of Panc-1 and Panc-28 pancreatic cancer cells. Activation of both receptor-dependent and receptor-independent (ER stress) pathways by DIM and DIM-C-pPhtBu in pancreatic cancer cells enhances the efficacy and potential clinical importance of these compounds for cancer chemotherapeutic applications."

*Dietary intake of lycopene is associated with reduced **pancreatic cancer** risk.* Nkondjock A, Ghadirian P, Johnson KC, Krewski D, Canadian Cancer Registries Epidemiology Research Group. J Nutr. 2005 Mar;135(3):592-7. **Key Finding:** "In this study, we investigated the possible association between dietary carotenoids and pancreatic cancer risk. A case-controlled study of 462 histologically confirmed pancreatic cancer cases and 4721 population-based controls in eight Canadian provinces took place. The results of this study suggest that a diet rich in tomatoes and tomato-based products with high lycopene content may help reduce pancreatic cancer risk."

*Potent chemopreventive agents against **pancreatic cancer**.* Nishikawa A, Furukawa F, Lee IS, Tanaka T, Hirose M. Curr Cancer Drug Targets. 2004 Jun;4(4):373-84. **Key Finding:** "Phenethyl isothiocyanate (PEITC) remarkably blocked the initiation phase of pancreatic as well as **lung carcinogenesis** in hamsters initiated with N-nitrosobis(2-oxopropyl)amine (BOP). However, PEITC failed to affect both pancreatic and lung carcinogenesis when given during the post-initiation (promotion) phase of carcinogenesis."

Inhibition of **pancreatic cancer** *growth by the dietary isoprenoids farnesol and geraniol.* Burke YD, Stark MJ, Roach SL, Sen SE, Crowell PL. Lipids. 1997 Feb;32(2):151-6. **Key Finding:** "Farnesol, geraniol, and perillyl alcohol suppress pancreatic tumor growth without significantly affecting blood cholesterol levels. These dietary isoprenoids warrant further investigation for pancreatic cancer prevention and treatment."

Prostate

Genistein-selenium combination induces growth arrest in **prostate cancer** *cells.* Kumi-Diaka J, Merchant K, Haces A, Hormann V, Johnson M. J Med Food. 2010 Aug;13(4):842-50. **Key Finding**: "Several in vitro studies together with animal models and epidemiological studies have indicated that phytochemicals can be antitumorigenic and may be protective against human cancers. In this study we investigated the effects of genistein-selenium combination on prostate cancer cells. This combination induced significant growth inhibition in both MMP-2 and LNCaP cell lines. The data obtained from the present study indicate that Gn-Se combination may have chemopreventive value for prostate tumors independent of hormonal status."

Tomato-based food products for prostate cancer prevention: what have we learned? Tan HL, Thomas-Ahner JM, Grainger EM, et al. Cancer Metastasis Rev. 2010 Sep;29(3):553-68. **Key Finding**: "Tomatoes are a source of bioactive phytochemicals. The opportunity [exists] to develop a highly consistent tomato-based food product rich in anticancer phytochemicals for clinical trials targeting specific cancers, particularly the **prostate**."

Isosilybin A induces apoptosis in human **prostate cancer** *cells via targeting Akt, NF-KB, and androgen receptor signaling.* Deep G, Gangar SC, Oberlies NH, Kroll DJ, Agarwal R. Mol Carcinog. 2010 Oct;49(10):902-12. **Key Finding**: "Our results demonstrated that isosilybin A activates apoptotic machinery in PCA cells via targeting, thereby indicating a promising role for this phytochemical in the management of clinical prostate cancer."

Proanthocyanidins from the American cranberry (vaccinium macrocarpon) inhibit matrix metalloproteinase-2 and matrix metalloproteinase-9 activity in **human pros-**

tate cancer *cells via alterations in multiple cellular signaling pathways.* Deziel BA, Patel K, Neto C, Gottschall-Pass K, Hurta RA. J Cell Biochem. 2010 Oct 15;111(3):742-54. **Key Finding**: "It is believed that an individual's diet affects his risk of developing prostate cancer. In this study we document the effects of proanthocyanidins from the American cranberry on MMP activity in DU145 human prostate cancer cells. Cranberry decreased cellular viability of DU145 cells at a concentration of 25 ug/ml by 30% after 6 hours of treatment."

Targeting CWR22Rv1 ***prostate cancer*** *cell proliferation and gene expression by combinations of the phytochemicals EGCG, genistein and quercetin.* Hsieh TC, Wu JM. Anticancer Res. 2009 Oct;29(10):4025-32. **Key Finding**: "These results demonstrate the feasibility of developing a diet-based combinatorial approach for prostate cancer prevention and treatment and raises the possibility that serum added to culture medium might affect uptake, bioavailability and biological efficacy of dietary phytochemicals."

Soy consumption and ***prostate cancer*** *risk in men: a revisit of a meta-analysis.* Yan L, Spitznagel EL. Am J Clin Nutr. 2009 Apr;89(4):1155-63. **Key Finding:** "We systematically reviewed studies and identified 15 epidemiologic publications on soy consumption and nine on isoflavones in association with prostate cancer risk. The results of this analysis suggest that consumption of soy foods is associated with a reduction in prostate cancer risk in men. This protection may be associated with the type and quantity of soy foods consumed."

A critical assessment of phytotherapy for ***prostate cancer.*** Perabo FG, Von Low EC, Siener R, et al. Urologe A. 2009 Mar;48(3):270-83. **Key Finding:** "The presented data show that at present there is no clinical evidence that phytochemicals might have a therapeutic use in prostate cancer in relation to reduction of tumor progression or improved survival. The question about an improved immune function or quality of life remains open."

W,w'-Diindolylmethane enhances taxotere-induced apoptosis in hormone-refractory ***prostate cancer*** *cells through surviving down-regulation.* Rahman KM, Banerjee S, Ali S, et al. Cancer Res. 2009 May 15;69(10):4468-75. **Key**

Finding: "Survivin, a member of inhibitor of apoptosis family, is associated with both prostate cancer progression and drug resistance. Therefore, we hypothesized that survivin may play a potentially important role in hormone-refractory prostate cancer and bone metastatic disease. We conclude that inactivation of survivin by 3,3'-Diindolylmethane (DIM) enhanced therapeutic efficacy of Taxotere in prostate cancer in general, which could be useful for the treatment of hormone-refractory prostate cancer and metastatic prostate cancer."

Radiation-induced HIF-1alpha cell survival pathway is inhibited by soy isoflavones in **prostate cancer** *cells.* Singh-Gupta V, Zhang H. Banerjee S, Kong D, et al. Int J Cancer. 2009 Apr 1;124(7):1675-84. **Key Finding:** "We previously showed that treatment of prostate cancer cells with soy isoflavones and radiation resulted in greater cell killing in vitro. We extended our studies to investigate the role of HIF-1alpha survival pathway and its upstream Src and STAT3 molecules in isoflavones and radiation interaction. Our novel findings suggest that the increased responsiveness to radiation mediated by soy isoflavones could be due to pleiotropic effects of isoflavones blocking cell survival pathways induced by radiation including Src/STAT3/HIF-1alpha, APE1/Ref-1 and NF-kappaB."

Phenethyl isothiocyanate inhibits STAT3 activation in **prostate cancer** *cells.* Gong A, He M, Kirshna Vanaja D, et al. Mol Nutr Food Res. 2009 Jul;53(7):878-86. **Key Finding:** "Our data demonstrated that phenethyl isothiocyanate (PEITC) can inhibit the activation of the JAK-STAT3 signal-cascade in prostate cancer cells and the underlying mechanism may be partially involved with blocking cellular ROS production during the early stage of the signaling activation by IL-6."

Dietary carotenoids and certain cancers, heart disease, and age-related macular degeneration: a review of recent research. Cooper DA, Eldridge AL, Peters JC. Nutr Rev. 2009 Apr 27;57(7):201-214. **Key Finding:** "Key epidemiologic studies show associations between high dietary intakes of certain carotenoid-containing fruits and vegetables and reduced risk of **prostate cancer**, **breast cancer**, **head and neck cancers**, **cardiovascular disease** and age-related **macular degeneration**, although overall the evidence is inconsistent. Little is known about the potential biochemical mechanisms whereby carotenoids might protect against disease, and human intervention trials are limited to high dose B-carotene, which is not protective against lung cancer or cardiovascular disease."

Luteolin inhibits invasion of **prostate cancer** *PC3 cells through E-cadherin.* Zhou Q, Yan B, Hu X, et al. J. Mol Cancer Ther. 2009 Jun;8(6):1684-91. **Key Finding:** "These findings provide a new sight into the mechanisms that luteolin has against cancer cells, and suggest that molecular targeting of E-cadherin by luteolin may be a useful strategy for treatment of invasive prostate cancer."

Prevention of **prostate cancer** *through custom tailoring of chemopreventive regimen.* Siddiqui IA, Afaq F, Adhami VM, Mukhtar H. Chem Biol Interact. 2008 Jan 30;171(2):122-32. **Key Finding:** "This review underscores the need to build an armamentarium of naturally occurring chemopreventive substances that could prevent or slow down the development and progression of prostate cancer. Thus, the new effective approach for cancer prevention 'building a customized mechanism-based chemoprevention cocktail of naturally occurring substances' is advocated."

Broccoli consumption interacts with GSTM1 to perturb oncogenic signaling pathways in the prostate. Traka M, Gasper AV, Melchini A, et al. PLoS One. 2008 Jul 2;3(7):e2568. **Key Finding:** "This study provides, for the first time, experimental evidence obtained in humans to support observational studies that diets rich in cruciferous vegetables may reduce the risk of **prostate cancer** and other chronic disease."

Lack of prospective associations between plasma and urinary phytoestrogens and risk of **prostate** *or* **colorectal cancer** *in the European Prospective Into Cancer Norfolk study.* Ward H, Chapelais G, Kuhnie GG, et al. Cancer Epidemiol Biomarkers Prev. 2008 Oct;17(10):2891-4. **Key Finding:** "Serum and urine samples were analyzed for seven phytoestrogens (daidzein, enterodiol, enterolactone, genistein, glycitein, O-desmethylangolensin, and equci) among 193 cases of prostate cancer and 828 controls, and 221 cases of colorectal cancer with 889 controls. There was no significant association between prostate cancer risk and total serum isoflavones, or between colorectal cancer risk and total serum isoflavones. Similarly, null associations were observed for individual serum phytoestrogens and for all urinary phytoestrogen biomarkers. In conclusion, we have found no evidence to support an inverse association between phytoestrogen exposure and prostate or colorectal cancer risk."

Plasma isoflavones and subsequent risk of **prostate cancer** *in a nested case-control study: the Japan Public Health Center.* Kurahashi N, Iwasaki M, Inoue M, Sasazuki S, Tsugane S. J Clin Oncol. 2008 Dec 20;26(36):5923-9. **Key Finding:** "The highest textile for plasma equoi, a metabolite of daidzein, was significantly associated with a decreased risk of total prostate cancer. We conclude that isoflavones may prevent the development of prostate cancer."

Fisetin, a novel dietary flavonoid, causes apoptosis and cell cycle arrest in human **prostate cancer** *LNCaP cells.* Khan N, Afaq F, Syed DN, Mukhtar H. Carcinogenesis. 2008 May; 29(5):1049-56. **Key Finding:** "These data provide the first evidence that fisetin could be developed as an agent against prostate cancer."

Green tea consumption and **prostate cancer** *risk in Japanese men: a prospective study.* Kurahashi N, Sasazuki S, Iwasaki M, Inoue M, Tsugane S. Am J Epidemiol. 2008 Jan 1;167(1):71-77. **Key Finding:** "Green tea was not associated with localized prostate cancer. However, consumption was associated with a dose-dependent decrease in the risk of advanced prostate cancer."

A novel dietary flavonoid fisetin inhibits androgen receptor signaling and tumor growth in athymic nude mice. Khan N, Asim M, Afaq F, Abu Zaid M, Mukhtar H. Cancer Res. 2008 Oct 15;68(20):8555-63. **Key Finding:** "These data identify fisetin as an inhibitor of androgen receptor signaling axis and suggest that it could be a useful chemopreventive and chemotherapeutic agent to delay progression of **prostate cancer**."

Transcription factors: molecular targets for **prostate cancer** *intervention by phytochemicals.* Kaur M, Agarwal R. Curr Cancer Drug Targets. 2007 Jun;7(4):355-67. **Key Finding:** "Recent research efforts are also directed on targeting the activity and activation of transcription factors, which ultimately control the expression of genes that are involved in almost all aspects of cell biology. One class of agents that is becoming increasingly successful, not only in targeting signaling cascades, but also transcription factors is phytochemicals present in diet and those consumed as supplement. The added advantage with these agents is that they are mostly non-toxic when compared to chemotherapeutic agents."

Chemopreventive efficacy of silymarin in skin and **prostate cancer**. Deep G, Agarwal R. Integr Cancer Ther. 2007 Jun;6(2):130-45. **Key Finding:** "The cancer chemopreventive role of silymarin has been extensively studied and has shown anticancer efficacy against various cancer sites, especially skin and prostate. In **skin cancer**, silymarin treatment inhibits ultraviolet B radiation or chemically initiated or promoted carcinogenesis. These effects of silymarin against skin carcinogenesis have been attributed to its strong antioxidant and anti-inflammatory action as well as its inhibitory effect on mitogenic signaling. Similarly, silymarin treatment inhibits 3,2-dimethyl-4-aminobiphenyl-induced prostate carcinogenesis and retards the growth of advanced prostate tumor xenograft in athymic nude mice."

Inhibition of **cancer** *cell proliferation and suppression of TNF-induced activation of NFkappaB by edible berry juice.* Boivin D, Blanchette M, Barrette S, Moghrabi A, Beliveau R. Anticancer Res. 2007 Mar-Apr;27(2):937-48. **Key Finding:** "The growth of various cancer cell lines, including those of **stomach, prostate, intestine and breast,** was strongly inhibited by raspberry, black currant, white currant, gooseberry, velvet leaf blueberry, low-bush blueberry, sea buckhorn and cranberry juice, but not (or only slightly) by strawberry, high-bush blueberry, serviceberry, red currant, or blackberry juice."

Review. Facts and fictions of phytotherapy for **prostate cancer**: *a critical assessment of preclinical and clinical data.* Von Low EC, Perabo FG, Siener R, Muller SC. In Vivo. 2007 Mar-Apr;21(2):189-204. **Key Finding:** "The objective of this work was to substantially review all preclinical and clinical data on phytochemicals, such as genistein, lycopene, curcumin, epigallocatechin-gallate, and resveratrol, in terms of their effects as a potential treatment of prostate cancer. The preclinical data for the phytochemicals presented in this review show a remarkable efficacy against prostate cancer cells in vitro, with molecular targets ranging from cell cycle regulation to induction of apotosis. In addition, well-conducted animal experiments support the belief that these substances might have a clinical activity on human cancer. However, it is impossible to make definite statements or conclusions on the clinical efficacy in cancer patients because of the great variability and differences of the study designs, small patient numbers, short treatment duration and lack of a standardised drug formulation. Although some results from these clinical studies seem encouraging, reliable or long-term data on tumor recurrence, disease progression and survival are unknown. At present, there is no convincing clinical proof or evidence that the cited phytochemicals might be used in an attempt to cure cancer of the prostate."

*Dietary isoflavones may protect against **prostate cancer** in Japanese men.* Nagata Y, Sonoda T, Mori M., et al. J Nutr. 2007 Aug;137:1974-79. **Key Finding:** "Isoflavone significantly decreased the risk of prostate cancer regardless of adjustment by PUFA, (n-6) fatty acids or magnesium. In conclusion, our findings indicate that isoflavones might be an effective dietary protective factor against prostate cancer in Japanese men."

*Inhibition of angiogenesis and invasion by 3,3'-diindolylmethane is mediated by the nuclear factor-kappaB downstream target genes MMP-9 and uPA that regulated bioavailability of vascular endothelial growth factor in **prostate cancer**.* Kong D, Li Y, Wang Z, Banerjee S, Sarkar FH. Cancer Res. 2007 Apr 1;67(7):3310-9. **Key Finding:** "Progression of prostate cancer is believed to be dependent on angiogenesis induced by tumor cells. 3,3'-Diindolylmethane (DIM) has been shown to repress neovascularization in a Matrigel plug assay and inhibit cell proliferation, migration, invasion, and capillary tube formation of cultured human umbilical vein endothelial cells. However, the molecular mechanism has not been fully elucidated. Our data suggest that inhibition of NF-kappaB DNA binding activity by B-DIM contributes to the regulated bioavailability of vascular endothelial growth factor by MMP-9 and uPA and, in turn, inhibits invasion and angiogenesis."

*Soy product and isoflavone consumption in relation to **prostate cancer** in Japanese men.* Kurahashi N, Iwasaki M, Sasazuki S, Otani T, Tsugane S. Cancer Epidemiol Biomarkers Prev. 2007 Mar;18(3):538-45. **Key Finding:** "We found that isoflavone intake was associated with a reduced risk of localized prostate cancer."

The citrus flavonoid naringenin stimulates DNA repair in **prostate cancer** *cells.* Gao K, Henning SM, Niu Y, et al.Nutr Biochem. 2006 Feb;17(2):89-95. **Key Finding:** "The cancer-preventive effects of citrus fruits demonstrated in epidemiological studies may be due in part to stimulation of DNA repair by naringenin, which by stimulating base excision repair processes may prevent mutagenic changes in prostate cancer cells."

Multiple, disparate roles for calcium signaling in apoptosis of **human prostate and cervical cancer** *cells exposed to diindolylmethane.* Savino JA, Evans JF, Rabinowitz D, Auborn KJ, Carter TH. Mol Cancer Therap. 2006 Mar 1;5,556. **Key Finding:** "Diindolylmethane (DIM) derived from indole-3-carbinol in cruciferous vegetables causes growth arrest and apoptosis of cancer cells in vitro. We asked whether elevated cytosolic free calcium [Ca2+] is required for cytotoxicity of DIM and thapsigargin in two cancer cell lines from cervix and prostate. Our results suggest that DIM induces apoptosis by different mechanisms in these two cell lines and/or that calcium mobilization also activates different survival pathways."

Down-regulation of androgen receptor by 3,3'-diindolylmethane contributes to inhibition of cell proliferation and induction of apoptosis in both hormone-sensitive LNCaP and insensitive C4-2B **prostate cancer** *cells.* Bhuiyan MR, Li Y, Banerjee S, et al. Cancer Res. 2006 Oct 15;66,10064. **Key Finding:** "These results suggest B-DIM-induced proliferation inhibition and apoptosis induction are partly mediated through the down-regulation of AR, AKt and NF-nB signaling. These observations provide a rationale for devising novel therapeutic approaches for the treatment of hormone-sensitive, but more importantly, hormone-refractory prostate cancer by using 3,3'-diindolylmethane alone or in combination with other therapeutics."

The citrus flavonoid naringenin stimulates DNA repair in **prostate cancer** *cells.* Gao K, Henning SM, Niu Y, et al. J Nutr Biochem. 2006 Feb;17(2):89-95. **Key Finding:** "The cancer-preventive effects of citrus fruits demonstrated in epidemiological studies may be due in part to stimulation of DNA repair by naringenin, which by stimulating base excision repair processes may prevent mutagenic changes in prostate cancer cells."

*Molecular signatures of soy-derived phytochemicals in androgen-responsive **prostate cancer** cells: a comparison study using DNA microarray.* Takahashi Y, Lavigne JA, Hursting SD, et al. Mol Carcinog. 2006 Dec;45(12):943-56. **Key Finding:** "These results provide the foundation for establishing molecular signatures for equoi, daidzein, and genistein. Moreover, these results also allow for the identification of candidate mechanisms by which soy phytochemicals and soy may act in prostate cancer cells."

Phase II study of pomegranate juice for men with rising prostate-specific antigen following surgery or radiation for prostate cancer. Pantuck AJ, Leppert JT, Zomorodian N, et al. Clin Cancer Res. 2006 Jul 1;12(13):4018-26. **Key Finding:** "We report the first clinical trial of pomegranate juice in patients with **prostate cancer**. The statistically significant prolongation of PSA doubling time, coupled with corresponding laboratory effects on **prostate cancer** in vitro cell proliferation and apoptosis as well as oxidative stress, warrant further testing in a placebo-controlled study."

*BRCA1 and BRCA2 as molecular targets for phytochemicals indole-3-carbinol and genistein in breast and **prostate cancer** cells.* Fan S, Meng Q, Auborn K, Carter T, Rosen EM. Br J Cancer. 2006 Feb 13;94(3):407-26. **Key Finding:** "We provide evidence suggesting that the phytochemical induction of BRCA1 expression is due, in part, to endoplasmic reticulum stress response signaling. These findings suggest that the BRCA genes are molecular targets for some of the activities of I3C and genistein."

Inhibition of CWR22Rnu1 tumor growth and PSA secretion in athymic nude mice by green and black teas. Siddiqui IA, Zaman N, Ariz MH, et al. Carcinogenesis. 2006 Apr;27(4):833-9. **Key Finding:** "Our data demonstrated that the treatment with all the tea ingredients resulted in (1) significant inhibition in growth of implanted **prostate tumors**, (2) reduction in the level of serum prostate specific antigen, (3) induction of apoptosis accompanied with upregulation in Bax and decrease in Bcl-2 proteins, and (4) decrease in the levels of VEGF protein. Furthermore, we also found that GTP (green tea polyphenols) (0.01 or 0.05% w/v; given after establishment of CWR22Rnu1 tumor) causes a significant regression of tumors suggesting therapeutic effects of GTP at human achievable concentrations."

*Inhibition of **prostate cancer** cell growth by an avocado extract:role of lipid-soluble bioactive substances.* Lu OY, Arteaga JR, Zhang Q, et al. J Nutr Biochem. 2005 Jan;16(1):23-30. **Key Finding:** "An acetone extract of avocado containing these carotenoids (zeaxanthin, alpha-carotene and beta carotene) and tocopherols was shown to inhibit the growth of both androgen-dependent and androgen-independent prostate cancer cell lines in vitro. Because the avocado also contains a significant amount of monounsaturated fat, these bioactive carotenoids are likely to be absorbed into the bloodstream, where in combination with other diet-derived phytochemicals they may contribute to the significant **cancer** risk reduction."

*Intakes of selected nutrients, foods, and phytochemicals and **prostate cancer** risk in western New York.* McCann SE, Ambrosone CB, Moysich KB, et al. Nutr Cancer. 2005;53(1):33-41. **Key Finding:** "We conducted a case-control study of diet and prostate cancer in western New York involving 433 men with primary histologically confirmed prostate cancer and 538 population-based controls. Our results support the hypothesis that a phytochemical-rich plant-based diet is of importance in reducing risks of hormone-related neoplasms."

*Phytoestrogens and **prostate cancer** risk.* Ganry O. Prev Med. 2005 Jul;41(1):1-6. **Key Finding:** "We decided to review analytical epidemiological studies providing data on soy and prostate cancer protection. Overall, the results of these studies do not show protective effects. Only four of these studies are prospective and none of them found statistically significant prostate cancer reductions."

*Meta-analysis of soy food and risk of **prostate cancer** in men.* Yan L, Spitznagel EL. Int J Cancer. 2005 Nov 20;117(4):667-9. **Key Finding:** "We identified two cohort and six case-control studies that met the criteria for this meta-analysis. In summary, results of the analysis showed that consumption of soy food was associated with a lower risk of prostate cancer in men."

*Relationship between plasma carotenoids and **prostate cancer**.* Chang S, Erdman JW, Clinton SK, et al. Nutr Cancer. 2005;53(2):127-34. **Key Finding:** "These findings suggest that, in these 118 men with nonmetastatic prostate cancer and 52 healthy men from the same area, higher circulating levels of alpha-cryptoxanthin, alpha-carotene, trans-beta-carotene, and lutein and zeaxanthin may contribute to lower prostate cancer risk but not to disease progression."

Potential mechanism of phytochemical-induced apoptosis in human **prostate adenocarcinoma cells***: Therapeutic synergy in genistein and beta-lapachone combination treatment.* Kumi-Diaka J, Saddler-Shawnette S, Aller A, Brown J. Cancer Cell Int. 2004 Aug 17;4(1):5. **Key Finding**: "The demonstrated synergism between genistein and beta-lapachone justifies consideration of these phytochemicals in chemotherapeutic strategic planning."

Targeting cell cycle machinery as a molecular mechanism of sulforaphane in **prostate cancer** *prevention.* Wang L, Liu D, Ahmed T, et al. Int J Oncol. 2004 Jan;24(1):187-92. **Key Finding:** "The regulators of cell cycle have thus been revealed as targets of sulforaphane for growth arrest and apoptosis induction. The potential of sulforaphane as an active dietary factor to inhibit initiation and post-initiation of prostate cancer carcinogenesis is discussed."

Phyto-estrogens and prostatic growth. Vij U, Kumar A. Natl Med J India. 2004 Jan-Feb;17(1):22-6. **Key Finding:** "Although phyto-estrogens have not yet been used in long-term trials to evaluate their ability to reduce the risk of prostate carcinoma, the evidence thus far suggests that they have a protective effect against the growth of **prostate tumours**."

Tomato phytochemicals and **prostate cancer** *risk.* Campbell JK, Canene-Adams K, Lindshield BL, et al. J Nutr. 2004 Dec;134(12 Suppl):34865-34925. **Key Finding:** "This paper reviews the epidemiological evidence evaluating the relationship between prostate cancer risk and tomato consumption, and presents experimental data from this and other laboratories that suppor the hypothesis that whole tomato and its phytochemical components reduce the risk of prostate cancer."

Targeting multiple signaling pathways as a strategy for managing **prostate cancer***: multifocal signal modulation therapy.* McCarty MF. Integr Cancer Ther. 2004 Dec;3(4):349-80. **Key Finding:** "Various nutrients and phytochemicals suspected to have potential utility in prostate cancer prevention and therapy, but whose key molecular targets are still unknown, might reasonably be incorporated into multifocal signal modulation therapy for prostate cancer; these include lycopene, selenium, green tea polyphenols, genistein, and silibinin."

*Indole-3-carbinol and **prostate cancer**.* Sarkar FH, Li Y. J Nutr. 2004 Dec;134(12 Suppl):3493S-3498S. **Key Finding:** "The results from our laboratory and from others provide ample evidence for the benefit of indole-3-carbinol and 3,3'-diindolylmethane for the prevention and the treatment of prostate cancer."

*Ingestion of an isothiocyanate metabolite from cruciferous vegetables inhibits growth of human **prostate cancer** cell xenografts by apoptosis and cell cycle arrest.* Chiao JW, Wu H, Ramaswamy G, et al. Carcinogenesis. 2004 Aug;25(8):1403-8. **Key Finding:** "This study demonstrates the first in vivo evidence of dietary phenethyl isothiocyanate inhibiting tumorigenesis of prostate cancer cells. PEITC-NAC may prevent initiation of carcinogenesis and modulate the post-initiation phase by targeting cell cycle regulators and apoptosis induction."

*Indole-3-carbinol and **prostate cancer**.* Sarkar FH, Li Y. J Nutr. 2004 Dec;134(12 Suppl):3493S-3498S. **Key Finding:** "The results from our laboratory and from others provide ample evidence for the benefit of indole-3-carbinol and 3,3'-diindolylmethane for the prevention and the treatment of prostate cancer."

*Soy phytochemicals and tea bioactive components synergistically inhibit androgen-sensitive human **prostate tumor** in mice.* Zhou JR, Yu L, Zhong Y, Blackburn G. J Nutr. 2003 Feb;133:516-521. **Key Finding:** The combination of soy phytochemical concentrate and green tea synergistically inhibited final tumor weight and metastasis and significantly reduced serum concentrations of both testosterone and DHT in vivo.

Prostate carcinogenesis in N-methyl-N-nitrosourea (NMU)-testosterone-treated rats fed tomato powder, lycopene, or energy-restricted diets. Boileau TW, Liao Z, Kim S. et al. J Natal Cancer Inst. 2003 Nov 5;95(21):1578-86. **Key Finding:** "Consumption of tomato powder but not lycopene inhibited prostate carcinogenesis, suggesting that tomato products contain compounds in addition to lycopene that modify **prostate carcinogenesis**. Diet restriction also reduced the risk of prostate cancer. Tomato phytochemicals and diet restriction may act by independent mechanisms."

Potential risks and benefits of phytoestrogen-rich diets. Cassidy A. Int J Vitam Nutr Res. 2003 Mar;73(2):120-6. **Key Finding:** "The limited studies conducted so far in humans clearly confirm that soya isoflavones can exert hormonal effects. These effects may be of benefit in the prevention of many of the common diseases observed in Western populations (such as **breast cancer, prostate cancer, menopausal symptoms, osteoporosis**) where the diet is typically devoid of these biologically active naturally occurring compounds."

*Inhibition of orthotopic growth and metastasis of androgen-sensitive human **prostate tumors** in mice by bioactive soybean components.* Zhou JR, Yu L, Zhong Y, et al. Prostate. 2002 Oct 1;53(2):143-53. **Key Finding:** "Taken together, these data suggest that the anti-prostate cancer activity of dietary soy protein, soy phytochemicals, and genistein use different molecular pathways. In addition, we have demonstrated that the animal model can be used in the design of dietary strategies for prostate cancer prevention and therapy."

*Tomato products, lycopene, and **prostate cancer** risk.* Miller EC, Giovannucci E, Erdman JW Jr, et al. Urol Clin North Am. 2002 Feb;29(1):83-93. **Key Finding:** "It is reasonable to recommend to the general population the consumption of tomato products at approximately one serving per day or five servings per week as part of an overall healthy dietary pattern that may reduce the risks of prostate cancer, other malignancies, or other chronic diseases."

*The role of soy phytoestrogens in **prostate cancer**.* Castle EP, Thrasher JB. Urol Clin North Am. 2002 Feb;29(1):71-81. **Key Finding:** "We reviewed the current literature on the epidemiology and effects of two soy phytoestrogens, genistein and daidzein, and would stress the need for controlled human trials to assess the true preventive and therapeutic effects of these compounds."

The action of dietary phytochemicals quercetin, catechin, resveratrol and naringenin on estrogen-mediated gene expression. Ratna WN, Simonelli JA. Life Sci. 2002

Feb 15;70(13):1577-89. **Key Finding:** "To determine whether dietary phytochemicals purported to prevent hormone-dependent **breast and prostate cancers, and atherosclerosis**, acted via the estrogen-cell-signaling pathway, roosters were administered increasing doses up to 1 mmole/kg of resveratrol, quercetin, catechin, or naringenin parenternally and tested for hepatic expression of E-RmRNASF. Besides estrogen, the expression of E-RmRNASF in the liver was stimulated by resveratrol and catechin, indicating these agents to be estrogenic. A lack of E-RmRNASF expression was seen with the roosters treated with the naringenin or quercetin."

*Sulforaphane and its metabolite mediate growth arrest and apoptosis in human **prostate cancer** cells.* Chiao JW, Chung FL, Kancheria R, et al. Int J Oncol. 2002 Mar;20(3):631-6. **Key Finding:** "Sulforaphane and its metabolite N-acetylcysteine were demonstrated for the first time to mediate a dose-dependent apoptosis and growth arrest in the prostate cancer cells. Caspases were activated and DNA strand breaks were detected in apoptotic cells."

Flavonoids-potent and versatile biologically active compounds interacting with cytochromes P450. Hodek P, Refil P, Stiborova M. Chem Biol Interact. 2002 Jan 22;139(1):1-21. **Key Finding:** "Flavonoids in human diet may reduce the risk of various cancers, especially hormone-dependent **breast and prostate cancers**, as well as preventing menopausal symptoms."

*Tomatoes, lycopene, and **prostate cancer**: progress and promise.* Hadley CW, Miller EC, Schwartz SJ, Clinton SK. Exp Biol Med. 2002 Nov;227(10):869-80. **Key Finding:** "In contrast to the pharmacologic approach with pure lycopene, many nutritional scientists direct their attention upon the diverse array of tomato products as a complex mixture of biologically active phytochemicals that together may have anti-prostate cancer benefits beyond those of any single constitutent."

*Detrimental effect of **cancer** preventive phytochemicals silymarin, genistein and epigallocatechin 3-gallate on epigenetic events in human prostate carcinoma DU145 cells.* Bhatia N, Agarwal R. Prostate. 2001 Feb 1;46(2):98-107. **Key Finding:** "These results suggest that similar to silymarin, genistein and EGCG also inhibit mitogenic signaling pathways and alter cell cycle regulators, albeit at different levels, leading to growth inhibition and death of advanced and androgen-independent **prostate carcinoma** cells. More studies are therefore needed with these agents to explore their anti-carcinogenic potential against human prostate cancer."

Indole-3-carbinol (I3C) induced cell growth inhibition, G1 cell cycle arrest and apoptosis in **prostate cancer** *cells.* Chinni SR, Li Y, Upadhyay S, Koppolu PK, Sarkar FH. Oncogene. 2001 May 24;20(23):2927-36. **Key Finding:** "From these results, we conclude that I3C inhibits the growth of PC-3 prostate cancer cells by inducing G1 cell cycle arrest leading to apoptosis, and regulates the expression of apotosis-related genes. These findings suggest that I3C may be an effective chemopreventive or therapeutic agent against prostate cancer."

Indole-3-carbinol (I3C) induced cell growth inhibition, G1 cell cycle arrest and apoptosis in **prostate cancer** *cells.* Chinni SR, Li Y, Upadhyay S, Koppolu PK, Sarkar FH. Oncogene. 2001 May 24;20(23):2927-36. **Key Finding:** "These findings suggest that I3C may be an effective chemopreventive or therapeutic agent against prostate cancer."

Synergistic effects of thearubigin and genistein on human **prostate tumor** *cell (PC-3) growth via cell cycle arrest."* Sakamoto K. Cancer Lett. 2000 Apr 3;151(1):103-9. **Key Finding:** "There is evidence that habitual consumption of green tea by Japanese men is correlated with a reduction in cancers, including prostate; soybean isoflavones are also associated with increased protection. The present study compared the anti-proliferative effect of black tea polyphenol, thearubigin, alone or combined, with the isoflavone genistein, on human prostate PC-3 carcinoma cells. Thearubigin administered alone did not result in any alteration of cell growth. When combined with genistein, however, it significantly inhibited cell growth and induced a G2/M phase cell cycle arrest in a dose dependent manner. These findings indicate the potential use of combined phytochemicals to provide protection against prostate cancer."

Soybean phytochemicals inhibit the growth of transplantable human **prostate carcinoma** *and tumor angiogenesis in mice.* Zhou JR, Gugger ET, Tanaka T, et al. J Nutr. 1999 Sep;129(9):1628-35. **Key Finding:** "Our data suggest that dietary soy products may inhibit experimental prostate tumor growth through a combination of direct effects on tumor cells and indirect effects on tumor neovasculature."

Vegetable and fruit consumption in relation to **prostate cancer** *risk in Hawaii: a reevaluation of the effect of dietary beta-carotene.* Le Marchand L, Hankin JH, Kolonel LN, Wilkens LR. Am J. Epidemiol. 1991 Feb 1;133(3):215-9. **Key Finding:** This further analysis of a case-controlled study of 452 prostate cancer cases suggest that "the positive association with beta-carotene intake among older men that the authors previously reported was essentially due to the greater papaya consumption of cases compared with controls; and, intake of beta-carotene, lycopene, lutein, indoles, phenols, or other phytochemicals is not associated with prostate cancer risk."

Renal

No association between fruit, vegetables, antioxidant nutrients and risk of **renal cell carcinoma**. Bertoia M, Albanes D, Mayne ST, et al. Int J Cancer. 2009 Aug 14 [Epub ahead of print]. **Key Finding:** "Our results indicate that diet may not play a large role in the etiology of renal cell carcinoma in male smokers, although further examination of these associations in non-smokers, women, and diverse racial populations is warranted."

Flavonoids and the risk of **renal cell carcinoma**. Bosetti C, Rossi M, McLaughlin JK, et al. Cancer Epidemiol Biomarkers Prev. 2007 Jan;16(1):98-101. **Key Finding:** "Flavonoids, and particularly flavones and flavonols, may account, at least in part, for the favorable role of plant foods on renal cell carcinoma."

Skin

5-deoxykaempferol plays a potential therapeutic role by targeting multiple signaling pathways in **skin cancer**. Lee KM, Lee KW, Byun S, et al. Cancer Prev

Res. 2010 Apr;3(4):454-65. **Key Finding**: "Dietary phytochemicals were shown to exhibit cancer-preventive effects attributed to their antioxidant capacities. In this report, we show that the natural compound 5-deoxy-kaempferol exerts a chemopreventive effect on UVB-induced skin carcinogenesis by targeting multiple signaling molecules."

The promise of natural products for blocking early events in **skin carcinogenesis**. Clifford JL, DiGiovanni J. Cancer Prev Res. 2010 Feb;3(2):132-5. **Key Finding**: "Studies comprise results of naturally occurring phytochemicals and green tea polyphenols in mouse models of UV-induced and chemically induced skin carcinogenesis and results of prillyl alcohol in a phase clinical trial, all pointing to the great promise of this exciting approach for beter understanding of and preventing skin cancer."

Differential effects of several phytochemicals and their derivatives on murine keratinocytes in vitro and in vivo: implications for **skin cancer** *prevention*. Kowalczyk MC, Walaszek Z, Kowalczyk P, et al. Carcinogenesis. 2009 Jun;30(6):1008-15. **Key Finding:** "Differential effects of tested phytochemicals on events and processes critical for the growth inhibition of keratinocytes in vitro and in vivo indicate that combinations of tested compounds may, in the future, better counteract both tumor initiation and tumor promotion/progression."

Phytochemicals as protectors against ultraviolet radiation: versatility of effects and mechanisms. Dinkova-Kostova AT. Planta Med. 2008 Oct;74(13):1548-59. **Key Finding:** "Because of growing concerns that the level of **UV radiation** is increasing as a result of depletion of the stratospheric ozone and climate change, the development of strategies for protection of the skin is an urgent need. Many phytochemicals that belong to various families of secondary metabolite, such as alkaloids, flavonoids, carotenoids and isothiocyanates, offer exciting platforms for the development of such protective strategies. Mechanistically, they affect multiple signaling pathways and protect against UV radiation-inflicted damage by their ability to act as direct and indirect antioxidants, as well as anti-inflammatory and immunomodulatory agents."

*Chemopreventive action of embilica officinalis on **skin carcinogenesis** in mice.* Sancheti G, Jindal A, Kumari R, Goyal PK. Asian Pac J Cancer Prev. 2005 Apr-Jun;6(2):197-201. **Key Finding:** "The present study demonstrates the chemopreventive potential of Emblica officinalis fruit extract on DMBA induced skin tumorigenesis in Swiss albino mice."

*Carotenoids and protection against solar **UV radiation**.* Stahl W, Sies H. Skin Pharmacol Appl Skin Physiol. 2002;15:291-296. **Key Finding:** "Protection against UV light-induced erythema can be achieved by ingestion of a commonly consumed dietary source of lycopene. Such protective effect of carotenoids were also demonstrated in cell culture."

*Oral consumption of bitter gourd and tomato prevents lipid peroxidation in liver associated with DMBA induced **skin carcinogenesis** in mice.* De S, Chakraborty J, Das S. Asian Pac J Cancer Prev. 2000;1(3):203-206. **Key Finding:** "The protective role of two commonly consumed natural dietary items–bitter gourd and tomato—against endogenous as well as 7,12-dimethylbenz(a) anthracene (DMBA) incued lipid peroxidation in the livers of mice was investigated. The rationale for such an approach is that lipid peroxidation has been suggested to play a key role in human cancer development. Our observations support the hypothesis that natural combinations of phytochemicals present in the fruit juices exert **cancer**-protective effects via a decrease in lipid peroxidation."

Stomach

*Inhibition of **cancer** cell proliferation and suppression of TNF-induced activation of NFkappaB by edible berry juice.* Boivin D, Blanchette M, Barrette S, Moghrabi A, Beliveau R. Anticancer Res. 2007 Mar-Apr;27(2):937-48. **Key Finding:** "The growth of various cancer cell lines, including those of **stomach, prostate, intestine and breast,** was strongly inhibited by raspberry, black currant, white currant, gooseberry, velvet leaf blueberry, low-bush blueberry, sea buckhorn and cranberry juice, but not (or only slightly) by strawberry, high-bush blueberry, serviceberry, red currant, or blackberry juice."

Phytoestrogens and human health effects: weighing up the current evidence. Humfrey CD. Nat Toxins. 1998;6(2):51-9. **Key Finding:** "Epidemiological studies suggest that foodstuffs containing phytoestrogens may have a beneficial role in protecting against a number of chronic diseases and conditions. For cancer of the **prostate, colon, rectum, stomach and lung,** the evidence is most consistent for a protective effect resulting from a high intake of grains, legumes, fruits and vegetables. Dietary intervention studies indicate that in women soya and linseed may have beneficial effects on the risk of **breast cancer** and may help to alleviate **postmenopausal symptoms**. For **osteoporosis**, tentative evidence suggests phytoestrogens may have similar effects in maintaining **bone density**. Soya also appears to have beneficial effects on blood lipids which may help to reduce the risk of **cardiosvascular disease** and **atherosclerosis**. Generally, however, little evidence exists to link these effects directly to phytoestrogens; many other components of soy and linseed are biologically active in various experimental systems and may be responsible for the observed effects in humans."

Cardiovascular disease

Diet-derived phytochemicals: from chemoprevention to cardio-oncological prevention. Ferrari N, Tosetti F, De Flora s, et al. Curr Drug Targets. 2010 Dec 15. [Epub ahead of print] **Key Finding**: "There is now increasing evidence that some phytochemicals can be protective for the heart, having the potential to reduce cancer, **cardiovascular disease** and even anticancer drug-induced cardiotoxicity."

Bioactive compounds in cranberries and their biological properties. Cote J, Cailet S, Doyon G, Sylvain JF, Lacroix M. Crit Rev Food Sci Nutr. 2010 Aug;50(7):666-79. **Key Finding**: "Numerous phytochemicals present in cranberries–the anthoycanins, the flavonols, the flaven-3-ols, the proanthocyanidins, and the phenolic acid derivatives. The presence of these phytochemicals appears to be responsible for the cranberry property of preventing many diseases and infections, including **cardiovascular diseases, various cancers, and infections** involving the urinary tract, dental health, and Helicobacter pylori-induced stomach ulcers and cancers."

*Nuts, blood lipids and **cardiovascular disease**.* Sabate J, Wien M. Asia Pac J Clin Nutr. 2010;19(1):131-6. **Key Finding**: "Over 40 dietary intervention studies have been conducted evaluating the effect of nut containing diets on blood lipids. These studies have demonstrated that intake of different kinds of nuts lower total and LDL **cholesterol a**nd the LDL:HDL ratio in healthy subjects or patients with moderate hypercholesterolaemia even in the context of healthy diets. Additional cardioprotective nutrients found in nuts include phytochemicals."

*Ellagitannins, ellagic acid and **vascular health**.* Larrosa M, Garcia-Conesa MT, Espin JC, et al. Mol Aspects Med. 2010 Dec;31(6):513-39. **Key Finding**: "Hydrolysable tannins are phenolic phytochemicals that show high antioxidant and free-radical scavenging activities. For this reason their potential effects preventing oxidative related diseases, such as cardiovascular diseases, have been largely studied. In vitro studies show that ellagitannins, at concentrations in the range 10-100 uM, show some relevant anti-atherogenic, anti-thrombotic, anti-inflammatory and anti-angiogenic effects, supporting the molecule mechanisms for the vascular health benefits."

*The potential role of green tea catechins in the prevention of the **metabolic syndrome** a review.* Thielecke F, Boschmann M. Phytochemistry. 2009 Jan;70(1):11-24. **Key Finding:** "The majority of human epidemiological and intervention studies demonstrate beneficial effects of green tea or green tea extracts, rich in EGCG on weight management, glucose control and **cardiovascular risk** factors. The optimal dose has not yet been established. The current body of evidence in humans warrants further attention."

*Spice active principles as the inhibitors of **human platelet aggregation** and thromboxane biosynthesis.* Raghavendra RH, Naidu KA. Prostaglandins Leukot Essent Fatty Acids. 2009 Jun 4 [Epub ahead of print] **Key Finding:** "Among the spice active principles tested, eugenol and capsaicin are found to be most potent inhibitors of AA-induced platelet aggregation with IC50 values of 0.5 and 14.6muM, respectively. These results clearly suggest that spice principles have beneficial effects in modulating human platelet aggregation."

Dietary carotenoids and certain cancers, heart disease, and age-related macular degeneration: A review of recent research. Cooper DA, Eldridge AL, Peters JC. Nutr Rev. 2009 Apr 27;57(7):201-214. **Key Finding:** "Key epidemiologic studies show associations between high dietary intakes of certain carotenoid-containing fruits and vegetables and reduced risk of **prostate cancer**, **breast cancer**, **head and neck cancers**, **cardiovascular disease** and age-related **macular degeneration**, although overall the evidence is inconsistent. Little is known about the potential biochemical mechanisms whereby carotenoids might protect against disease, and human intervention trials are limited to high dose B-carotene, which is not protective against lung cancer or cardiovascular disease."

*The health benefits of berry flavonoids for menopausal women: **cardiovascular disease, cancer and cognition**.* Huntley AL, Mautritas. 2009 Aug 20;63(4):297-301. **Key Finding:** "Limited data from a combination of pre-clinical and clinical studies suggest that the addition of berry flavonoids to the diet has moderate effects in cardiovascular function in subjects at risk and potential preventative effects in oesophageal cancer. Evidence for cognitive benefits is limited to animal data but shows promise."

*Flavonoids, vascular function and **cardiovascular** protection.* Grassi D, Desideri G, Croce G, et al. Curr Pharm Des. 2009;15(10):1072-84. **Key Finding:** "The review of epidemiological and mechanistic studies supports the role of flavonoids, particularly cocoa and tea flavanols, in protecting the cardiovascular system against cardiovascular disease. Long term clinical trials are needed to definitively clarify the benefits deriving from long-term consumption of flavanol-rich foods."

Phytochemicals of cranberries *and cranberry products: characterization, potential health benefits, and processing stability.* Pappas E, Schaich KM. Crit Rev Food Sci Nutr. 2009 Oct;49(9):741-81. **Key Finding**: "Emerging evidence is elucidating how non-nutrient phytochemicals underlie the health promotion afforded by fruits and vegetables. This review focuses on the American cranberry compiling a comprehensive list of its known phytochemical components. Evidence for protection from several **bacterial pathogens, cancer, cardiovascular disease, and inflammation** is compelling, while **neuroprotection and anti-viral activity** also have begun to draw new consideration."

Fruit, vegetable, and fish consumption and heart rate variability: the Veterans Administration Normative Aging Study. Park SK, Tucker KL, O'Neill MS, et al. Am J Clin Nutr. 2009 Mar;89(3):778-86. **Key Finding:** "We examined whether high consumption of fruit, vegetables, and dark fish would be associated with beneficial changes in heart rate variability among 586 older men. Intake of green leafy vegetables was positively associated with normalized high-frequency power and inversely associated with normalized low-frequency power. No significant association was seen between heart rate variability measures and intakes of other fruit and vegetables, vitamin C, carotenoids, tuna and dark-meat fish, or n-3 fatty acids. These findings suggest that higher intake of green leafy vegetables may reduce the risk of **cardiovascular disease** through favorable changes in cardiac autonomic function."

Dietary green tea extract lowers plasma and hepatic triglycerides and decreases the expression of sterol regulatory element-binding protein-1c mRNA and its responsive genes in fructose-fed, ovariectomized rats. Shrestha S, Ehlers SJ, Lee JY, Fernandez ML, Koo SI. J Nutr. 2009 Apr;139(4):640-5. **Key Finding:** "The results suggest that the lipid-lowering effect of green tea is mediated partly by its inhibition of hepatic lipogenesis involving SREBP-1c and its responsive genes without affecting lipoprotein assembly."

Carotenoids and **cardiovascular disease**. Riccioni G. Curr Atheroscler Rep. 2009 Nov;11(6):434-9. **Key Finding:** "The aim of this review is to examine the published studies about the use of carotenoids, especially lycopene and asta-xanthin, in the treatment of cardiovascular disease."

Enhancement of a modified Mediterranean-style, low glycemic load diet with specific phytochemicals improves cardiometabolic risk factors in subjects with metabolic syndrome and hypercholesterolemia in a randomized trial. Lerman RH, Minich DM, Darland G, et al. Nutr Metab. 2008 Nov 4;5:29. **Key Finding:** "These results demonstrate that specific phytochemical supplementation (soy protein, phytosterols, rho iso-alpha acids, and proanthocyanidins) increased the effectiveness of the modified Mediterranean-style low-glycemic load dietary program on variables associated with metabolic syndrome and **cardiovascular disease**."

Phytochemical composition of nuts. Chen CY, Blumberg JB. Asia Pac J Clin Nutr. 2008; 17 Suppl 1:329-32. **Key Finding:** Tree nuts and peanuts contain numerous phytochemicals that "may contribute to promoting health and reducing the risk of chronic disease," including **cardiovascular disease** and **cancer**. "While many of these bioactive constituents remain to be fully identified and characterized, broad classes include carotenoids, phenols, and phytoesterols." Walnuts are particularly rich in total phenols.

*Flavonoids, flavonoid-rich foods, and **cardiovascular** risk: a meta-analysis of randomized controlled trials.* Hooper L, Kroon PA, Rimm EB, et al. Am J Clin Nutr. 2008 Jul;88(1):38-50. **Key Finding:** This assessment included 133 trials, but no randomized controlled trial studied effects on cardiovascular disease morbidity or mortality. Soy protein isolate (but not other soy components) was found to significantly reduce diastolic blood pressure and LDL cholesterol. Green tea reduced LDL. "To date, the effects of flavonoids from soy and cocoa have been the main focus of attention. Future studies should focus on other commonly consumed subclasses (eg, anthiocyanins and flavanones.)"

Macrophage as a target of quercetin glucronides in human atherosclerotic arteries: implication in the anti-atherosclerotic mechanism of dietary flavonoids. Kawai Y, Nishikawa T, Shiba Y, et al. J Biol Chem. 2008 Apr 4;283(14):9424-34. **Key Finding:** "These results suggest that injured/inflamed arteries with activated macrophages are the potential targets of the metabolites of dietary quercetin. Our data provide a new insight into the bioavailability of dietary flavonoids and the mechanism for the prevention of **cardiovascular diseases**."

Flavonoid intake and the risk of ischaemic stroke and CVD mortality in middle-aged Finnish men: the Kuopio Ischaemic Heart Disease Risk Factor Study. Mursu J, Voutilainen S, Nurmi T, et al. Br J Nutr. 2008 Oct;100(4):890-5. **Key Finding:** "The present study results suggest that high intakes of flavonoids may be associated with decreased risk of ischaemic **stroke** and possibly with reduced **cardiovascular disease** mortality."

Cardioprotective actions of grape polyphenols. Leifert WR, Abeywardena MY. Nutr Res. 2008 Nov;28(11):729-37. **Key Finding:** Consumption of grape and grape extracts may be beneficial in preventing the development of chronic degenerative diseases such as **cardiovascular disease**.

Macrophage as a target of quercetin glucuronides in human atherosclerotic arteries: implication in the anti-atherosclerotic mechanism of dietary flavonoids. Kawai Y, Nishikawa T, Shiba Y, et al. J Biol Chem. 2008 Apr 4;283(14):9424-34. **Key Finding:** "These results suggest that injured/inflamed arteries with activated macrophages are the potential targets of the metabolite of dietary quercetin. Our data provide a new insight into the bioavailability of dietary flavonoids and the mechanism for the prevention of **cardiosvascular diseases**."

(Vaccinium macrocarpon) and **cardiovascular disease** *risk factors.* **Cranberries** McKay DL, Blumberg JB. Nutr Rev. 2007 Nov;65(11):490-502. **Key Finding:** "A growing body of evidence suggests that polyphenols, including those found in cranberries, may contribute to reducing the risk of cardiovascular disease by increasing the resistance of LDL to oxidation, inhibiting platelet aggregation, reducing blood pressure, and via other anti-thrombotic and anti-inflammatory mechanisms."

Nutrition, physical activity, and **cardiovascular disease**: *an update.* Ignarro LJ, Balestrieri ML, Napoli C. Cardiovasc Res. 2007 Jan 15;73(2):326-40. **Key Finding:** "Novel findings and critical appraisal regarding antioxidants, dietary fibers, omega-3 polyunsaturated fatty acids, nutraceuticals, vitamins and minerals, are presented here in support of the current dietary habits together with physical exercise recommendations for prevention and treatment of cardiovascular disease."

Evidence of the cardioprotective potential of fruits: the case of cranberries. Ruel G, Couillard C. Mol Nutr Food Res. 2007 Jun;51(6):692-701. **Key Finding:** "Consumption of cranberries or their related products could be of importance not only in the maintenance of health but also in preventing **cardiovascular disease**. This review presents evidence supported for the most part by clinical observations that cranberries can exert potentially healthy effects for your heart."

Dietary fibre, nuts and **cardiosvascular diseases**. Salas-Salvado J, Bullo M, Perez-Heras A, Ros E. Br J Nutr. 2006 Nov;96 Suppl 2:S46-51. **Key Finding:** "Surprisingly, the consumption of insoluble fibre from whole grains, though metabolically inert, has been associated with a reduction in the risk of developing coronary heart disease and diabetes in epidemiological studies. The likely reason is that whole grains, like nuts, legumes and other edible seeds, contain many bioactive phytochemicals and various antioxidants. After cereals, nuts are the vegetable foods that are richest in fibre, which may partly explain their benefit on the lipid profile and cardiovascular health."

Local food and **cardioprotection**: *the role of phytochemicals*. Visioli F, Bogani P, Grande S, et al. Forum Nutr. 2006;59:116-29. **Key Finding:** "The data uniformly demonstrate that phytochemical components of the Mediterranean diet exert cardioprotective effects whose mechanisms are being progressively elucidated."

Vegetarian diets: what are the advantages? Leitzmann C. Forum Nutr. 2005;(57):147-56. **Key Finding:** "In most cases, vegetarian diets are beneficial in the prevention and treatment of certain diseases, such as **cardiovascular disease, hypertension, diabetes, cancer, osteoporosis, renal disease and dementia**, as well as **diverticular disease, gallstones, and rheumatoid arthritis**."

Sorghum phytochemicals and their potential impact on human health. Awika JM, Rooney LW. Phytochemistry. 2004 May;65(9):1199-221. **Key Finding:** "Sorghum is a rich source of various phytochemicals including tannins, phenolic acids, anthocyanins, phytoesterols and policosanols. This paper reviews available information on sorghum phytochemicals, how the information relates to current phytonutrient research and how it has potential to combat common nutrition-related diseases, including **cancer, cardiosvascular disease** and **obesity**."

Vegetables, fruits and phytoestrogens in the prevention of diseases. Heber D. J Postgrad Med. 2004 Apr-Jun;50(2):145-9. **Key Finding:** "Consumers are advised to ingest one serving of each of the seven colour groups daily. For instance, red foods contain lycopene which may be involved in maintaining **prostate** health and which has been linked to a decreased risk of **cardiosvascular disease**. Green foods, including broccoli, brussels sprouts and kale, have been associated with a decreased risk of cancer. White-green foods such as garlic may inhibit cancer cell growth. Grouping plant foods by colour provides simplification, but it is also important as a method to help consumers make wise food choices and promote health."

Fruit and vegetable intake and risk of major chronic disease. Hung JC, Joshipura KJ, Jiang R, et al. J Natl C Inst. 2004;96(21):1577-1584. **Key Finding:** "A total of 71,910 female participants in the Nurses' Health Study and 37,725 male participants in the Health Professionals' Follow-up Study completed food-frequency questionnaires in 1984 and 1986. Total fruit and vegetable intake was inversely associated with risk of cardiosvascular disease but not with overall cancer incidence. Of the food groups analyzed, green leafy vegetable intake showed the strongest inverse association with major chronic disease and **cardiovascular disease**."

*Flavonoid intake and the risk of **cardiovascular disease** in women.* Sesso HD, Gaziano JM, Liu S, Buring JE. Am J Clin Nutr. 2003 Jun;77(6): 1400-6. **Key Finding:** "Women free of CVD and cancer participated in a prospective study using a food frequency questionnaire. Flavonoid intake was not strongly associated with a reduced risk of cardiovascular disease. The nonsignificant inverse associations for broccoli, apples, and tea with CVD were not mediated by flavonoids and warrant further study."

*Whole grains protect against atherosclerotic **cardiovascular disease**.* Anderson JW. Proc Nutr Soc. 2003 Feb;62(1):135-42. **Key Finding:** "Diets rich in wholegrain foods tend to decrease serum LDL-cholesterol and triacylglycerol levels as well as blood pressure while increasing serum HDL-cholesterol levels. Whole-grain intake may also favorably alter antioxidant status, serum homocysteine levels, vascular reactivity and the inflammatory state. Whole-grain components that appear to make major contributions to these protective effects are: dietary fibre, vitamins, minerals, antioxidants, phytosterols, and other phytochemicals."

*Dietary intake of fruits and vegetables and risk of **cardiovascular disease***. Bazzano LA, Serdula MK, Liu S. Curr Atheroscler Rep. 2003 Nov;5(6): 492-9. **Key Finding:** "In this review, we examine the scientific evidence in support of current dietary recommendations to increase fruit and vegetable intake for cardiovascular disease prevention. Many nutrients and phytochemicals in fruits and vegetables, including fiber, potassium, and folate, could be independently, or jointly, responsible for the apparent reduction in CVD risk. Functional aspects of fruits and vegetables, such as their low dietary glycemic load and energy density, may also play a significant role."

*Plant-based foods and prevention of **cardiovascular disease**: an overview.* Hu FB. Am J Clin Nutr. 2003 Sep;78(3 Suppl):544S-551S. **Key Finding:** "Evidence from prospective cohort studies indicates that a high consumption of plant-based foods such as fruit and vegetables, nuts, and whole grains is associated with a significantly lower risk of coronary artery disease and stroke."

*Bioactive compounds in foods: their role in the prevention of **cardiovascular disease and cancer***. Kris-Etherton PM, Hecker KD, Bonanome A, et al.Am J Med. 2002 Dec 30;113, Suppl 98:715-885. **Key Finding:** Many epidemiological studies have shown protective effects of plant-based diets on cardiosvascular disease and cancer. "There is sufficient evidence to recommend consuming food sources rich in bioactive compounds...this translates to recommending a diet rich in a variety of fruits, vegetables, whole grains, legumes, oils, and nuts."

Interactions of flavones and other phytochemicals with adenosine receptors. Jacobson KA, Moro S, Manthey JA, West PL, Ji XD. Adv Exp Med Biol. 2002;505:163-71. **Key Finding:** "Adenosine receptors are involved in the homeostasis of **the immune, cardiovascular, and central nervous systems**. The affinity of flavonoids and other phytochemicals to adenosine receptors suggests that a wide range of natural substances in the diet may potentially block the effects of endogenous adenosine."

*A prospective study of dietary fiber intake and risk of **cardiovascular disease** among women.* Liu S, Buring JE, Sesso HD, et al. J Am Coll Cardiol. 2002 Jan 2;39(1):49-56. **Key Finding:** "A higher intake of dietary fiber was associated with a lower risk of cardiovascular disease and myocardial infarction, although the association was not statistically significant after further adjusting for multiple confounding factors. Nevertheless, these prospective data generally support current dietary recommendations to increase the consumption of fiber-rich whole grains and fruits and vegetables as a primary preventive measure against CVD."

Phytoestrogens and human health effects: weighing up the current evidence. Humfrey CD. Nat Toxins. 1998;6(2):51-9. **Key Finding:** "Epidemiological studies suggest that foodstuffs containing phytoestrogens may have a beneficial role in protecting against a number of chronic diseases and conditions. For cancer of the **prostate, colon, rectum, stomach and lung,** the evidence is most consistent for a protective effect resulting from a high intake of grains, legumes, fruits and vegetables. Dietary intervention studies indicate that in women soya and linseed may have beneficial effects on the risk of **breast cancer** and may help to alleviate **postmenopausal symptoms**. For **osteoporosis**, tentative evidence suggests phytoestrogens may have similar effects in maintaining **bone density**. Soya also appears to have beneficial effects on blood lipids which may help to reduce the risk of **cardiovascular disease** and **atherosclerosis**. Generally, however, little evidence exists to link these effects directly to phytoestrogens; many other components of soy and linseed are biologically active in various experimental systems and may be responsible for the observed effects in humans."

Phyto-oestrogens: where are we now? Bingham SA, Atkinson C, Liggins J, Bluck L, Coward A. Br J Nutr. 1998 May;79(5):393-406. **Key Finding:** "Evidence is beginning to accrue that they may begin to offer protection against a wide range of human conditions, including **breast, bowel, prostate** and other cancers, **cardiovascular disease**, brain function, alcohol abuse, **osteoporosis** and **menopausal symptoms.** There are few indications of harmful effects at present, although possible proliferative effects have been reported."

*Phytochemicals and **cardiovascular disease**.* Howard BV, Kritchevsky D. Circulation. 1997;95:2591. **Key Finding:** A substantial body of evidence about the lowering of risk for heart disease has accumulated in three areas: plant sterols, flavonoids, and plant sulfur compounds. This review summarizes the state of knowledge to date in these three areas.

Beta-carotene, carotenoids, and disease prevention in humans. Mayne ST. FASEB J. 1996 May;10(7):690-701. **Key Finding:** "Researchers should now seek explanations for the apparently discordant findings of observational studies vs. intervention trials. The most pressing research issues include studies of interactions of carotenoids with themselves and with other phytochemicals and mechanistic studies of the actions of beta-carotene in **lung carcinogenesis** and **cardiovascular disease**."

Cataracts

*Oxidants, antioxidants, and the degenerative diseases of **aging**.* Ames BN, Shigenaga MK, Hagen TM. Proc Natl Acad Sci. 1993 Sep 1;90(17):7915-22. **Key Finding:** "Metabolism, like other aspects of life, involves tradeoffs. Oxidant by-products of normal metabolism cause extensive damage to DNA, protein, and lipid. We argue that this damage (the same as that produced by radiation) is a major contributor to aging and to degenerative diseases of aging such as cancer, cardiovascular disease, immune-system decline, brain dysfunction, and cataracts. Antioxidant defenses against this damage include ascorbate, tocopherol, and carotenoids. Dietary fruits and vegetables are the principal source. Low dietary intake of fruits and vegetables doubles the risk of most types of **cancer** and also markedly increase the risk of **heart disease** and **cataracts**."

Cerebrovascular disease

Flavonoid intake and risk of chronic diseases. Knekt P, Kumpulainen J, Jarvinen R, et al. Am J Clin Nutr. 2002 Sep;76(3):560-68. **Key Finding:** "The total dietary intakes of 10,054 men and women were determined with a dietary history method. Persons with higher quercetin intakes had lower mortality from ischemic **heart disease**. The incidence of **cerebrovascular disease** was lower at higher kaempferol, naringenin, and hesperetin intakes. Men with higher quercetin intakes had a lower **lung cancer** incidence and men with higher myricetin intakes had a lower **prostate cancer** risk. **Asthma** incidence was lower at higher quercetin, naringenin, and hesperetin. A trend toward a reduction in risk of **type 2 diabetes** was associated with higher quercetin and myricetin intakes."

*Quercetin intake and the incidence of **cerebrovascular disease**.* Knekt P, Isotupa S, Rissanen H, et al. Eur J Clin Nutr. 2000 May;54(5):415-7. **Key Finding:** "The results suggest that the intake of apples is related to a decreased risk of thrombotic stroke. This association apparently is not due to the presence of the antioxidant flavonoid quercetin."

Cholesterol

Nuts and berries for heart health. Ros E, Tapsell LC, Sabate J. Curr Atheroscler Rep. 2010 Nov;12(6):397-406. **Key Finding**: "Nuts are likely to beneficially impact heart health. Epidemiologic studies have associated nut consumption with a reduced incidence of **coronary heart disease** in both genders and **diabetes** in women. Limited evidence also suggests beneficial effects on hypertension and inflammation. Intervention studies consistently show that nut intake has a **cholesterol-lowering effect** and there is emerging evidence of beneficial effects on oxidative stress, **inflammation**, and vascular reactivity. **Blood pressure**, visceral adiposity, and glycemic control also appear to be positively influenced by frequent nut consumption without evidence of undue weight gain. Berries are another plant food rich in bioactive phytochemicals, particularly flavonoids, for which there is increasing evidence of benefits on cardiometabolic risk that are linked to their potent antioxidant power."

*Nuts, blood lipids and **cardiovascular disease**.* Sabate J, Wien M. Asia Pac J Clin Nutr. 2010;19(1):131-6. **Key Finding**: "Over 40 dietary intervention studies have been conducted evaluating the effect of nut containing diets on blood lipids. These studies have demonstrated that intake of different kinds of nuts lower total and LDL **cholesterol** and the LDL:HDL ratio in healthy subjects or patients with moderate hypercholesterolaemia even in the context of healthy diets. Additional cardioprotective nutrients found in nuts include phytochemicals."

*Soy isoflavones lower serum total and **LDL cholesterol** in humans: a meta-analysis of 11 randomized controlled trials.* Taku K, Umegaki K, Sato Y, Teki Y, Watanabe S. Am J Clin Nutr. 2007 Apr;85(4):1148-56. **Key Finding:** Soy isoflavones significantly reduced serum total and LDL cholesterol but did not change HDL cholesterol and triacylglycenol."

*Cranberries inhibit **LDL** oxidation and induce LDL receptor expression in hepatocytes.* Chu YF, Liu RH. Life Sci. 2005 Aug 26;77(15):1892-901. **Key Finding:** "Cranberries were evaluated for their potential roles in dietary prevention of cardiosvascular disease. Cranberry extracts were found to have potent antioxidant capacity preventing in vitro LDL oxidation with increasing delay and suppression of LDL oxidation in a dose dependent manner. We propose that additive or synergistic effects of phytochemicals in cranberries are responsible for the inhibition of LDL oxidation, the induced expression of LDL receptors, and the increased uptake of cholesterol in hepatocytes."

Soy isoflavones affect sterol regulatory element binding proteins (SREBPs) and SREBP-regulated genes in HepG2 cells. Mullen E, Brown RM,. Osborne TF, Shay NF. J Nutr. 2004 Nov;134(11):2942-7. **Key Finding:** "Soy intake reduces **cholesterol** levels. We propose that the isoflavone component of soy mediates this effect, at least in part, by affecting cellular sterol homeostasis."

*Serum plant sterols and cholesterol precursors reflect **cholesterol** absorption and synthesis in volunteers of a randomly selected male population.* Miettinen TA, Tilvis RS, Kesaniemi YA. Am J Epidemiol. 1990;131(1):20-31. **Key Finding:** "To investigate the regulation of serum levels of cholesterol precursor sterols and plant sterols, these noncholesterol sterols, fatty acids, and various parameters of cholesterol metabolism were analyzed in 63 volunteers from a randomly selected Finnish male population. The serum noncholesterol sterols are significant indicators of cholesterol absorption and synthesis even under basal conditions."

*Serum plant sterols and their relation to **cholesterol** absorption.* Tilvis RS, Miettinen TA. Am J Clin Nutr. 1986;43:92-97. **Key Finding:** "Our findings suggest that, in general, serum levels of noncholesterol sterols are effectively determined by the absorption which in turn is proportionate to the fractional absorption of cholesterol."

*Optimizing the effect of plant sterols on **cholesterol** absorption in man.* Mattson FH, Grundy SM, Crouse JR. A J Clin Nutr. 1982;35:697-700. **Key Finding:** Nine adults were fed three meals containing 500 mg of cholesterol as a component of scrambled eggs. The addition of beta-sitosterol to their meal resulted in a 42% decrease in cholesterol absorption; the addition of beta-sitosteryl oleate caused a 33% reduction.

*Plant sterols as **cholesterol**-lowering agents: clinical trials in patients with **hypercholesterolemia** and studies of sterol balance.* Lees AM, Mok HY, Lees RS, McCluskey MA, Grundy SM. Atherosclerosis. 1977 Nov;28(3):325-38. **Key Finding:** "We have evaluated the efficacy of plant sterol preparations from two different sources and in two different physical forms in lowered the plasma cholesterol of a total of 46 patients with type II hyperlipoproteinemia when given in addition to appropriate diet therapy. The maximal mean cholesterol lowering in response to any preparation was 12 percent, although it was much greater in some individual patients."

Health effects of vegetables and fruit: assessing mechanisms of action in human experimental studies. Lampe JW. Am J Clin Nutr. 1999 Sep;70 (3 Suppl):475S-490S. **Key Finding:** "Phytochemicals can have complementary and overlapping mechanisms of action, including modulation of detoxification enzymes, stimulation of the immune system, reduction of platelet aggregation, modulation of **cholesterol** synthesis and hormone metabolism, reduction of **blood pressure**, and **antioxidant, antibacterial, and antiviral** effects. Although these effects have been examined primarily in animal and cell-culture models, experimental dietary studies in humans have also shown the capacity of vegetables and fruit and their constitutents to modulate some of these potential disease-preventive mechanisms."

*Do dietary phytochemicals with cytochrome P-450 enzyme-inducing activity increase high-density **lipoprotein** concentrations in humans?* Nanjee MN, Verhagen H, van Poppel G, et al. Am J Clin Nutr. 1996 Nov;64(5):706-11. **Key Finding:** "Low plasma concentrations of high-density lipoprotein are associated with increased risk of coronary heart disease. To test the hypothesis that phytochemicals with cytochrome P-450-inducing activity may also increase plasma HDL concentrations in humans, two controlled dietary trials were undertaken in healthy nonsmoking males. One study examined the effect of replacing 300 g glucosinolate-free vegetables with 300 g brussels sprouts for 3 wk. The other study examined the effects of 150 mg eugenol in capsule form. There was no significant increases in plasma apo A-1, apo A-II, HDL cholesterol, or HDL phospholipids. These results suggest that dietary phytochemicals that induce members of the cytochrome P-450 system do not necessarily raise plasma HDL concentrations in humans."

Cognition

Flavonoids: modulators of brain function? Spencer JP. Br J Nutr. 2008 May;99 E Suppl 1:ES60-77. **Key Finding:** A review of "emerging evidence that suggests dietary phytochemicals, in particular flavonoids, may exert beneficial effects on the **central nervous system** by protecting **neurons** against stress-induced injury, by suppressing neuroinflammation and by improving cognitive function."

Flavonoid fisetin promotes ERK-dependent long-term potentiation and enhances memory. Maher P, Akaishi T, Abe K. Proc Natl Acad Sci. 2006 Oct 31;103(44):16568-73. **Key Finding:** "Small molecules that activate signaling pathways used by neurotrophic factors could be useful for treating CNS disorders. Here we show that the flavonoid fisetin activates ERK and induces cAMP response element-binding protein (CREB) phosphorylation in rat hippocampal slices, facilitates long-term potentiation in rat hippocampal slices, and enhances object recognition in mice. Together, these data demonstrate that the natural product fisetin can facilitate long-term memory, and therefor it may be useful for treating patients with **memory disorders**."

Sweet and sour cherry phenolics and their protective effects on **neuronal cells**. Kim DQ, Heo HJ, Kim YJ, Yang HS, Lee CY. J Agric Food Chem. 2005 Dec 28;53(26):9921-7. **Key Finding:** "Cherry phenolics protected neuronal cells (PC 12) from cell-damaging oxidative stress in a dose-dependent manner mainly due to anthocyanins. Overall results showed that cherries are rich in phenolics, especially in anthocyanins, with a strong antineurodegenerative activity and that they can serve as a good source of biofunctional phytochemicals in our diet."

Strawberry and its anthocyanins reduce oxidative stress-induced apoptosis in PC12 cells. Heo HJ, Lee CY. J Agric Food Chem. 2005 Mar 23;53(6):1984-9. **Key Finding:** "Strawberry showed the highest cell protective effects among the fresh fruit samples. The overall relative **neuronal** cell protective activity of three fruits (strawberry, banana and orange) by three tests followed the decreasing order strawberry>banana>orange. The protective effects appeared to be due to the higher phenolic contents including anthocyanins, and anthocyanins in strawberries seemed to be the major contributors."

Vegetarian diets: what are the advantages? Leitzmann C. Forum Nutr. 2005;(57):147-56. **Key Finding:** "In most cases, vegetarian diets are beneficial in the prevention and treatment of certain diseases, such as **cardiovascular disease, hypertension, diabetes, cancer, osteoporosis, renal disease and dementia**, as well as **diverticular disease, gallstones, and rheumatoid arthritis**."

Potential impact of strawberries on human health: a review of the science. Hannum SM. Crit Rev Food Sci Nutr. 2004;44(1):1-17. **Key Finding:** "Individual compounds in strawberries have demonstrated **anticancer** activity in several different experimental systems, blocking initiation of carcinogenesis, and suppressing progression and proliferation of tumors. Preliminary animal studies have indicated that diets rich in strawberries may also have the potential to provide benefits to the **aging brain**."

*Natural extracts as possible protective agents of **brain aging**.* Bastianetto S. Quirion R. Neurobiol Aging. 2002 Sep-Oct;23(5):891-97. **Key Finding:** "These results support the hypothesis that dietary intake of natural substances may be beneficial in normal aging of the brain."

Long-term dietary strawberry, spinach, or vitamin E supplementation retards the onset of age-related neuronal signal-transduction and cognitive behavioral deficits. Joseph JA, Shukitt-Hale B, Denisova NA, et al. J Neurosci. 1998 Oct 1;18(19):8047-55. **Key Finding:** "Phytochemicals present in antioxidant-rich foods such as spinach may be beneficial in retarding functional age-related

CNS and **cognitive behavioral deficits** and, perhaps, may have some benefit in **neurodegenerative disease**."

Coronary artery disease

Nuts and berries for heart health. Ros E, Tapsell LC, Sabate J. Curr Atheroscler Rep. 2010 Nov;12(6):397-406. **Key Finding**: "Nuts are likely to beneficially impact heart health. Epidemiologic studies have associated nut consumption with a reduced incidence of **coronary heart disease** in both genders and **diabetes** in women. Limited evidence also suggests beneficial effects on hypertension and inflammation. Intervention studies consistently show that nut intake has a **cholesterol-lowering effect** and there is emerging evidence of beneficial effects on oxidative stress, **inflammation**, and vascular reactivity. **Blood pressure**, visceral adiposity, and glycemic control also appear to be positively influenced by frequent nut consumption without evidence of undue weight gain. Berries are another plant food rich in bioactive phytochemicals, particularly flavonoids, for which there is increasing evidence of benefits on cardiometabolic risk that are linked to their potent antioxidant power."

Increased consumption of fruit and vegetables is related to a reduced risk of ***coronary heart disease****: meta-analysis of cohort studies.* He FJ, Nowson CA, Lucas M, MacGregor GA. J Hum Hypertens. 2007 Sep;21(9):717-28. **Key Finding:** "We quantitatively assessed the relation between fruit and vegetable intake and incidence of coronary heart disease by carrying out a meta-analysis of cohort studies. Our meta-analysis demonstrates that increased consumption of fruit and vegetables from less than 3 to more than 5 servings a day is related to a 17% reduction in coronary heart disease risk."

Fruit and vegetable consumption and risk of ***coronary heart disease****: a meta-analysis of cohort studies.* Dauchet L, Amouyel P, Hercberg S, Dallongeville J. J Nutr. 2006 Oct;136(10):2588-93. **Key Finding:** "Nine studies were eligible for inclusion in the meta-analysis that consisted of 91,379 men, 129,701 women, and 5,007 coronary heart disease events. This meta-analysis of cohort studies shows that fruit and vegetable consumption is inversely associated with the risk of CHD. The causal mechanism of this association, however, remains to be demonstrated."

Cardioprotective effects of dietary polyphenols. Zern TL, Fernandez ML. J Nutr. 2005 Oct;135(10):2291-4. **Key Finding:** "It is the purpose of this review to examine recent information on the multiple functions of dietary polyphenols, with an emphasis on grape polyphenols, in decreasing the risk of **coronary heart disease** by improving plasma lipid profiles and reducing inflammation."

*Dietary intake and **coronary heart disease**: a variety of nutrients and phytochemicals are important.* Tucker KL. Curr Treat Options Cardiovasc Med. 2004 Aug;6(4):291-302. **Key Finding:** "Many new studies have shown a link between intake of fruit and vegetables and whole grains and protection against coronary heart disease. This has been ascribed to their fiber, vitamin, mineral, and phytochemical content. In particular, there is accumulating evidence of protective effects for folate, vitamin B_6, vitamin B_{12}, vitamin E, vitamin C, flavonoids and phytoestrogens."

Bioactive phytochemicals in Indian foods and their potential in health promotion and disease prevention. Rao BN. Asia Pac J Clin Nutr. 2003;12(1):9-22. **Key Finding:** "Studies carried out during the past 2-3 decades have shown that phytochemicals have an important role in preventing chronic diseases like **cancer**, **diabetes, coronary heart disease** and hyper-cholesterolaemia. The major classes of phytochemicals with disease-preventing functions are dietary fibre, antioxidants, detoxifying agents, immunity-potentiating agents and neuropharmacological agents."

*Optimal diets for prevention of **coronary heart disease**.* Hu FB, Willett WC. JAMA. 2002 Nov 27;288(20):2569-78. **Key Finding:** "Substantial evidence indicates that diets using nonhyrogenated unsaturated fats as the predominant form of dietary fat, whole grains as the main form of carbohydrates, an abundance of fruits and vegetables, and adequate omega-3 fatty acids can offer significant protection against coronary heart disease."

*The effect of fruit and vegetable intake on risk for **coronary heart disease**.* Joshipura KJ, Hu FB, Manson JE, et al. Ann Intern Med. 2001 Jun

19;134(12):1106-14. **Key Finding:** "Participants included 84,251 women 34 to 59 years of age who were followed for 14 years and 42,148 men 40 to 75 years who were followed for 8 years. Consumption of fruits and vegetables, particularly green leafy vegetables and vitamin C-rich fruits and vegetables, appears to have a protective effect against coronary heart disease."

Dietary catechins in relation to **coronary heart disease** *death among postmenopausal women.* Arts IC, Jacobs DR, Harnack LJ, Gross M, Folsom AR. Epidemiology. 2001 Nov;12(6):668-75. **Key Finding:** "There was a strong inverse association between the intake of (+)-catechin and (-)-epicatechin and coronary heart disease death among the 34,492 participants. A high intake of gallates, catechins typical of tea, was not associated with coronary heart disease death. Our data suggest that preventive effects might be limited to certain types of catechins."

Intake of vegetables rich in carotenoids and risk of **coronary heart disease** *in men: The Physicians' Health Study.* Liu S, Lee IM, Ajani U, et al. J Epdemiol. 2001;30:130-135. **Key Finding:** "Our results suggest an inverse association between vegetable intake and risk of coronary heart disease. These prospective data support current dietary guidelines to increase vegetable intake for the prevention of CHD."

Diet and prevention of **coronary heart disease:** *the potential role of phytochemicals.* Visioli F, Borsani L, Galli C. Cardiovasc Res. 2000 Aug 18;47(3):419-25. **Key Finding:** This article reviews the evidence that links a high dietary intake of phytochemicals with a reduced incidence of coronary heart disease.

Dietary intakes of flavonols, flavones and isoflavones by Japanese women and the inverse correlation between quercetin intake and plasma LDL cholesterol concentration. Arai Y, Watanabe S, Kimira M, et al. J Nutr. 2000 Sep;130(9):2243-50. **Key Finding:** Subjects were 115 women volunteers. The major source of flavonoids was onions and that of isoflavones was tofu. "These results suggest that a high consumption of both flavonoids and isolfavones by Japanese women may contribute to their low incidence of **coronary heart disease** compared with women in other countries."

*Antioxidant potentials of vitamin A and carotenoids and their relevance to **heart disease**.* PalaceVP, Khaper N, Qin Q, Singal PK. F Rad Biol Med. 1999 Mar;26(5-6):746-761. **Key Finding:** "This review assembles information regarding the basic structure and metabolism of vitamin A and carotenoids as related to their antioxidant activities. Epidemiological intervention trials and experimental evidence about the effectiveness of vitamin A and carotenoids for reducing cardiosvascular disease is also reviewed."

Flavonoid intake and coronary mortality in Finland: a cohort study. Knekt P, Jarvinen R, Reunanen A, Maatela J. BMJ. 1996;312:478-481. **Key Finding:** Data was collected on 5,133 Finnish men and women aged 30-69 years of age. "The results suggest that people with very low intakes of flavonoids have higher risks of **coronary disease**."

*Flavonoid intake and long-term risk of **coronary heart disease** and **cancer** in the Seven Countries Study.* Hertog MG, Kromhout D, Aravanis C, et al. Arch Int Med. 1995 Feb;155(4):381-386. **Key Finding:** "Average flavonoid intake may partly contribute to differences in coronary heart disease mortality across populations, but it does not seem to be an important determinant of cancer mortality."

*Dietary antioxidant flavonoids and risk of **coronary heart disease**: the Zutphen Elderly Study.* Hertog MG, Feskens EJ, Hollman PC, Katan MB, Kromhout D. Lancet.1993 Oct 23;342(8878):1007-11. **Key Finding:** The flavonoid intake of 805 men aged 65-84 years was measured. The major sources of intake were tea, onions and apples. "Flavonoid intake was significantly inversely associated with mortality from coronary heart disease. Flavonoids in regularly consumed foods may reduce the risk of death from coronary heart disease in elderly men."

Diabetes

Nuts and berries for heart health. Ros E, Tapsell LC, Sabate J. Curr Atheroscler Rep. 2010 Nov;12(6):397-406. **Key Finding**: "Nuts are likely to beneficially impact heart health. Epidemiologic studies have associated nut consumption with a reduced incidence of **coronary heart disease** in both genders and **diabetes** in women. Limited evidence also suggests beneficial effects on hypertension and inflammation. Intervention studies consistently show that nut intake has a **cholesterol-lowering effect** and there is emerging evidence of beneficial effects on oxidative stress, **inflammation**, and vascular reactivity. **Blood pressure**, visceral adiposity, and glycemic control also appear to be positively influenced by frequent nut consumption without evidence of undue weight gain. Berries are another plant food rich in bioactive phytochemicals, particularly flavonoids, for which there is increasing evidence of benefits on cardio-metabolic risk that are linked to their potent antioxidant power."

Antioxidant phytochemicals against **type 2 diabetes**. Dembinska-Kiec A, Mykkanen O, Kiec-Wilk B, Mykkanen H. Br J Nutr. 2008 May;99 E Suppl 1:ES109-17. **Key Finding:** "This article presents an overview of how phytochemicals, especially polyphenols in fruits, vegetables, berries, beverages and herbal medicines, may modify imbalanced lipid and glucose homeostatis thereby reducing the risk of the metabolic syndrome and type 2 diabetes complications."

Phytochemical composition and metabolic performance-enhancing activity of dietary berries traditionally used by Native North Americans. Burns Kraft TF, Dev M, Rogers RB, et al. J Agric Food Chem. 2008 Feb 13;56(3):654-60. **Key Finding:** Four wild berry species, Amelanchier ainifolia, Viburnum trilobum, Prunus virginiana, and Shepherdia argentea, all integral to the traditional subsistence diet of Native American tribal communities, were evaluated to elucidate phytochemical composition and bioactive properties related to performance and human health. "The results demonstrate that these berries contain a rich array of phytochemicals that have the capacity to promote health and protect against chronic diseases, such as **diabetes.**"

*Chronic administration of Satsuma mandarin fruit (Citrus unshiu Marc.) improves oxidative stress in streptozocin-induced **diabetic** rat liver.* Sugiura M, Ohshima M, Ogawa K, Yang M. Biol Pharm Bull. 2006 Mar;29(3):588-91. **Key Finding:** "In this study, we investigated the effects of the chronic administration of Satsuma mandarin fruit on an antioxidant defense system in streptozotocin-induced diabetic rat liver. These results suggest that Satsuma mandarin may act as a suppressor against liver cell damage and inhibit the progression of liver dysfunction induced by chronic hyperglycemia."

Role of antioxidants, essential fatty acids, carnitine, vitamins, phytochemicals and trace elements in the treatment of **diabetes** *mellitus and its chronic complications.* Triggiani V, Resta F, Guastamacchia E, et al. Endocr Metab Immune Disord Drug Targets. 2006 Mar;6(1):77-93. **Key Finding:** "We have attempted to review the current concepts dealing with the usefulness of these complementary therapies in treating diabetic patients."

Epigallocatechin gallate supplementation alleviates **diabetes** *in rodents.* Wolfram S, Raederstorff D, Preller M, et al. J Nutr. 2006 Oct;136:2512-2518. **Key Finding:** "This study shows that EGCG beneficially modifies glucose and lipid metabolism in H4IIE cells and markedly enhances glucose tolerance in diabetic rodents. Dietary supplementation with EGCG could potentially contribute to nutritional strategies for the prevention and treatment of type 2 diabetes mellitus."

Vegetarian diets: what are the advantages? Leitzmann C. Forum Nutr. 2005;(57):147-56. **Key Finding:** "In most cases, vegetarian diets are beneficial in the prevention and treatment of certain diseases, such as **cardiovascular disease, hypertension, diabetes, cancer, osteoporosis, renal disease and dementia**, as well as **diverticular disease, gallstones, and rheumatoid arthritis**."

Associations of dietary flavonoids with risk of **type 2 diabetes**, *and markers of insulin resistance and systemic inflammation in women: a prospective study and cross-sectional analysis.* Song Y, Manson JE, Buring JE, Sesso HD, Liu S. J Am Coll Nutr. 2005 Oct;24(5):376-84. **Key Finding:** "The aim of this study was to examine the association of dietary flavonol and flavone intake with type 2 diabetes, and biomarkers of insulin resistance and systemic inflammation. These results do not support the hypothesis that high intake of flavonols and flavones reduces the development of type 2 diabetes, although we cannot rule out a modest inverse association with intake of apples and tea."

Bioactive phytochemicals in Indian foods and their potential in health promotion and disease prevention. Rao BN. Asia Pac J Clin Nutr. 2003;12(1):9-22. **Key**

Finding: "Studies carried out during the past 2-3 decades have shown that phytochemicals have an important role in preventing chronic diseases like **cancer**, **diabetes, coronary heart disease** and hyper-cholesterolaemia. The major classes of phytochemicals with disease-preventing functions are dietary fibre, antioxidants, detoxifying agents, immunity-potentiating agents and neuropharmacological agents."

A mixed fruit and vegetable concentrate increases plasma antioxidant vitamins and folate and lowers plasma homocysteine in men. Samman S, Sivarajah G, Man JC, et al. J Nutr. 2003 Jul;133(7):2188-93. **Key Finding:** "In the absence of dietary modification, supplementation with a fruit and vegetable concentrate produced responses consistent with a reduction in **coronary heart disease** risk."

Flavonoid intake and risk of chronic diseases. Knekt P, Kumpulainen J, Jarvinen R, et al. Am J Clin Nutr. 2002 Sep;76(3):560-68. **Key Finding:** "The total dietary intakes of 10,054 men and women were determined with a dietary history method. Persons with higher quercetin intakes had lower mortality from ischemic **heart disease**. The incidence of **cerebrovascular disease** was lower at higher kaempferol, naringenin, and hesperetin intakes. Men with higher quercetin intakes had a lower **lung cancer** incidence and men with higher myricetin intakes had a lower **prostate cancer** risk. **Asthma** incidence was lower at higher quercetin, naringenin, and hesperetin. A trend toward a reduction in risk of **type 2 diabetes** was associated with higher quercetin and myricetin intakes."

Diarrhea

*Phytochemicals from traditional medicinal plants used in the treatment of **diarrhea**:modes of action and effects on intestinal function.* Palombo EA. Phytother Res. 2006 Sep;20(9):717-24. **Key Finding:** "Of the numerous phyotchemicals (such as alkaloids, tannins, flavonoids and terpenes) present in active extracts, tannins and flavonoids are thought to be responsible for antidiarrheal activity by increasing colonic water and electrolyte reabsorption. Others act by inhibiting intestinal motility."

Eye diseases

*Phytochemicals and age-related **eye diseases**.* Rhone M, Basu A. Nutr Rev. 2008 Aug;66(8):465-72. **Key Finding:** "Observational and clinical trials support the safety of higher intakes of the phytochemicals lutein and zeaxanthin and their association with reducing risks of cataracts in healthy postmenopausal women and improving clinical features of age-related macular degeneration in patients. Additional phytochemicals of emerging interest, like green tea catechins, anthocyanins, resveratrol, and Ginkgo biloba, shown to ameliorate ocular oxidative stress, deserve more attention in future clinical trials."

Flavonoids protect human retinal pigment epithelial cells from oxidative-stress-induced death. Hanneken A, Lin FF, Johnson J, Maher P. Invest Ophthalmol Vis Sci. 2006 Jul;47(7):3164-77. **Key Finding:** "The effective flavonoids included the dietary flavonoids fisetin, luteolin, quercetin, eriodictyoi, baicalein, galangin and EGCG. The results identify a select group of flavonoids that protect RPE cells from oxidative-stress-induced death with a high degree of potency and low toxicity. This group of flavonoids and the foods that contain high levels of these compounds may have some clinical benefit for patients with **retinal diseases**."

Chemistry, distribution, and metabolism of tomato carotenoids and their impact on human health. Khachik F, Carvalho L, Bernstein PS, et al. Exp Biol Med. 2002 Nov;227(10):845-51. **Key Finding:** "In this review we identified and quantified the complete spectrum of carotenoids from pooled human retinal pigment epithelium, ciliary body, iris, lens, and the unveal tract and in other tissues of the human eye to gain a better insight into the metabolic pathways of ocular carotenoids. Lycopene and a wide range of dietary carotenoids have been detected in high concentrations in ciliary body and retinal pigment epithelium. The possible role of lycopene and other dietary carotenoids in the prevention of age-related macular degeneration and other **eye diseases** is discussed."

Helicobacter pylori infection

*Phytoceuticals: mighty but ignored weapons against **Helicobacter pylori** infection.* Lee SY, Shin YW, Hahm KB. J Dig Dis. 2008 Aug;9(3):129-39. **Key Finding:** "Helicobacter pylori infection causes peptic ulcer disease, mucosa-associated tissue lymphomas and gastric adenocarcinomas, for which the pathogenesis of chronic gastric inflammation prevails. Phytoceuticals such as Korean red ginseng, green tea, flavonoids, broccoli sprouts, garlic, probiotics are known to inhibit H. pylori colonization, decrease gastric inflammation by inhibiting cytokine and chemokine release, and repress precancerous changes by inhibiting nuclear factor-kappa B DNA binding, inducing profuse levels of apoptosis and inhibiting mutagenesis."

Hepatitis

Phytochemicals from Phyllanthus niruri Linn. and their pharmacological properties: a review. Bagalkotkar G, Sagineedu SR, Saad MS, Stanslas J. J Pharm Pharmacol. 2006 Dec;58(12):1559-70. **Key Finding:** "This review discusses the medicinal plant Phyllanthus niruri Linn. (Euphorbiaceae), its wide variety of phytochemicals and their pharmacological properties. The active phytochemicals, flavonoids, alkaloids, terpenoids, lignans, polyphenols, tannins, coumarins and saponins, have been identified from various parts of P. niruri. Extracts of this herb have been proven to have therapeutic effects in many clinical studies. Some of the most intriguing therapeutic properties include anti-hepatotoxic, anti-lithic, anti-hypertensive, anti-**HIV** and anti-**hepatitis B.**"

HIV infection

*The main green tea polyphenol epigallocatechin-3-gallate counteracts semen-mediated enhancement of **HIV infection**.* Hauber I, Hohenberg H, Holstermann B, Hunstein W, Hauber J. Proc Natl Acad Sci. 2009 Jun 2;106(22):9033-8. **Key Finding:** "Peptide fragments, derived from psotatic acidic phosphatase, are secreted in large amounts into human semen and form amyloid fibrils. These fibrillar structures, termed semen-derived enhancer of virus infaction (SEVI), capture HIV virions and direct them to target cells. Thus, SEVI appears to be an important infectivity factor of HIV during sexual transmission. Here, we are able to demonstrate that epigallocatechin-3-gallate (EGCG), the major active constitutent of green tea, targets SEVI for degradation. Furthermore, it is shown that EGCG inhibits SEVI activity and abrogates semen-mediated enhancement of HIV-1 infection in the absence of cellular toxicity. Therefore, EGCG appears to be a promising supplement to antiretroviral microbicides to reduce sexual transmission of HIV-1."

Phytochemicals from Phyllanthus niruri Linn. and their pharmacological properties: a review. Bagalkotkar G, Sagineedu SR, Saad MS, Stanslas J. J Pharm Pharmacol. 2006 Dec;58(12):1559-70. **Key Finding:** "This review discusses the medicinal plant Phyllanthus niruri Linn. (Euphorbiaceae), its wide variety of phytochemicals and their pharmacological properties. The active phytochemicals, flavonoids, alkaloids, terpenoids, lignans, polyphenols, tannins, coumarins and saponins, have been identified from various parts of P. niruri. Extracts of this herb have been proven to have therapeutic effects in many clinical studies. Some of the most intriguing therapeutic properties include anti-hepatotoxic, anti-lithic, anti-hypertensive, anti-**HIV** and **anti-hepatitis B.**"

Natural antimutagenic agents may prolong efficacy of **human immunodeficiency virus** *drug therapy.* McCarty MF. Med Hypotheses. 1997 Mar;48(3):215-20. **Key Finding:** "Ample but safe intakes of selenium, green-tea polyphenols, and cruciferous vegetables, in the context of a diet low in fat and assimilable iron, can be expected to prolong the efficacy of drug therapy in subjects infected with the human immunodeficiency virus. These measures can also be recommended for cancer prevention in the general population."

Hypercolesterolemia

Dietary a-linolenic acid inhibits proinflammatory cytokine production by peripheral blood mononuclear cells in **hypercholesterolemic** *subjects.* Zhao G, Etherton TD, Martin KR, et al. Am J Clin Nutr. 2007 Feb;85(2):385-391. **Key Finding:** "Increased intakes of dietary a-linolenic acid (ALA) elicit anti-inflammatory effects by inhibiting IL-6, IL-1B, and INF-a production in cultured PBMCs. The **cardioprotective** effects of ALA are mediated in part by a reduction of **inflammatory** cytokines."

*Effect of raw garlic vs commercial garlic supplements on plasma lipid concentrations in adults with moderate **hypercholesterolemia**: a randomized clinical trial.* Gardner CD, Lawson LD, Block E, et al. Arch Intern Med. 2007 Feb 26;167(4):346-53. **Key Finding:** "None of the forms of garlic used in this study, including raw garlic, when given at an approximate dose of a 4-g clove per day, 6 d/wk for 6 months, had statistically or clinically significant effects on LDL-C or other plasma lipid concentrations in adults with moderate hypercholesterolemia."

*A combination therapy including psyllium and plant sterols lowers LDL cholesterol by modifying lipoprotein metabolism in **hypercholesterolemic** individuals.* Shrestha S, Volek JS, Udani J, et al. J Nutr. 2006 Oct;136:2492-2497. **Key Finding:** "We conducted a randomized, double blind, crossover, placebo-controlled study to determine the effects of a combination therapy including plant sterols and psyllium on plasma lipids and on the size and subfraction distribution of VLDL, LDL, and HDL. Plasma total cholesterol concentrations were significantly reduced for all subjects, from 5.65=0.72 mmol/L after the placebo period to 5.28=0.76 mmoI/L after the combination period. These reductions were primarily in LDL-C. We conclude that the combination therapy resulted in a less atherogenic lipoprotein profile."

*Plant sterols as **cholesterol**-lowering agents: clinical trials in patients with **hypercholesterolemia** and studies of sterol balance.* Lees AM, Mok HY, Lees RS, McCluskey MA, Grundy SM. Atherosclerosis. 1977 Nov;28(3):325-38. **Key Finding:** "We have evaluated the efficacy of plant sterol preparations from two different sources and in two different physical forms it lowered the plasma cholesterol of a total of 46 patients with type II hyperlipoproteinemia when given in addition to appropriate diet therapy. The maximal mean cholesterol lowering in response to any preparation was 12 percent, although it was much greater in some individual patients."

*Prune suppresses ovariectomy-induced **hypercholesterolemia** in rats.* Lucas EA, Juma S, Stoecker BJ, Arimandi BH. J Nutr Biochem. 2000 May;11(5):255-9.

Key Finding: "Elevated cholesterol among women who have experienced natural or surgical menopause has been linked to ovarian hormone deficiency. The purpose of this study was to investigate the efficacy of prune, a good source of dietary fiber and phytochemicals, on lowering cholesterol in 48 rats. The findings of this study showed that prune exhibits hypocholesterolemic properties in ovarian hormone deficiency."

Hyperglycemia

Health benefits of traditional corn, beans, and pumpkin: in vitro studies for **hyperglycemia** *and* **hypertension** *management.* Kwon YI, Apostolidis E, Kim YC, Shetty K. J Med Food. 2007 Jun;10(2):266-75. **Key Finding:** "In this study antidiabetic and antihypertension relevant potentials of phenolic phytochemicals were confirmed in select important traditional plant foods of indigenous communities such as pumpkin, beans and maize. Pumpkin showed the best overall potential."

Hypertension

Nuts and berries for heart health. Ros E, Tapsell LC, Sabate J. Curr Atheroscler Rep. 2010 Nov;12(6):397-406. **Key Finding**: "Nuts are likely to beneficially impact heart health. Epidemiologic studies have associated nut consumption with a reduced incidence of **coronary heart disease** in both genders and **diabetes** in women. Limited evidence also suggests beneficial effects on hypertension and inflammation. Intervention studies consistently show that nut intake has a **cholesterol-lowering effect** and there is emerging evidence of beneficial effects on oxidative stress, **inflammation**, and vascular reactivity. **Blood pressure**, visceral adiposity, and glycemic control also appear to be positively influenced by frequent nut consumption without evidence of undue weight gain. Berries are another plant food rich in bioactive phytochemicals, particularly flavonoids, for which there is increasing evidence of benefits on cardiometabolic risk that are linked to their potent antioxidant power."

Chronic intake of a phytochemical-enriched diet reduces cardiac fibrosis and diastolic dysfunction caused by prolonged salt-sensitive hypertension. Seymour EM, Singer AA, Bennink MR, et al. J Gerontol A Biol Sci Med Sci. 2008 Oct;63(10):1034-

42. **Key Finding:** "Physiologically relevant phytochemical intake reduced salt-sensitive **hypertension** and diastolic dysfunction."

Health benefits of traditional corn, beans, and pumpkin: in vitro studies for **hyperglycemia** *and* **hypertension** *management.* Kwon YI, Apostolidis E, Kim YC, Shetty K. J Med Food. 2007 Jun;10(2):266-75. **Key Finding:** "In this study antidiabetic and antihypertension relevant potentials of phenolic phytochemicals were confirmed in select important traditional plant foods of indigenous communities such as pumpkin, beans and maize. Pumpkin showed the best overall potential."

A phytochemical in the edible Tamogi-take mushroom (Pleurotus cornucopiae), D-mannitol, inhibits ACE activity and lowers the blood pressure of spontaneously **hypertensive** *rats.* Hagiwara SY, Takahashi M, Shen Y, et al. Biosci Biotechnol Biochem. 2005 Aug;69(8):1603-5. **Key Finding:** "D-mannitol, one of the main phyotchemicals of the edible Tamogi-take mushroom, was found to inhibit an angiotensin I converting enzyme ACE. The antihypertensive effect of D-mannitol and a hot water extract of Tamogi-take mushroom was demonstrated in spontaneously hypertensive rats by oral administration."

Garlic supplementation prevents oxidative DNA damage in essential **hypertension.** Dhawan V, Jain S. Mol Cell Biochem. 2005 Jul;275(1-2):85-94. **Key Finding:** "These findings point out the beneficial effects of **garlic** supplementation in reducing blood pressure and counteracting oxidative stress, and thereby, offering cardioprotection in essential hypertensives."

Vegetarian diets: what are the advantages? Leitzmann C. Forum Nutr. 2005;(57):147-56. **Key Finding:** "In most cases, vegetarian diets are beneficial in the prevention and treatment of certain diseases, such as **cardiovascular disease, hypertension, diabetes, cancer, osteoporosis, renal disease and dementia**, as well as **diverticular disease, gallstones, and rheumatoid arthritis**."

Effects of fruit and vegetable consumption on plasma antioxidant concentrations and **blood pressure**: *a randomized controlled trial.* John J, Ziebland S, Yudkin P, Roe L, Neil H. The Lancet. 2002;359(9322):1969-1974. **Key Finding:**

"Plasma concentrations of a-carotene, B-carotene, lutein, B-cryptoxanthin, and ascorbic acid increased by more in the intervention group than in controls. The effects of the intervention on fruit and vegetable consumption, plasma antioxidants, and blood pressure would be expected to reduce cardiovascular disease in the general population."

Health effects of vegetables and fruit: assessing mechanisms of action in human experimental studies. Lampe JW. Am J Clin Nutr. 1999 Sep;70 (3 Suppl):4755-4905. **Key Finding:** "Phytochemicals can have complementary and overlapping mechanisms of action, including modulation of detoxification enzymes, stimulation of the immune system, reduction of platelet aggregation, modulation of **cholesterol** synthesis and hormone metabolism, reduction of **blood pressure**, and **antioxidant, antibacterial, and antiviral** effects. Although these effects have been examined primarily in animal and cell-culture models, experimental dietary studies in humans have also shown the capacity of vegetables and fruit and their constituents to modulate some of these potential disease-preventive mechanisms."

Immune system

Complementary and alternative medicine: herbs, phytochemicals and vitamins and their immunologic effects. Mainardi T, Kapoor S, Bielory L. J Allergy Clin Immunol. 2009 Feb;123(2):283-94. **Key Finding:** "This article reviews the history of complementary and alternative medicine and its use among patients, paying special attention to new research focusing on herbals, phytochemicals, and vitamins and their potential interaction with the **immune system**."

Interactions of flavones and other phytochemicals with adenosine receptors. Jacobson KA, Moro S, Manthey JA, West PL, Ji XD. Adv Exp Med Biol. 2002;505:163-71. **Key Finding:** "Adenosine receptors are involved in the homeostatis of **the immune, cardiovascular, and central nervous systems**. The affinity of flavonoids and other phytochemicals to adenosine receptors suggests that a wide range of natural substances in the diet may potentially block the effects of endogenous adenosine."

Infertility

Toxic potential of dietary genistein isoflavone and beta-lapachone on capacitation and acrosome reaction of epididymal spermatozoa. Kumi-Diaka J, Townsend J. J Med Food. 2003 Fall;6(3):201-8. **Key Finding:** "It is concluded that, in view of the fact that acrosome reaction is a physiological prerequisite for fertilization of most mammalian eggs, both genistein and beta-lapachone could potentially suppress male fertility via suppression of acrosome reaction at higher doses, but could enhance fertility by promoting acrosome reaction at lower doses. This bimodal mode of action of both phytochemicals could offer a potentially new dimension in the search for causes of **male infertility** and possibly for male contraceptive development."

Inflammation

Phytochemicals of cranberries *and cranberry products: characterization, potential health benefits, and processing stability.* Pappas E, Schaich KM. Crit Rev Food Sci Nutr. 2009 Oct;49(9):741-81. **Key Finding**: "Emerging evidence is elucidating how non-nutrient phytochemicals underlie the health promotion afforded by fruits and vegetables. This review focuses on the American cranberry compiling a comprehensive list of its known phytochemical components. Evidence for protection from several **bacterial pathogens, cancer, cardiovascular disease, and inflammation** is compelling, while **neuroprotection and anti-viral activity** also have begun to draw new consideration."

Luteolin reduces IL-6 production in microglia by inhibiting JNK phosphorylation and activation of AP-1. Jang S, Kelley KW, Johnson RW. Proc Natl Acad Sci. 2008 May 27;105(21):7534-9. **Key Finding:** "These data suggest luteolin inhibits LPS-induced IL-6 production in the brain by inhibiting the JNK signaling pathway and activation of AP-1 in microglia. Thus, luteolin may be useful for mitigating **neuroinflammation.**"

Serum C-reactive protein concentrations are inversely associated with dietary flavonoid intake in U.S. adults. Chun OK, Chung SJ, Claycombe KJ, Song WO. J Nutr. 2008 Apr;138(4):753-60. **Key Finding:** "Our findings demonstrate that intake of dietary flavonoids is inversely associated with serum CRP concentrations in U.S. adults. Intake of flavonoid-rich foods may thus reduce **inflammation-mediated chronic diseases**."

Availability of blueberry phenolics for microbial metabolism in the colon and the potential **inflammatory** *implications.* Russell WR, Labat A, Scobbie L, Duncan SH. Mol Nutr Food Res. 2007 Jun;51(6):726-31. **Key Finding:** "These results suggest that any potential protective effect of blueberry phenolics as anti-inflammatory agents in the colon is a likely result of microbial metabolism."

Dietary PUFA and flavonoids as deterrents for environmental pollutants. Watkins BA, Hannon K, Ferruzzi M, Li Y. J Nutr Biochem. 2007 Mar;18(3):196-205. **Key Finding:** "The purpose of this review is to introduce the concept for studying food components that influence **inflammation** and how long-chain omega-3 polyunsaturated fatty acids and flavonoids could be used therapeutically against inflammation that is mediated by environmental pollutants."

Anti-inflammatory *and anti-***arthritic** *effects of Yucca schidigera: a review.* Cheeke PR, Piacente S, Oleszek W. J Inflamm (Lond). 2006 Mar 29;3:6. **Key Finding:** "Yucca schidigera is a medicinal plant native to Mexico. Yucca phenolics are anti-oxidants and free-radical scavengers, which may aid in suppressing reactive oxygen species that stimulate inflammatory responses. Based on these findings, further studies on the anti-arthritic effects of Yucca schidigera are warranted."

Divergent responses of chondrocytes and endothelial cells to shear stress: cross-talk among COX-2, the phase 2 response, and apoptosis. Healy ZR, Lee NH, Gao X, et al. Proc Natl Acad Sci. 2005 Sep 27;102(39):14010-5. **Key Finding:** Based on experiments with human cells, phytochemicals found in cruciferous plants were seen to block the activity of an enzyme that triggers **inflammation** in joints which could lead to new **arthritis** treatments.

Rocaglamide derivatives are immunosuppressive phytochemicals that target NF-AT activity in T cells. Proksch P, Giaisi M, Treiber MK, et al. J Immunol. 2005 Jun 1;174(11):7075-84. **Key Finding:** "Aglaia plants are used in traditional medicine (e.g., in Vietnam) for the treatment of **inflammatory skin diseases** and allergic inflammatory disorders such as asthma. In this study we show that rocaglamides are potent immunosuppressive phytochemicals that suppress IFN-gamma, INF-alpha, IL-2, and IL-4 production in peripheral blood T cells at nanomolar concentrations. Our study suggests that rocaglamide derivatives may serve as a new source of NF-AT-specific inhibitors for the treatment of certain inflammatory diseases."

Menopause

*Role of phytochemicals in the prevention of **menopausal bone loss**: evidence from in vitro and in vivo, human interventional and pharmacokinetic studies.* Sharan K, Siddiqui JA, Swarnkar G, Maurya R, Chattopadhyay N. Curr Med Chem. 2009;16(9):1138-57. **Key Finding:** "As phytochemicals have multiple beneficial influences on bone cells, making analogues of the most potent molecule for developing synthetic series with rational drug design approach could pay rich dividends in menopausal osteoporosis therapy."

Health effects of phytoestrogens. Branca F, Lorenzetti S. Forum Nutr. 2005;(57):100-11. **Key Finding:** "For the relief of **menopausal symptoms** a consumption of 60 mg aglycones/day has been suggested; for cancer prevention a consumption between 50 and 110 mg aglycones/day is considered beneficial to reduce risks of breast, colon and prostate cancer; to decrease cardiovascular risk a minimum intake of 40-60 mg aglycones/day, together with about 25 g of soy protein has been suggested. For improvement in bone mineral desnity, 60-100 mg aglycones/day for a period of at least 6-12 months could be beneficial."

Potential risks and benefits of phytoestrogen-rich diets. Cassidy A. Int J Vitam Nutr Res. 2003 Mar;73(2):120-6. **Key Finding:** "The limited studies conducted so far in humans clearly confirm that soya isoflavones can exert hormonal effects. These effects may be of benefit in the prevention of many of the common diseases observed in Western populations (such as **breast cancer, prostate cancer, menopausal symptoms, osteoporosis**) where the diet is typically devoid of these biologically active naturally occurring compounds."

Phyto-oestrogens: where are we now? Bingham SA, Atkinson C, Liggins J, Bluck L, Coward A. Br J Nutr. 1998 May;79(5):393-406. **Key Finding:**

"Evidence is beginning to accrue that they may begin to offer protection against a wide range of human conditions, including **breast, bowel, prostate** and other cancers, **cardiovascular disease**, brain function, alcohol abuse, **osteoporosis** and **menopausal symptoms.** There are few indications of harmful effects at present, although possible proliferative effects have been reported."

Multiple Sclerosis

Oral flavonoids delay recovery from experimental autoimmune encephalomyelitis in SJL mice. Verbeek R, van Tol EA, Van Noort JM. Biochem Pharmacol. 2005 Jul 15;70(2):220-8. **Key Finding:** "Previously, we demonstrated that in vitro flavonoids including luteolin and apigenin, inhibit proliferation and IFN-gamma production by murine and human autoimmune T cells. In the present study, we examined the effects of oral flavonoids as well as of curcumin on autoimmune T cell reactivity in mice and on the course of experimental autoimmune encephalomyelitis, a model for **multiple sclerosis**. Our results indicate that oral curcumin had overall mild but beneficial effects, but oral flavonoids fail to beneficially influence the course of EAE in mice, but, instead, suppress recovery from acute inflammatory damage."

Neurodegenerative diseases

Neuroprotective effects *of naturally occurring polyphenols on quinolinic acid-induced excitotoxicity in human neurons.* Braidy N, Grant R, Adams S, Guillemin GJ. FEBS J. 2010 Jan;277(2):368-82. **Key Finding**: "The inhibitory effect of some natural phytochemicals on specific excitotoxic processes, such as Ca(2+) influx, provides additional evidence for the beneficial health effects of polyphenols in excitable tissue, particularly within the central nervous system."

Recent trends and advances in berry health benefits research. Seeram NP. J Agric Food Chem. 2010 Apr 14;58(7):3869-70: **Key Finding**: "Recent advances have been made in our scientific understanding of how berries promote human health and prevent chronic illnesses such as some

cancers, heart disease, and neurodegenerative diseases. Berry bioactives encompass a wide diversity of phytochemicals."

Phytochemicals of cranberries and *cranberry products: characterization, potential health benefits, and processing stability.* Pappas E, Schaich KM. Crit Rev Food Sci Nutr. 2009 Oct;49(9):741-81. **Key Finding**: "Emerging evidence is elucidating how non-nutrient phytochemicals underlie the health promotion afforded by fruits and vegetables. This review focuses on the American cranberry compiling a comprehensive list of its known phytochemical components. Evidence for protection from several **bacterial pathogens, cancer, cardiovascular disease, and inflammation** is compelling, while **neuroprotection and anti-viral activity** also have begun to draw new consideration."

Emerging role of polyphenolic compounds in the treatment of neurodegenerative diseases: A review of their intracellular targets. Ramassamy C. Eur J Pharmacol. 2006 Sep;545(1):51-64. **Key Finding: "Aging** is the major risk factor for neurodegenerative diseases such as **Alzheimer's** and **Parkinson's** diseases. A large body of evidence indicates that oxidative stress is involved in the pathophysiology of these diseases. Oxidative stress can induce neuronal damages, modulate intracellular signaling, ultimately leading to neuronal death by apoptosis or necrosis. Thus antioxidants have been studied for their effectiveness in reducing these deleterious effects and neuronal death in many in vitro and in vivo studies. Increasing number of studies demonstrated the efficacy of polyphenolic antioxidants from fruits and vegetables to reduce or to block neuronal death."

Blueberry and spirulina-enriched diets enhance striatal dopamine recovery and induce a rapid, transient microglia activation after injury of the rat nigrostriatal dopamine system. Stromberg I, Gemma C, Vila J, Bickford PC. Exp Neurol. 2005 Dec;196(2):298-307. **Key Finding:** "Neuroinflammation plays a critical role in loss of dopamine neurons during brain injury and in **neurodegenerative diseases**. Adult rats were treated with a diet enriched in blueberry or spirulina after being injected to cause a progressive loss of dopamine neurons. Enhanced striatal dopamine recovery appeared in animals treated with diet enriched antioxidants and anti-inflammatory phytochemicals and coincided with an early, transient increase in OX-6-positive microglia."

A possible emerging role of phytochemicals in improving age-related **neurological dysfunctions***: a multiplicity of effects.* Youdim KA, Joseph JA. Free Radic Biol Med. 2001 Mar 15;30(6):583-94. **Key Finding:** It is "extremely important to explore methods to retard or reverse age-related neuronal deficits as well as their subsequent, behavioral manifestations. In this regard, a new role in which certain dietary components may play important roles in alleviating certain disorders are beginning to receive increased attention, in particular those involving phytochemicals found in fruits and vegetables."

Long-term dietary strawberry, spinach, or vitamin E supplementation retards the onset of age-related neuronal signal-transduction and cognitive behavioral deficits. Joseph JA, Shukitt-Hale B, Denisova NA, et al. J Neurosci. 1998 Oct 1;18(19):8047-55. **Key Finding:** "Phytochemicals present in antioxidant-rich foods such as spinach may be beneficial in retarding functional age-related CNS and **cognitive behavioral deficits** and, perhaps, may have some benefit in **neurodegenerative disease**."

Obesity

Phytochemicals and adipogenesis. Andersen C, Rayalam S, Della-Fera MA, Baile CA Biofactors. 2010 Nov-Dec;36(6):415-22. **Key Finding**: "**Obesity** is an increasing health problem all over the world. Phytochemicals are potential agents to inhibit differentiation of preaipocytes, stimulate lipolysis, and induce apoptosis of existing adipocytes, thereby reducing the amount of adipose tissue. Flavonoids and stilbenoids represent the most researched groups of phytochemicals with regards to their effect on adipogenesis."

Higher dietary flavones, flavonol, and catechin intakes are associated with less of an increase in BMI over time in women: a longitudinal analysis from the Netherlands Cohort Study. Hughes LA, Arts IC, Ambergen T, et al. Am J Clin Nutr. 2008 Nov;88(5):1341-52. **Key Finding:** "Women with the highest intake of total flavonols/flavones and total catechins experienced a signficiantly lower increase in body mass index. Our results suggest that flavonoid intake may contribute to maintaining **body weight** in the general female population."

Active spice-derived components can inhibit inflammatory responses of adipose tissue in **obesity** *by suppressing inflammatory actions of macrophages and release of mono-cyte chemoattractant protein-1 from adipocytes.* Woo HM, Kang JH, Kawada T, et al. Life Sci. 2007 Feb 13;80(10):926-31. **Key Finding:** "Raw 264.7 macrophages were treated with the adipose-tissue-conditioned medium with or without active spice-derived components (diallyl disulfide, allyl isothiocyanate, piperine, zingeroen and curcumin. Our finding suggest that the spice-derived components can suppress obesity-induced inflammatory responses by suppressing adipose tissue macrophase accumulation or activation and inhibiting MCP-1 release from adipocytes. These spice-derived components may have a potential to improve chronic inflammatory conditions in obesity."

Effect of genistein with carnitine administration on lipid parameters and **obesity** *in C57Bl/6J mice fed a high-fat diet.* Yang JY, Lee SJ, Park HW, Cha YS. J Med Food. 2006 Winter;9(4):459-67. **Key Finding:** "We investigated the effect of dietary genistein (the principal soy isoflavone) alone and combined with L-carnitine to evaluate possible synergistic effects on the intentionally induced prediabetic state characterized by insulin resistance and obesity. Especially in liver, the results showed that genistein with carnitine transcriptionally up-regulated expressions of acyl-coenzyme A synthetase (ACS) and carnitine palmitoyltransferase-I (CPT-I) by approximately 50% and 40%, respectively, compared with genistein alone."

Genistein, EGCG, and capsaicin inhibit adipocyte differentiation process via activating AMP-activated protein kinase. Hwang JT, Park IJ, Shin JI, et al. Biochem Biophys Res Commun. 2005 Dec 16;338(2):694-9. **Key Finding:** "Phytochemicals such as soy isoflavone genistein have been reported to possess therapeutic effects for obesity, diabetes, and cardiovascular diseases. In the present study, the molecular basis of selective phytochemicals with emphasis on their ability to control intracellular signaling cascades of AMP-activated kinase AMPK responsible for the inhibition of adipogenesis was investigated. We suggest that AMPK is a novel and critical component of both inhibition of adiopocyte differentiation and apoptosis of mature adiopocytes by genistein or EGCG or capsaicin further implying AMPK as a prime target of **obesity** control."

Sorghum phytochemicals and their potential impact on human health. Awika JM, Rooney LW. Phytochemistry. 2004 May;65(9):1199-221. **Key Finding:** "Sorghum is a rich source of various phytochemicals including tannins, phenolic acids, anthocyanins, phytoesterols and policosanols. This paper reviews available information on sorghum phytochemicals, how the information relates to current phytonutrient research and how it has potential to combat common nutrition-related diseases, including **cancer, cardiovascular disease** and **obesity**."

Inhibitory effects of grape seed extract on lipases. Moreno DA, Ilic N, Poulev A, et al. Nutrition. 2003 Oct;19(10):876-9. **Key Finding:** "The grape seed extract compounds that inhibit lipases may provide a safe, natural, and cost-effective **weight control** treatment."

Obstructive pulmonary disease

*Chronic **obstructive pulmonary disease** and intake of catechins, flavonols, and flavones: the MORGEN Study.* Tabak C, Arts IC, Smit HA, Heekerik D, Kromhout D. Am J Respir Crit Care Med. 2001 Jul 1;164(1):61-4. **Key Finding:** "Total catechin, flavonol, and flavones intake was positively associated with pulmonary function and inversely associated with chronic cough and breathlessness, but not chronic phlegm. Our results suggest a beneficial effect of a high intake of catechins and solid fruits against chronic obstructive pulmonary disease."

Osteoporosis

Phase 2 enzyme inducer sulphoraphane blocks matrix metalloproteinase production in articular chondrocytes. Kim HA, Yeo Y, Kim WU, Kim S. Rheumatology. 2009 Aug;48(8):932-8. **Key Finding:** "Sulphoraphane was found to inhibit MMP production in pro-inflammatory cytokine-stimulated chondrocytes. Delineation of the biochemical mechanism regulating cartilage catabolism by SPN may identify safe and effective therapeutic targets for the inhibition of **cartilage degradation.**"

Phenolic phytochemicals and bone. Habauzit V, Horcajada MN. Phytochemistry Reviews. 2008 July; vol 7, no 2:313-344. **Key Finding:** "To date, investigations providing some evidence of a positive impact of some phytochemicals on bone metabolism are accumulating, but further studies, notably clinical trials, are needed to explore the various bioactivities offered by such compounds. It may be postulated that increased consumption of plant-derived foods may be positive in the prevention of **osteoporosis.**"

Vegetarian diets: what are the advantages? Leitzmann C. Forum Nutr. 2005;(57):147-56. **Key Finding:** "In most cases, vegetarian diets are beneficial in the prevention and treatment of certain diseases, such as **cardiovascular disease, hypertension, diabetes, cancer, osteoporosis, renal disease and dementia**, as well as **diverticular disease, gallstones, and rheumatoid arthritis**."

Potential risks and benefits of phytoestrogen-rich diets. Cassidy A. Int J Vitam Nutr Res. 2003 Mar;73(2):120-6. **Key Finding:** "The limited studies conducted so far in humans clearly confirm that soya isoflavones can exert hormonal effects. These effects may be of benefit in the prevention of many of the common diseases observed in Western populations (such as **breast cancer, prostate cancer, menopausal symptoms, osteoporosis**) where the diet is typically devoid of these biologically active naturally occurring compounds."

Phytoestrogens and human health effects: weighing up the current evidence. Humfrey CD. Nat Toxins. 1998;6(2):51-9. **Key Finding:** "Epidemiological studies suggest that foodstuffs containing phytoestrogens may have a beneficial role in protecting against a number of chronic diseases and conditions. For cancer of the **prostate, colon, rectum, stomach and lung,** the evidence is most consistent for a protective effect resulting from a high intake of grains, legumes, fruits, and vegetables. Dietary intervention studies indicate that in women, soya and linseed may have beneficial effects on the risk of **breast cancer** and may help to alleviate **postmenopausal**

symptoms. For **osteoporosis**, tentative evidence suggests phytoestrogens may have similar effects in maintaining **bone density**. Soya also appears to have beneficial effects on blood lipids which may help to reduce the risk of **cardiovascular disease** and **atherosclerosis**. Generally, however, little evidence exists to link these effects directly to phytoestrogens; many other components of soy and linseed are biologically active in various experimental systems and may be responsible for the observed effects in humans."

Phyto-oestrogens: where are we now? Bingham SA, Atkinson C, Liggins J, Bluck L, Coward A. Br J Nutr. 1998 May;79(5):393-406. **Key Finding:** "Evidence is beginning to accrue that they may begin to offer protection against a wide range of human conditions, including **breast, bowel, prostate** and other cancers, **cardiovascular disease**, brain function, alcohol abuse, **osteoporosis** and **menopausal symptoms.** There are few indications of harmful effects at present, although possible proliferative effects have been reported."

Parkinson's disease

Emerging role of polyphenolic compounds in the treatment of neurodegenerative diseases: A review of their intracellular targets. Ramassamy C. Eur J Pharmacol. 2006 Sep;545(1):51-64. **Key Finding: "Aging** is the major risk factor for neurodegenerative diseases such as **Alzheimer's** and **Parkinson's** diseases. A large body of evidence indicates that oxidative stress is involved in the pathophysiology of these diseases. Oxidative stress can induce neuronal damages, modulate intracellular signaling, ultimately leading to neuronal death by apoptosis or necrosis. Thus antioxidants have been studied for their effectiveness in reducing these deleterious effects and neuronal death in many in vitro and in vivo studies. Increasing number of studies demonstrated the efficacy of polyphenolic antioxidants from fruits and vegetables to reduce or to block neuronal death."

Dietary supplementation with blueberry extract improves survival of transplanted dopamine neurons. McGuire SO, Sortwell CE, Shukitt-Hale B, et al. Nutr Neurosci. 2006 Oct-Dec;9(5-6):251-8. **Key Finding:** "These findings provide support for the potential of dietary phytochemicals as an easily administered and well-tolerated therapy that can be used to improve the effectiveness of dopamine neuron replacement in the treatment of **Parkinson's disease.**"

Periodontal disease

An extract of green tea, epigallocatechin-3-gallate, reduces periapical lesions by inhibiting cysteine-rich 61 expression in osteoblasts. Lee YL, Hong CY, Kok SH, et al. J Endod. 2009 Feb;35(2):206-11. **Key Finding:** "EGCG suppresses the progression of apical **periodontitis,** possibly by diminishing Cyr61 expression in osteoblasts and, subsequently, macrophage chemotaxis into the lesions."

Prostate

*Role of lycopene and tomato products in **prostate** health.* Stacewicz-Sapuntzakis M, Bowen PE. Biochem Biophys Acta. 2005 May 30;1740(2):202-5. **Key Finding:** "We conducted a small intervention trial among patients diagnosed with prostate adenocarcinoma. Tomato sauce pasta was consumed daily for 3 weeks. Oxidative DNA damage in leukocytes and prostate tissues was significantly diminished, the latter mainly in the tumor cell nuclei, possibly due to the antioxidant properties of lycopene. Quite surprising was the decrease in blood prostate-specific antigen, which was explained by the increase in apoptotic death of prostate cells, especially in carcinoma regions. Other phytochemicals in tomato may act in synergy with lycopene to potentiate protective effects and to help in the maintenance of prostate health."

Vegetables, fruits and phytoestrogens in the prevention of diseases. Heber D. J Postgrad Med. 2004 Apr-Jun;50(2):145-9. **Key Finding:** "Consumers are advised to ingest one serving of each of the seven colour groups daily. For instance, red foods contain lycopene which may be involved in maintaining **prostate** health and which has been linked to a decreased risk of **cardiovascular disease**. Green foods, including broccoli, brussels sprouts and kale, have been associated with a decreased risk of cancer. White-green foods such as garlic may inhibit cancer cell growth. Grouping plants foods by colour provides simplification, but it is also important as a method to help consumers make wise food choices and promote health."

Sepsis

*Polyphenols in the prevention and treatment of **sepsis** syndromes: rationale and preclinical evidence.* Shapiro H, Lev S, Cohen J, Singer P. Nutrition. 2009 Jun 5. [Epub ahead of print] **Key Finding:** "Sepsis is the overwhelming systemic response to infection. Whether delivered alone or in combination with nutritional formulas, polyphenols may help to prevent and treat sepsis."

Sexual dysfunction

*Phytochemicals and the breakthrough of traditional herbs in the management of **sexual dysfunctions**.* Adimoelia A. Int J Androl. 2000;23 Suppl 2:82-4. **Key Finding:** "Phytochemicals manage erectile dysfunction in the frame of sexual dysfunction as a whole entity. Protodioscin is a phytochemical agent derived from Tribulus terrestris L. plant, which has been clinically proven to improve sexual desire and enhance erection via the conversion of protdioscine to DHEA."

Stroke

Flavonoid intake and the risk of ischaemic stroke and CVD mortality in middle-aged Finnish men: the Kuopio Ischaemic Heart Disease Risk Factor Study. Mursu J, Voutilainen S, Nurmi T, et al. Br J Nutr. 2008 Oct;100(4):890-5. **Key Finding:** "The present study results suggest that high intakes of flavonoids may be associated with decreased risk of ischaemic **stroke** and possibly with reduced **cardiovascular disease** mortality."

*Cranberry and blueberry: evidence for protective effects against **cancer** and vascular diseases.* Neto CC. Mol Nutr Food Res. 2007 Jun;51(6):652-64. **Key Finding:** "Growing evidence from tissue culture, animal, and clinical models suggests that the flavonoid-rich fruits of the North American cranberry and blueberry have the potential ability to limit the development and severity of certain cancers and vascular diseases including **atheroscle-**

rosis, ischemic stroke, and neurodegenerative diseases of aging. Cranberry and blueberry constituents are likely at act by mechanisms that counteract oxidative stress, decrease inflammation, and modulate macromolecular interactions and expression of genes associated with disease processes."

*Fruit and vegetable consumption and **stroke**: meta-analysis of cohort studies.* He FJ, Nowson CA, MacGregor GA. Lancet. 2006 Jan 28;367(9507):320-6. **Key Finding:** "Eight studies, consisting of nine independent cohorts, met the inclusion criteria. Subgroup analyses showed that fruit and vegetables had a significant protective effect on both ischaemic and haemorrhagic stroke. Our results provide strong support for the recommendations to consume more than five servings of fruit and vegetables per day, which is likely to cause a major reduction in strokes."

***Antioxidant** health effects of aged garlic extract.* Borek C. J Nutr. 2001 Mar;131(3s):1010S-5S. **Key Finding:** "Although additional observations are warranted in humans, compelling evidence supports the beneficial health effects attributed to aged garlic extract, i.e., reducing the risk of **cardiovascular disease, stroke, cancer and aging**, including the oxidant-mediated brain cell damage that is implicated in **Alzheimer's disease**."

Thrombosis (blood clots)

The effect of vegetarian diet, plant foods, and phytochemicals on hemostasis and thrombosis. Rajaram S. Am J Clin Nutr. 2003 Sep;78(3 Suppl):552S-558S. **Key Finding:** "Although this review suggests that a plant-based diet with sufficient n-3 fatty acids and certain fruits and vegetables may have a favorable impact on hemostasis and **thrombosis,** the evidence is neither sufficient nor conclusive at this time to warrant specific recommendations for the public."

*On the mechanism of **antithrombotic** action of flavonoids.* Gryglewski RJ, Korbut R, Robak J, Swies J. Biochem Pharmacol. 1987 Feb 1;36(3):317-22. **Key Finding:** Flavonols (quercetin and rutin) and flavanes (cyanidol and meciadonol) were studied for their effect on non-enzymatic lipid peroxidation and other activities. All four flavonoids inhibited the ascorbate-stimulated formation of malondiaidhyde by boiled rat liver microsomes.

Tuberculosis

Successful use of an inhalational phytochemical to treat pulmonary **tuberculosis**: *a case report.* Sherry E, Warnke PH. Phytomedicine. 2004 Feb;11(2-3): 95-7. **Key Finding:** "The aim of this case report is to describe a potential new method for treating those with primary pulmonary tuberculosis using phytochemicals via inhalation. We report the first case of using inhaled phytochemicals in treating primary pulmonary tuberculosis. A 28-year-old female presented with symptoms suggestive of primary pulmonary tuberculosis and she was found to be positive via chest X-ray and sputum culture. She subsequently underwent treatment with conventional DOTS treatment. Ten days post-inhalation of the phytochemical, the patient is tuberculosis negative with no clinical symptoms."

CHAPTER TWO

Evidence for the Healing Effects of Nutrient Synergies

OUTSTANDING SCIENTIFIC MEDICAL EVIDENCE has surfaced documenting the essential effect that combined nutrients have in fighting premature aging and disease. Quite simply put, a chemical synergy is a combination of two or more chemical ingredients—in this case, nutrients—that have an impact much greater than any one ingredient can have on its own.

In the same ways that we see the necessity of symbiosis in our general world, we find this process deep in the cells of plant fiber. Like the domino effect or stepping stones leading to success, one nutrient and another must combine to create the maximum health benefit. As nutritional science further delves into this team effect, researchers find that nature has created an infinite web of supporting casts that ultimately creates a pristine product.

This knowledge offers us insight into how wrong we have been in the field of nutritional supplementation. Most manufacturers produce isolated chemicals in high amounts, yet they remain completely naïve to the damaging results. Isolated chemicals alone cause havoc in a body that needs and anticipates a symphonic orchestra, not a soloist.

At the Hippocrates Health Institute, on an ongoing basis, we have observed the powerful nutritional synergistic effects that whole foods and their related supplements have on strengthening the immune system and overall health. We have also observed the ill effect that the long-term use of isolates has on the anatomy and health maintenance.

Although we are all in the beginning stages of understanding nutrient synergies, the one thing that has been well established is that you and all other life forms are dependent upon the utilization and ingestion of a wide and potentially endless gathering of supporting elements.

Human health benefits associated with the synergistic or additive impact of phytochemical combinations has been a focus for mainstream medical and nutrition research for only a decade or so. Of the thousands of phytochemicals in plants identified in laboratories thus far, just a few dozen combinations have been studied for their synergistic potential to address health problems as preventive or healing agents.

But in my own observations and work with people facing health challenges, a cause and effect pattern has been apparent, linking synergies to successful treatment strategies. Here are just two representative examples, from among hundreds that I know of, where a nutrient-dense diet of phytochemicals stimulated synergistic reactions to benefit health once the nutrients are absorbed in the human body.

Erin DeNardo, 23, of New Jersey was a beautiful fashion model traveling the world on modeling assignments. She appeared on the TV series "Project Runway" and her image graced the advertising campaigns of Levi's jeans and Ban deodorant. In 2007 she began to experience migraines that blurred her vision and inflicted severe pressure in her head.

Erin had a CAT scan that showed a brain tumor the size of a golf ball. She went through a seven-hour surgery to have the tumor removed. Still, a second surgery had to be performed to remove even more of the tumor. When she had a three-month follow-up MRI, the tumor had reappeared and physicians wanted her to undergo a third surgery with chemotherapy and/or radiation therapy. After serious consideration, she decided not to undergo the third surgery but would instead explore nutritional treatments.

She adopted a 100-percent raw vegan foods diet that consisted primarily of consuming green drinks made from fresh organic vegetables, along with drinking wheatgrass juice several times a day. Erin's next MRI revealed, to her physician's amazement, that the tumor had dramatically decreased in size and appeared to be gone. He encouraged her to continue whatever it was she had been doing because it seemed to be working. Today, Erin is a proud poster girl for what a nutrient-dense dietary regimen can achieve.

David Strong is a Florida resident and irrigation contractor who faced a similar health challenge and made the same treatment decision. He was diagnosed with prostate cancer and given the options of surgery or radiation treatment. In 2006, his PSA reading had reached more than 16, when a normal reading was 4. He decided to try a living-foods diet with green juices and wheatgrass juice.

David describes what happened: "By the third week on this diet, I had lost 40 pounds and my PSA was cut in half. It was the first time in years that I felt in control of my life. It's now been two years of living this lifestyle and my health is under control. I feel better every day and I'm happy."

The field of nutritional science is poised on a new frontier of discoveries which draw new links between nutrient synergies and human health. Here is the lineup of medical studies that support the important role that combinations of foods and their nutrient synergies play in promoting human health and healing.

Aging

Neurobehavioral aspects of antioxidants in **aging**. Cantuti-Castelvetri I, Shukitt-Hale B, Joseph JA. Int J Dev Neurosci. 2000 Jul-Aug;18(4-5):367-81. **Key Finding:** This paper reviews studies concerning the influence of antioxidants on age-related, reactive oxygen species-induced behavioral changes in humans and animals. The antioxidants reviewed may have synergistic effects among them.

Antioxidation

Antioxidant *effect of trans-resveratrol, pterostilbene, quercetin, and their combinations in human erythrocytes in vitro.* Mikestacka R, Rimando AM, Ignatowicz E. Plant Foods Hum Nutr. 2010 Mar;65(1):57-63. **Key Finding:** "At lower concentrations, resveratrol with quercetin or pterostilbene inhibited synergistically the oxidative injury of membrane lipids. These protective effects may partially explain the health benefit of these bioactive microcomponents when together in the diet."

Comparative **antioxidant** *activities and synergism of resveratrol and oxyresveratrol.* Aftab N, Likhitwitayawuid K, Vieira A. Nat Prod Res. 2010 Nov;24(18):1726-33. **Key Finding**: "Resveratrol and oxyresveratrol are phytoalexins with antioxidant activities and proposed effects against several pathological processes. Our results indicate that they can synergise in combination or with another phytochemical antioxidant, curcumin."

A novel dietary supplement containing multiple phytochemicals and vitamins elevates hepatorenal and **cardiac antioxidant** *enzymes in the absence of significant serum chemistry and genomic changes.* Bulku E. Zinkovsky D, Patel P, et al. Oxid Med Cell Longev. 2010 Mar-Apr;3(2):129-44. **Key Finding**: "A novel dietary supplement composed of three well-known phytochemicals, namely, Salvia officinalis (sage) extract, Camellia sinensis (oolong tea) extract, and Paullinia cupana (guarana) extract, and two prominent vitamins (thiamine and niacin) was designed to provide nutritional support by enhancing metabolism and maintaining healthy weight and energy. The present study evaluated the safety of this dietary supplement and assessed changes in target organ antioxidant enzymes (liver, kidneys and heart), serum chemistry profiles and organ histopathology in Fisher 344 rats. Results suggest that dietary supplement exposure produces normal serum chemistry coupled with elevated antioxidant capacity and does not adversely influence any of the vital target organs. This study reiterates the potential benefits of exposure to a pharmacologically relevant **combination of phytochemicals** compared to a single phytochemical entity."

Antioxidant activities of curcumin and combinations of this curcuminoid with other phytochemicals. Aftab N, Vieira A. Phytother Res. 2009 Nov 19. [Epub ahead of print] **Key Finding:** "Curcumin shows significantly greater synergism with resveratrol than with quercetin. Curcumin and resveratrol together (5 muM each) resulted in a synergistic antioxidant effect: 15.5 +/- 1.7% greater than an average of individual activities. This synergy was significantly greater ($p < 0.05$; about 4-fold) than that of curcumin together with the flavonol quercetin."

In vitro activity of almond skin polyphenols for scavenging free radicals and inducing quinone reductase. Chen O, Blumberg J. J Agric. Food Chem. 2008; 56(12):4427-34. **Key Finding:** "The interaction between ASP-GI (almond skin polyphenols) plus VC (vitamins C or E) promoted their radical scavenging activity."

Dietary botanical diversity affects the reduction of **oxidative** *biomarkers in women due to high vegetable and fruit intake.* Thompson HJ, Heimendinger J, Diker A, et al. J Nutr. 2006 Aug;136(8):2207-12. **Key Finding:** "The objective of this study was to determine whether the botanical diversity of high vegetables and fruit diets alters the response in oxidative biomarkers for lipid peroxidation and DNA oxidation. Two diets were developed. The high botanical diversity diet included foods from the 18 botanical families that induced a reduction in oxidative damage or lipids or DNA. The low botanical diversity diet emphasized five of these botanical families. A total of 106 women completed the study. Only the high botanical diversity diet induced a significant reduction in DNA oxidation. Both the high and low diets were associated with a reduction in lipid peroxidation. These findings indicate that botanical diversity plays a role in determining the bioactivity of high vegetable/fruit diets and that smaller amounts of many phytochemicals may have greater beneficial effects than larger amounts of fewer phytochemicals."

Antioxidant activities of curcumin and combinations of this curcuminoid with other phytochemicals. Aftab N, Vieira A. Phytother Res. 2009 Nov 19. [Epub ahead of print] **Key Finding:** "The main goal of the present study was to compare antioxidant activities of curcumin with those of resveratrol. Combination of the two were examined for potential synergism in a heme-enhanced oxidation reaction. Curcumin and resveratrol together (5 muM each) resulted in a synergistic antioxidant effect: 15.5 +/- 1.7% greater than an average of individual activities. This synergy was significantly greater than that of curcumin together with the flavonol quercetin."

Safety and whole-body **antioxidant** *potential of a novel anthocyanin-rich formulation of edible berries.* Bagchi D, Roy S, Patel V, et al. Mol Cell Biochem. 2006 Jan;281(1-2):197-209. **Key Finding:** "Six berry extracts (wild blueberry, bilberry, cranberry, elderberry, raspberry seeds and strawberry) singly and in combinations, were studied in our laboratories for **antioxidant** efficacy, cytotoxic potential, cellular uptake and anti-angiogenic properties. Combinations of edible berry extracts were evaluated to develop a synergistic formula, OptiBerry, which exhibited high oxygen radical absorbance capacity (ORAC) value, low cytotoxicity and superior **anti-angiogenic** properties compared to the other combinations tested."

Turmeric and curcumin enriched beverages for educing the risk for oxidation linked chronic diseases. Vattem D, Crixell S. Research Enhancement Program Final Reports. Paper 61. 2005. Available at: http://ecommons.txstate.edu/osp_regs/61. Accessed May 17, 2011. **Key Finding:** "Results strongly suggest that the functionality of fruit extracts can be significantly increased by creating novel synergies with turmeric. We were able to show that **antioxidant** activity of these synergies was significantly higher than the pure extracts alone."

Flavonoids from almond skins are bioavailable and act synergistically with vitamins C and E to enhance hamster and human LDL resistance in oxidation. Chung-Yen C, Milbury P, Lapsley K, Blumberg J. J Nutr. 2005;135(6):1366-73. **Key Finding:** Almond skin flavonoids "possess antioxidant capacity in vitro, they are bioavailable and act in synergy with vitamins C and E to protect LDL against **oxidation.**"

*Effect of resveratrol and beta-sitosterol in combination on **reactive oxygen species** and prostaglandin release by PC-3 cells.* Awad AB, Burr AT, Fink CS. Prostaglandins Leukot Essent Fatty Acids. 2005 Mar;72(3):219-26. **Key Finding:** "Phytochemical supplementation resulted in inhibition in cell growth. Beta-sitosterol was more potent than resveratrol and the combination of the two resulted in greater inhibition than supplementation with either alone."

Anti-angiogenic, antioxidant, and anti-carcinogenic properties of a novel anthocyanin-rich berry extract formula. Bagchi D, Sen CK, Bagchi M, Atalay M. Biochemistry. 2004 Jan;69(1):75-80. **Key Finding:** "Six berry extracts (wild blueberry, bilberry, cranberry, elderberry, raspberry seeds and strawberry) were studied for antioxidant efficacy, cytotoxic potential, cellular uptake, and anti-angiogenic (the ability to reduce unwanted growth of blood vessels, which can lead to varicose veins and tumor formation) properties. We evaluated various combinations of edible berry extracts and developed a synergistic formula, OptiBerry IH141, which exhibited high ORAC (oxygen-radical absorbing capacity) value, low cytotoxicity, and superior anti-angiogenic properties compared to the other combinations tested. Anti-angiogenic approaches to treat cancer represent a priority area in vascular tumor biology. OptiBerry significantly inhibited both H_2O_2- and TNF-alpha-induced VEGF (Vascular Endothelial Growth Factor) expression by human keratinocytes. VEGF is a key regulator of tumor angiogenesis. Matrigel assay using human microvascular endothelial cells showed that OptiBerry impaired angiogenesis. Endothelioma cells pretreated with OptiBerry showed a diminished ability to form hemangioma and markedly decreased tumor growth by more than 50%."

Antioxidant capacity of different broccoli, (brassica oleracea) genotypes using the oxygen radical absorbance capacity (ORAC) assay. Kurilich AC, Jeffery EH, Juvik JA, Wallig MA, Klein BP. J Agric Food Chem. 2002 Aug 28;50(18):5053-7. **Key Finding:** "Ascorbic acid and flavonoid content of the hydrophilic extracts did not explain the total variation in antioxidant capacity of these extracts, suggesting either the presence of other antioxidant components that have yet to be identified or that the known antioxidants are producing synergistic effects."

*The synergistic upregulation of phase II **detoxification** enzymes by glucosinolate breakdown products in cruciferous vegetables.* Nho CW, Jeffery E. Toxicol Appl Pharmacol. 2001 Jul 15;174(2):146-52. **Key Finding:** "The mixture of crambene and indole-3-carbinol caused induction of glutathione S-transferase and quinine reductase that was significantly greater than the sum of the induction by individual treatments. We had previously shown that a mixture of four major glucosinolate breakdown products from brussels sprouts interact to produce a synergistic induction of phase II detoxification enzymes."

*Synergistic activity of catechin and other **antioxidants**.* Saucier CT, Waterhouse AL. J Agric Food Chem. 1999 Oct. 2;47(11):4491-4. **Key Finding:** Interaction studies showed simple additive effects in all cases except with the catechin/SO2 mixture "which showed a remarkable synergistic effect in both assays."

*Carotenoid mixtures protect multilamellar liposomes against **oxidative damage:** synergistic effects of lycopene and lutein.* Slahla W, Junghansa A, de Boerb B, et al. FEBS Letters. 1998 May 8;427(2):305-8. **Key Finding:** The antioxidant activity of carotenoids was more effective in combinations than in single compounds. This synergistic effect was most pronounced when lycopene or lutein was present.

Antiviral/Antibacterial

*Phytochemical screening and modulation of **antibiotic** activity by Ocimum gratissimum L.* Matias EF, Santos KK, Almeida TS, Costa JG, Coutinho HD. Biomed Pharmacother. 2010 Oct 23 [epub ahead of print]. **Key Finding:** "This study is the first test of change in resistance of antibiotic activity by Ocimum gratissimum L. against multiresistant strains of E. coli and Staphylococcus aureus. The synergy of the methanolic and hexane were verified. A synergistic effect of both extracts combined with the aminoglycosides was demonstrated."

*Antimicrobial activity of phenolics and glucosinolate hydrolysis products and their synergy with streptomycin against **pathogenic bacteria**.* Saavedra MJ, Borges A, Dias C, et al. Med Chem. 2010 May 1;6(3):174-83. **Key Finding:** "The results showed that all of the isothiocyanates had significant antimicrobial activities. The application of dual combinations demonstrated synergy between streptomycin and gallic acid, ferulic acid, chlorogenic acid, allylisothiocyanate and 2-phenylethylisothiocyanate against the gram-negative bacteria."

Effects of a nutrient mixture on infectious properties of the highly pathogenic strain of avian influenza virus A/H5N1. Deryabin PG, Lvov DK, Botikov AG, et al. Biofactors. 2008;33(2):85-97. **Key Finding:** "A unique nutrient mixture (NM) containing lysine, proline, ascorbic acid demonstrated high **antiviral** activity even at prolonged periods after infection."

Indole and (E)-2-hexenal, phytochemical potentiators of polymyxins against Pseudomonas aeruginosa and Escherichia coli. Kubo A, Lunde CS, Kubo I. Antimicrob Agents Chemother. 1996 June;Vol. 40, No. 6:1438-1441. **Key Finding:** Phytochemical combinations with antibiotics enhance total biological activity in **antimicrobial** tests against two types of bacteria.

Arthritis

Synergistic effect of Kalpaamruthaa on anti-arthritic and anti-inflammatory properties—its mechanism of action. Mythilypriya R, Shanthi P,

Sachdanandam P. Inflammation. 2008 Dec;31(6):391-8. **Key Finding:** The nut milk extract combined with honey and Emblica officinalis, Kalpa-amruthaa (KA), "exhibited enhanced effect on **anti-inflammatory** and **anti-arthritic** properties than sole nut milk extract treatment and the collective effect might be due to the combined interactions of the phytochemicals such as flavonoids, tannins, and other compounds such as vitamin C present in KA."

Atherosclerosis

Plant-derived micronutrients suppress monocyte adhesion to cultured human aoertic endothelial cell layer by modulating its extracellular matrix composition. Ivanov V, Ivanova S, Kalinovsky T, Niedzwiecki A, Rath M. J Cardiovasc Pharmacol. 2008 Jul;52(1):55-65. **Key Finding:** A mixture of the micronutrients ascorbic acid, quercetin, gotu kola extract, and green tea extract reduced ECM capacity to bind monocytes in a dose dependent manner, which could be important in treating **atherosclerosis**.

Anti-atherogenic effects of a mixture of ascorbic acid, lysine, proline, arginine, cysteine, and green tea phenolics in human aortic smooth muscle cells. Ivanov V, Roomi MW, Kalinvosky T, Niedzwiecki A, Rath M. J Cardiovasc Pharmacol. 2007 Mar;49(3):140-45. **Key Finding:** "These data suggest that the nutrient mixture has potential in blocking the development of **atherosclerotic lesions** by inhibiting atherogenic responses of vascular SMC to pathologic stimuli."

Synergistic inhibition of low-density lipoprotein oxidation by rutin, yterpinene, and ascorbic acid. Mildea J, Elstnera EP, Grabmann J. Phytomedicine. 2004;11(2):105-113. **Key Finding:** "Low-density lipoprotein LDL oxidation may play a significant role in **atherogenesis**. We investigated the combination of rutin with a hydrophilic (ascorbate) and a lipophilic antioxidant (y-terpinene) in copper-mediate LDL oxidation. In both cases we found a synergistic effect on lag phase prolongation."

Cancer

Modulation of CXCR4, CXCL12, and tumor cell invasion potential in vitro by phytochemicals. Hsu EL, Chen N, Westbrook A, et al. J Oncol. 2009:491985. Epub 2009 Mar 24. **Key Finding:** "Our data suggest a novel mechanism for the protective effects of phytochemicals against **cancer** progression and indicate that in combination, these compounds may prove even more efficacious."

*Synergistic potentiation of D-fraction with vitamin C as possible alternative approach for **cancer** therapy.* Konno S. Int J Gen Med. 2009 Jul 30;2:91-108. **Key Finding**: "Maitake mushroom D-fraction in numerous studies performed in vitro and in vivo or in clinical settings showed that it was capable of modulating immunologic and hematologic parameters, inhibiting or regressing the cancer cell growth. Synergistic potentiation of Maitake D-fraction with vitamin C demonstrated in vitro may have clinical implication because such combination therapy appears to help improve the efficacy of currently ongoing cancer therapies."

Mechanisms of combined action of different chemopreventive dietary compounds: a review. De Kok TM, Van Breda SG, Manson MM. Eur J Nutr. 2008 May;47 (Suppl 2):51-9. **Key Finding:** "We discuss the molecular mechanisms that are likely to be involved in **cancer** chemoprevention and summarize the most important findings of those studies that report synergistic chemopreventive effects of dietary compounds."

Interactive effects of polymethoxy flavones from citrus on cell growth inhibition in human neuroblastoma SH-SYSY cells. Akao Y, Itoh T, Ohguchi K, Iinuma M, Nozawa Y. Bioorg Med Chem. 2008 Mar 15;16(6):2803-10. **Key Finding:** The interactive effects of polymethoxy flavones from citrus on cell growth were investigated. "These results indicate the relevance of the combination of phytochemicals for the enhancement of the **anticancer** effect."

*Fractionation of polyphenol-enriched apple juice extracts to identify constituents with **cancer** chemopreventive potential.* Zessner H, Pan L, Will F, et al. Mol Nutr Food Res. 2008 Jun;52 (Suppl 1):528-44. **Key Finding:** Apple juice extract was fractionated to determine which constituents contribute to potential chemopreventive activities. "Overall, apple juice constituents belonging to different structural classes have distinct profiles of biological activity in these in vitro test systems. Since carcinogenesis is a complex process, combination of compounds with complementary activities may lead to enhanced preventive effects."

*Nutritional interactions: credentialing of molecular targets for **cancer** prevention.* Davis CD. Expl Biol Med. 2007; 232:176-83. **Key Finding:** "Evidence suggests that the cancer protective effects of an individual's diet may reflect the combined effects of various vitamins, minerals, and other bioactive components such as flavonoids, isothiocyanates, and/or allium compounds rather than from the effect of a single ingredient."

*Ins and outs of dietary phytochemicals in **cancer** chemoprevention.* Russo GL. Biochem Pharmacol. 2007 Aug 15;74(4):533-44. **Key Finding:** The bioavailability of phytochemical compounds is discussed, as is whether purified phytochemicals have the same protective effects as whole food mixtures of the compounds; also, the synergistic effects of compounds present in the diet.

*Molecular basis for **chemoprevention** by sulforaphane: a comprehensive review.* Judge N, Mithen RF, Traka M. Cell Mol Life Sci. 2007 May;64(9):1105-27. **Key Finding:** "It is becoming clear that there are multiple mechanisms activated in response to sulforaphane, including suppression of cytochrome P450 enzymes, induction of apoptotic pathways, suppression of cell cycle progression, inhibition of angiogenesis and **anti-inflammatory** activity. Moreover, these mechanisms seem to have some degree of interaction to synergistically afford chemoprevention."

*Cranberry and its phytochemicals: a review of in vitro **anticancer** studies.* Neto CC. J Nutr. 2007 Jan;137(1 Suppl):186S-193S. **Key Finding:** "The unique combination of phytochemicals found in cranberry fruit may produce synergistic health benefits. Possible chemopreventive mechanisms of action by cranberry phytochemicals include induction of apoptosis in tumor cells, reduced ornithine decarboxylase activity, decreased expression of matrix metalloproteinases associated with prostate tumor metastasis, and anti-inflammatory activities including inhibition of cyclooxygenases."

Pre-exposure to a novel nutritional mixture containing a series of phytochemicals prevents acetaminophen-induced programmed and unprogrammed cell deaths by enhancing BCL-XL expression and minimizing oxidative stress in the liver. Ray SD, Patel N, Shah N, et al. Mol Cell Biochem. 2006 Dec;293(1-2):119-36. **Key Finding:** "We proposed that the additive and synergistic effects of phytochemicals in fruits and vegetables are responsible for these potent antioxidant and **anticancer** activities, and that the benefit of a diet rich in fruits and vegetables is attributed to the complex mixture of phytochemicals present in plants. Our investigation suggests that a mixture containing an assortment of phytochemicals/nutraceuticals may serve as a much more powerful blend in preventing drug or chemical-induced organ injuries than a single phytochemical or nutraceutical entity."

*Potential synergism of natural products in the treatment of **cancer**.* Hemalswarya S, Dobie M. Phytother Res. 2006 Apr;20(4):239-49. **Key Finding:** "This review focuses on a number of reports of herb-drug interactions, their mechanism of action with a special emphasis on dietetic phytochemicals such as quercetin, genistein, curcumin, and catechins. All phytochemicals tend to increase the therapeutic effect by blocking one or more targets of the signal transduction pathway, by increasing the bioavailability of the other drug or, by stabilizing the other drug in the system."

*Activation of coupled Ah receptor and Nrf2 gene batteries by dietary phytochemicals in relation to **chemoprevention**.* Kohle C, Bock KW. Biochem Pharmacol. 2006 Sep 28;72(7):795-805. **Key Finding:** "This finding offers the possibility that distinct but partially overlapping AhR and Nrf2 gene batteries of Phase II xenobiotic-metabolizing enzymes can be synergistically activated by a number of phytochemicals, acting as selective or mixed activators of target genes."

Synergy among phytochemicals within crucifers: does it translate into **chemoprotection?** Wallig M, Heinz-Taheny K, Epps D, Gossman T. J Nutr. Dec. 2005; 135:2972S-77S. **Key Finding:** Two derivatives, indole-3-carbinol and 1-cyano-2-hydroxy-3-butene (crambene) have been shown in rats to induce a synergistic enhancement of detoxification enzyme activity. High combination dietary doses also demonstrated enhanced protection from short-term carcinogenicity using aflatoxin B1.

Black raspberry extract and fractions contain angiogenesis inhibitors. Liu Z, Schwimer J, Liu D, et al. J Agric Food Chem. 2005 May 18;53(10):3909-15. **Key Finding:** "These findings suggest that an active black raspberry fraction may be a promising complementary **cancer** therapy. It is natural and potent enough for manageable dosing regimens. These extracts contain multiple active ingredients that may be additive or synergistic in their antiangiogenic effects. These observations warrant further investigations in animals and human trials."

Potential synergy of phytochemicals in **cancer** *prevention: mechanism of action.* Liu RH. J Nutr. Dec. 2004; 134(12 Suppl):3479S-3485S. **Key Finding:** "Work performed by our group and others has shown that fruits and vegetable phytochemical extracts exhibit strong antioxidant and antiproliferative activities and that the major part of total antioxidant activity is from the combination of phytochemicals. We proposed that the additive and synergistic effects of phytochemicals in fruits and vegetables are responsible for these potent antioxidant and anticancer activities and that the benefit of a diet rich in fruits and vegetables is attributed to the complex mixture of phytochemicals present in whole foods."

Cancer prevention with food factors: along and in combination. Ohigashia H, Murakami A. Biofactors. 2004;22(1-4):49-55. **Key Finding:** "Cancer prevention strategies making use of combined agents with distinct molecular mechanisms, rather than individual agents, are considered promising for higher efficacy and lower toxicity. The present review briefly highlights the potential effectiveness of combinations of several agents, such as EGCG from green tea and genistein, with anti-oxidative and anti-inflammatory properties for **cancer** preventive strategies."

Anti-angiogenic, antioxidant, and anti-carcinogenic properties of a novel anthocyanin-rich berry extract formula. Bagchi D, Sen CK, Bagchi M, Atalay M. Biochemistry. 2004 Jan;69(1):75-80. **Key Finding:** "Six berry extracts (wild blueberry, bilberry, cranberry, elderberry, raspberry seeds and strawberry) were studied for antioxidant efficacy, cytotoxic potential, cellular uptake, and anti-angiogenic (the ability to reduce unwanted growth of blood vessels, which can lead to varicose veins and tumor formation) properties. We evaluated various combinations of edible berry extracts and developed a synergistic formula, OptiBerry IH141, which exhibited high ORAC (oxygen-radical absorbing capacity) value, low cytotoxicity, and superior anti-angiogenic properties compared to the other combinations tested. Anti-angiogenic approaches to treat cancer represent a priority area in vascular tumor biology. OptiBerry significantly inhibited both H202- and TNF-alpha-induced VEGF (vascular endothelial growth factor) expression by human keratinocytes. VEGF is a key regulator of tumor angiogenesis. Matrigel assay using human microvascular endothelial cells showed that OptiBerry impaired angiogenesis. Endothelioma cells pretreated with OptiBerry showed a diminished ability to form hemangioma and markedly decreased tumor growth by more than 50%."

Synergistic capsicum-tea mixtures with **anticancer** *activity.* Morre DJ, Morre DM. J Pharm-Pharmacol. 2003 Jul; 55(7): 987-94. **Key Finding:** Green tea and capsicum preparations were synergistic in their inhibition of the target cancer cells in culture.

Synergistic suppression of superoxide and nitric-oxide generation from inflammatory cells by combined food factors. Murakami A, Takahashi D, Koshimizu K, Ohigashi H. Mutat Res. 2003 Feb-Mar;523-524:151-61. **Key Finding:** "The present findings suggest that individual food phytochemicals have complex interactions that can be antagonistic, additive, and/or synergistic in biological systems, depending upon certain environmental factors including concentrations. Further, these results support and emphasize the concept that combinations of different types of chemicals at low concentrations are one of the essential areas of study for chemopreventive strategies."

Cruciferous vegetables and **cancer** *prevention.* Murillo G, Mehta RG. Nutr Cancer. 2001;41(1-2):17-28. **Key Finding:** "Results clearly point toward a positive correlation between cancer prevention of many target organs and consumption of cruciferous vegetable or their active constitutents. Yet we are still far from complete understanding of the effects of combinations of chemopreventive phytochemicals present in these cruciferous vegetables and their overall mechanisms of action in providing protective effects."

Apoptosis and cell-cycle arrest in human and **murine tumor** *cells are initiated by isoprenoids.* Mo H, Elson CE. J Nutr. 1999 Apr;129(4):804-13. **Key Finding:** "The additive and potentially synergistic actions of isoprenoids in the suppression of tumor cell proliferation and initiation of apoptosis coupled with the mass action of the diverse isoprenoid constitutents of plant products may explain, in part, the impact of fruit, vegetable and grain consumption on cancer risk."

Phytochemicals as modulators of **cancer** *risk.* Bradlow HL, Telang NT, Sepkovic DW, Osborne MP. Adv Exp Med Biol. 1999;472:207-21. **Key Finding:** "Dietary changes could play a role in decreasing the incidence of a variety of tumors. 13C and the other compounds discussed may well be only prototypes for other as yet unexplored phytochemicals present in the diet. There have been no attempts to explore the possibilities of synergistic action among the various phytochemicals, 13C, limonene, curcumin, epigallocatechin gallate, sulforaphene, or genistein. Mixtures of these compounds might well show potency at lower doses for each of the compounds and show even greater promise than that already demonstrated."

Isoprenoid-mediated inhibition of mevalonate synthesis: potential application to **cancer**. Elson CE, Peffley DM, Hentosh P, Mo H. Proc Soc Exp Biol Med.

1999 Sep;221(4):294-311. **Key Finding:** "Isoprenoid-mediated activities are additive, and, sometimes synergistic. Therefore, the combined actions of the estimated 23,000 isoprenoid constituents of plant materials, acting in concert with other chemopreventive phytochemicals, may explain the lowered cancer risk associated with a diet rich in plant products."

Antimutagenic activity of carotenoids in green peppers against some nitroarenes. Gonzalez de Mejia E, Quintanar-Hernandez A, Loarca-Pina G. Mutat Res. 1998 Aug 7;416(1-2):11-9. **Key Finding**: "These results suggest that each one of the pepper extracts have more than one **antimutagenic** compound (e.g., beta-carotene and xanthophylls) and those functional nutrients apparently have a synergistic effect."

Alimentary

*New approaches to the role of diet in the prevention of **cancers of the alimentary tract**.* Johnson IT. Mutat Res. 2004 Jul 13;551(1-2):9-28. **Key Finding:** "Plant foods contain a variety of components including micronutrients, polyunsaturated fatty acids, and secondary metabolites such as glucosinolates and flavonoids, many of which can inhibit cell proliferation and induce apoptosis, and which may well act synergistically when combined in the human diet. The future challenge is to fully characterize and evaluate these effects at the cellular and molecular level, so as to exploit their full potential as protective mechanisms for the population as a whole."

Bladder

Antitumor effect of ascorbic acid, lysine, proline, arginine, and green tea extract on bladder cancer cell line T-24. Roomi MW, Ivanov V, Kalinovsky T, Niedzwiecki A, Rath M. Int J Urol. 2006 Apr;13(4):415-9. **Key Finding:** "Our results suggest that our nutrient mixture is an excellent candidate for therapeutic use in the treatment of **bladder cancer**, by inhibiting critical steps in cancer development and spread, such as MMP secretion and invasion."

Breast

*Synergistic effect of apple extracts and quercetin 3-beta-d-glucoside combination on antiproliferative activity in MCF-7 human **breast cancer** cells in vitro.* Yang J, Liu RH. J Agric Food Chem. 2009 Sep 23;57(18):8581-6. **Key Finding:** "The results suggest that the apple extracts plus Q3G combination possesses a synergistic effect in MCF-7 cell proliferation. The two-way combination of apple plus Q3G was conducted. In this two-way combination, the EC(5) values of apple extracts and Q3G were 2- and 4-fold lower, respectively, than those of apple extracts and Q3G alone. The combination index (Ci) values at 50 and 95% inhibition rates were 0.76 +/- 0.39-fold, respectively."

*Dietary intakes of mushrooms and green tea combine to reduce the risk of **breast cancer** in Chinese women.* Zhang M, Huang J, Xie X, Holman CD. Int J Cancer. 2009 Mar 15;124(6):1404-8. **Key Finding:** "We conclude that higher dietary intake of mushrooms decreased breast cancer risk in pre- and post-menopausal Chinese women and an additional decreased risk of breast cancer from joint effect of mushrooms and green tea was observed."

*Suppression of cell proliferation and gene expression by combinatorial synergy of EGCG, resveratrol and gamma-tocotrienol in estrogen receptor-positive MCF-7 **breast cancer** cells.* Hsieh TC, Wu JM. Int J Oncol. 2008 Oct;33(4):851-9. **Key Finding:** "These results suggest that diet-based protection against breast cancer may partly derive from synergy amongst dietary phytochemicals directed against specific molecular targets in responsive breast cancer cells, and provide support for the feasibility of the development of a diet-based combinatorial approach in the prevention and treatment of breast cancer."

*Soy phytochemicals synergistically enhance the preventive effect of tamoxifen on the growth of estrogen-dependent human **breast carcinoma** in mice.* Mai Z, Blackburn GL, Zhou JR. Carcinogenesis. 2007 Jun;28(6):1217-23. **Key Finding:** "**Genistein** and tamoxifen combination synergistically delayed the growth of breast tumor which decreased estrogen level and activity, and down-regulation of EGFR expressions. The results from our studies suggest that further investigations may be warranted to determine if the combination of tamoxifen and bioactive soy components may be used for prevention and/or treatment of estrogen-dependent **breast cancer**."

Cranberry phytochemical extracts induce cell cycle arrest and apoptosis in human MCF-7 **breast cancer** *cells.* Sun J, Hai Liu R. Cancer Lett. 2006 Sep 8;241(1):124-34. **Key Finding:** "Epidemiological studies have consistently suggested the inverse association between cancer risk and intake of fruits and vegetables. These health benefits have been linked to the additive and synergistic combination of phytochemicals in fruits and vegetables. Our results suggest that cranberry phytochemical extracts possess the ability to suppress the proliferation of human breast cancer MCF-7 cells and this suppression is at least partly attributed to both the initiation of apoptosis and the G1 phase arrest."

In vitro and in vivo antitumorigenic activity of a mixture of lysine, proline, ascorbic acid, and green tea extract on human **breast cancer** *lines MDA-MB-231 and MCF-7.* Roomi MW, Ivanov V, Kalinovsky T, Niedzwiecki A, Rath M. Med Oncol. 2005;22(2):129-38. **Key Finding:** "The results of this study demonstrated that the nutrient mixture tested significantly suppressed tumor growth of breast cancer cells in female athymic nude mice and significantly inhibited MMP expression, angiogenesis, and invasion in breast cancer cells in vitro, offering promise for therapeutic use in the treatment of breast cancer."

Extracts from organically and conventionally cultivated strawberries inhibit **cancer** *cell proliferation in vitro.* Olsson ME, Andersson SC, Berglund RH, Gustavsson KE, Oredsson S. Acta Hort. 2007 (ISHS) 744:189-94. Available at: http://www.actahort.org/books/744/744_19.htm. Accessed on May 19, 2011. **Key Finding:** "The strawberry extracts inhibited cell proliferation in **colon cancer** cells HT29 and **breast cancer** cells MCF-7 in a concentration dependent way. Extracts from organically grown strawberries inhibited cell proliferation to a higher extent than conventionally grown at the two highest concentrations. The content of ascorbate was 36% higher and the ratio of ascorbate to dehydroascorbate were eight-fold higher in the organically grown strawberries than in the conventionally grown. Ascorbate is suggested to act synergistically with other substances in the extracts."

Dietary factors modifying **breast cancer** *risk and relation to time of intake.* Tsubura A, Uehara N, Kiyozuka Y, Shikata N. J Mammary Gland Biol

Neoplasia. 2005 Jan;10(1):87-100. **Key Finding:** "Some phytochemicals present in fruits and vegetables are protective. Time of intake appears to be important: lifetime protection may be achieved if one is exposed to a dietary factor that lowers breast cancer risk early in life. Synergistic and antisynergistic interactions between dietary factors can modify breast cancer risk. The available evidence suggests that breast cancer risk can be reduced by early dietary intervention."

Combined inhibition of estrogen-dependent human **breast carcinoma** *by soy and tea bioactive components in mice.* Zhou JR, Yu L, Mai Z, Blackburn GL. Int J Cancer. 2004 Jan 1;108(1):8-14. **Key Finding:** "Breast cancer is significantly less prevalent among Asian women, whose diets contain high intake of soy products and tea. The objective of our present study was to identify the combined effects of dietary soy phytochemicals and tea components on breast tumor progression in a clinically relevant in vivo model of MCF-7-androgen-dependent human breast tumor in female SCID mice. Analysis of serum and tumor biomarkers showed that the combined effects of SPC (soy phytochemical concentrate) and GT (green tea) inhibited tumor angiogenesis and reduced estrogen receptor (ER)-alpha and serum levels of insulin-like growth factor. Our study suggests that dietary SPC plus GT may be used as a potential effective dietary regimen for inhibiting progression of estrogen-dependent breast cancer."

Synergistic anti-cancer effects of grape seed extract and conventional cytotoxic agent doxorubicin against human **breast carcinoma** *cells.* Sharma G, Tyagi AK, Singh RP, Chan DC, Agarwal R. Breast Cancer Res Treat. 2004 May;85(1):1-12. **Key Finding:** "We investigated the efficacy of chemotherapy agents against breast cancer treatment, here, we investigated the anti-cancer effects of grape seed extract (GSE) and doxorubicin (Dox), either alone or in combination, in estrogen receptor-positive MCF-7 and receptor-negative MDA-MB468 human breast carcinoma cells. In both MCF-7 and MDA-MB468 cells, a combination of 100 micro g/ml GSE with 25-75 nM Dox treatment for 48 h showed a strong synergistic effect in cell growth inhibition, but mostly an additive effect in cell death."

Catechins and the treatment of **breast cancer**: *possible utility and mechanistic targets.* Rosengren RJ. IDrugs. 2003 Nov;6(11):1073-8. **Key Finding:** In vitro studies have demonstrated that the combination of the catechin epigallocatechin gallate and tamoxifen is synergistically cytotoxic to ERalpha-breast cancer cells. These results suggest that the catechins have significant potential in the treatment of breast cancer.

Combined inhibition of estrogen-dependent human **breast carcinoma** *by soy and tea bioactive components in mice.* Zhou JR, Yu L, Mai Z, Blackburn G. Int J Cancer. 2003;108(1):8-14. **Key Finding:** The combined effects of soy phytochemical concentrate and green tea inhibited tumor angiogenesis and reduced estrogen receptor (ER)-a and serum levels of insulin-like growth factor. This combination is a potential effective dietary regimen for inhibiting the progression of estrogen-dependent breast cancer.

The inhibition of the estrogenic effects of pesticides and environmental chemicals by curcumin and isoflavonoids. Verma SP, Goldin BR, Lin PS. Environ Health Perspect. 1998 Dec;106(12):807-12. **Key Finding:** The inhibitory action of curcumin and a combination of curcumin and isoflavonoids were studied in ER-positive (estrogen receptor-positive) human **breast cancer cells** induced by a pesticide and environmental pollutants. "A combination of curcumin and isoflavonoids was able to inhibit the induced growth of ER-positive cells up to 95%. These data suggest that combinations of natural plant compounds may have preventive and therapeutic applications against the growth of breast tumors induced by environmental estrogens."

Curcumin and genistein, plant natural products, show synergistic inhibitory effects on the growth of human **breast cancer** *MCF-7 cells induced by estrogenic pesticides.* Verma SP, Salamone E, Goldin B. Biochem Biophys Res Commun. 1997 Apr 28;233(3):692-6. **Key Finding:** "When curcumin and genistein were added together to MCF-7 cells, a synergistic effect resulting in a total inhibition of the induction of MCF-7 cells by the highly estrogenic activity of endosulfane/chlordane/DDT mixtures was noted. The inclusion of turmeric and soybeans in the diet to prevent hormone-related cancers deserves consideration."

Cervical

*Concurrent sulforaphane and eugenol induces differential effects on human **cervical cancer** cells.* Hussain A, Priyani A, Sadrieh L, et al. Integr. Cancer Ther. 2011 Mar 7 [epub ahead of print]. **Key Finding**: "Simultaneous treatment with variable dose combinations of sulforaphane and eugenol resulted in differential effects with an antagonistic effect at lower and synergistic at higher sub-lethal doses as reflected in cell cytotoxicity and apoptosis induction. Sulforaphane and eugenol combinations at synergistic dose significantly downregulated the expression of Bci-2, COX-2 and IL-Bbut but not the antagonistic combinations."

*Anti-carcinogenic effects of sulforaphane in association with its apoptosis-inducing and anti-inflammatory properties in human **cervical cancer** cells.* Sharma C, Sadrieh L, Priyani A, et al. Cancer Epidemiol. 2010 Oct 16 [epub ahead of print]. **Key Finding**: "Our results suggest that sulforaphane exerts its anticancer activities via apoptosis induction and anti-inflammatory properties and provides the first evidence demonstrating synergism between sulforaphane and gemcitabine, which may enhance the therapeutic index of prevention and/or treatment of cervical cancer."

Colon

*Curcumin synergizes with resveratrol to inhibit **colon cancer**.* Majumdar AP, Banerjee S, Nautiyal J, et al. Nutr Cancer. 2009;61(4):544-53. **Key Finding:** "Our current data suggest that the combination of curcumin and resveratrol could be an effective preventive/therapeutic strategy for colon cancer. The combination of curcumin and resveratrol was found to be more effective in inhibiting growth of p53-positive (wt) and p53-negative colon cancer HCT-116 cells in vitro and in vivo in SCID xenografts of colon cancer HCT-116 (wt) cells than either agent alone."

*Concomitant supplementation of lycopene and eicosapentaenoic acid inhibits the proliferation of human **colon cancer** cells.* Tang FY, Cho HJ, Pai MH, Chen YH. Nutr Biochem. 2009 Jun;20(6):426-34. **Key Finding**: "Our novel findings suggest that lycopene and EPA synergistically inhibited the growth of human colon cancer HT-29 cells even at low concentrations."

Synergistic effects of a combination of dietary factors sulforaphane and (-) epigal-locatechin-3-gallate in HT-29 AP-1 human **colon carcinoma** *cells.* Nair S, Hebbar V, Shen G, et al. Pharm Res. 2008 Feb;25(2):387-99. **Key Finding:** "The combinations of SFN and EGCG dramatically enhanced transcriptional activation of AP-1 reporter in HT-29 cells. Isobologram analysis showed synergistic activation for the combinations with combination index, CI<1. Taken together, the synergistic activation of AP-1 by the combination of SFN and EGCG that was potentiated by HDAC inhibitors TSA and attenuated by free radical scavenger SOD point to a possible multifactorial control of colon carcinoma that may involve a role for HDACs, inhibition of cellular senescence, and SOD signaling."

Quantitative combination effects between sulforaphane and 3,3'-diindolylmethane on proliferation of human **colon cancer** *cells in vitro.* Pappa G, Strathmann J, Lowinger M, Bartsch H, Gerhauser C. Carcinogenesis. 2007 Jul;28(7):1471-7. **Key Finding:** "Our results indicate that cytotoxic concentrations of SFN/DIM combinations affect cell proliferation synergistically. At low total concentrations (below 20 microM), which are physiologically more relevant, the combined broccoli compounds showed antagonistic interactions in terms of cell growth inhibition. These data stress the need for elucidating mechanistic interactions for better predicting beneficial health effects of bioactive food components."

Combination treatment with curcumin and quercetin of adenomas in familial adenomatous polyposis. Cruz-Correa M, Shoskes DA, Sanchez P. Clin Gastroenterol Hepatol. 2006 Aug; 4(8):1035-8. **Key Finding:** The phytochemical combination of curcumin and quercetin reduced the number of **colon polyps** in test subjects by 60 percent and caused some polyps to shrink.

Extracts from organically and conventionally cultivated strawberries inhibit **cancer** *cell proliferation in vitro.* Olsson ME, Andersson SC, Berglund RH, Gustavsson KE, Oredsson S. Acta Hort. 2007 (ISHS) 744: 189-94. Available at: http://www.actahort.org/books/744/744_19.htm. Accessed on May 19, 2011. **Key Finding:** "The strawberry extracts inhibited cell proliferation in **colon cancer** cells HT29 and **breast cancer** cells MCF-7 in a concentration dependent way. Extracts from organically grown strawberries inhibited cell proliferation to a higher extent than conventionally grown at the two highest concentrations. The content of ascorbate was 36% higher and the ratio of ascorbate to dehydroascorbate were eight-fold higher in the organically grown strawberries than in the conventionally grown. Ascorbate is suggested to act synergistically with other substances in the extracts."

Total cranberry extract versus its phytochemical constituents: antiproliferative and synergistic effects against human **tumor cell** *lines.* Seeram NP, Adams LS, Hardy ML, Heber D. J Agric Food Chem. 2004 May 5;52(9):2512-7. **Key Finding:** "All cranberry fractions were evaluated against human **oral, colon, and prostate cancer** cell lines. The total polyphenol fractions was the most effective against all cell lines with 96.1% and 95% inhibition of KB and CAL27 oral cancer cells, respectively. For the colon cancer cells, the antiproliferative activity of this fraction was greater against HCT116 (92.1%) than against HT-29 (61.1%), SW480 (60%) and SW620 (63%). The enhanced antiproliferative activity of total polyphenols compared to total cranberry extract and its individual phytochemicals suggests synergistic or additive antiproliferative interactions of the anthoycyanins, proanthocyanidins, and flavonol glycosides within the cranberry extract."

In vitro antiproliferative, apoptotic and antioxidant activities of punicalagin, ellagic acid and a total pomegranate tannin extract are enhanced in combination with other polyphenols as found in pomegranate juice. Seeram NP, Adams LS, Henning SM, et al. J Nutr Biochem. 2005 Jun;16(6):360-7. **Key Finding:** "Pomegranate juice showed greatest antiproliferative activity against all **colon cancer** cell lines by inhibiting proliferation from 30% to 100%. The superior bioactivity of pomegranate juice compared to its purified polyphenols illustrated the multifactorial effects and chemical synergy of the action of multiple compounds compared to single purified active ingredients."

Synergistic effect of combination of lysine, proline, arginine, ascorbic acid, and epigallocatechin gallate on **colon cancer** *cell line HCT 116.* Roomi MW, Ivanov V, Kalinovsky T, Niedzwiecki A, Rath M. JANA. 2004;7(2):40-43. **Key Finding:** "Individual nutrients are not as powerful as nutrient synergy. Our previous studies demonstrated that the synergistic anticancer effect of ascorbic acid, proline, lysine and EGCG on several cancer cell lines in tissue culture studies was greater than that of the individual nutrients.

The results of this study suggest the formulation of lysine, proline, arginine, ascorbic acid, and epigallocatechin gallate tested as a valuable and promising candidate for therapeutic use in the treatment of colon cancer, by inhibiting cell proliferation, MMP expression, and invasion."

Some perspectives on dietary inhibition of carcinogenesis: studies with curcumin and tea. Conney AH, Lou YR, Xie JG, et al. Proc Soc Exp Biol Med. 1997 Nov;216(2):234-45. **Key Finding:** "Topical application of curcumin inhibits chemically induced carcinogenesis on mouse skin, and oral administration of curcumin inhibits chemically induced **oral, forestomach, duodenal, and colon carcinogenesis**. Although curcumin alone had little or no effect on cellular differentiation in the human promyelocytic HL-60 **leukemia** cell model system, when it was combined with all-trans retinolic acid or 1alpha,25-dihydroxyvitamin D3 a synergistic effect was observed. It is possible that many dietary chemicals in fruits, vegetables, and other edible plants can prevent cancer by synergizing with endogenously produced stimulators of differentiation."

Fibrosarcoma

In vivo and in vitro antitumor effect of ascorbic acid, lysine, proline, arginine, and green tea extract on human fibrosarcoma cells HT-1080. Roomi W, Ivanov V, Kalinovsky T, Niedzwiecki A. Rath M. Med Oncol. 2006;23(1):105-11. **Key Finding:** "These results offer promise in the therapeutic use of the nutrient mixture of lysine, proline, arginine, ascorbic acid, and green text extract tested in the treatment of **fibrosarcoma** (an aggressive cancer of the connective tissue.)"

Synergistic antitumor effect of ascorbic acid, lysine, proline, and epigallocatechin gallate on human fibrosarcoma cells HT-1080. Roomi W, Ivanov V, Niedzwiecki A, Rath M. Ann Canc Res Ther. 2004. 12(1,2):146-56. **Key Finding:** "Our results suggest that the synergistic effect of lysine, proline, and EGCG, is an effective, yet safe agent for adjunctive therapeutic use in the treatment of **fibrosarcoma,** by inhibiting cell proliferation, MMP expression, and matrigel invasion."

Gastric

Sulforaphane inhibits extracellular, intracellular, and antibiotic-resistant strains of He-licobacter pylori and prevents benzo (a)pyrene-induced stomach tumors. Fahey JW, Haristoys X, Dolan PM, et al. Proc Natl Acad Sci USA. 2002 May 28;99(11):7610-5. **Key Finding:** Sulforaphane isolated from broccoli seeds is bactericidal to both extracellular and intracellular forms of H. pylori by mechanisms that are not yet understood. "The dual proper-ties of sulforaphane as an antibiotic and **anticancer** agent provide a two-tiered, and possibly synergistic approach to eliminating H. pylori and reducing the incidence of **gastric disease**."

Glioma

*Resveratrol and quercetin cooperate to induce senescence-like growth arrest in C6 rat **glioma cells**.* Zamin LL, Filippi-Chiela EC, Dillenburg-Pilla P, et al. Cancer Sci. 2009 Sep;100(9):1655-62. **Key Finding:** "Resveratrol and quercetin chronically administered presented a strong synergism in induc-ing senescence-like growth arrest. These results suggest that the combina-tion of polyphenols can potentialize their **antitumoral** activity, thereby reducing the therapeutic concentration needed for glioma treatment."

Leukemia

*Ellagic acid and quercetin interact synergistically with resveratrol in the induction of apoptosis and cause transient cell cycle arrest in human **leukemia** cells.* Mertens-Talcott SU, Percival SS. Cancer Lett. 2005 Feb 10;218(2):141-51. **Key Finding:** "Results showed a more than additive interaction for the com-bination of ellagic acid with resveratrol and furthermore, significant al-terations in cell cycle kinetics induced by single compounds and combina-tions were observed. Results indicate that the anticarcinogenic potential of foods containing polyphenols may not be based on the effects of in-dividual compounds, but may involve a syngeristic enhancement of the anticancer effects."

*Low concentration of quercetin and ellagic acid synergistically influence proliferation, cytotoxicity and apoptosis in MOLT-4 human **leukemia** cells.* Mertens-Talcott S, Talcott S, Percival S. J Nutr. 2003;133:2669-2674. **Key Finding:** "The interaction of ellagic acid and quercetin, two polyphenolics that are present predominantly in small fruits, demonstrated an enhanced anti-carcinogenic potential of polyphenol combinations, which was not based solely on the additive effect of individual compounds, but rather on synergistic biochemical interactions."

Some perspectives on dietary inhibition of carcinogenesis: studies with curcumin and tea. Conney AH, Lou YR, Xie JG, et al. Proc Soc Exp Biol Med. 1997 Nov;216(2):234-45. **Key Finding:** "Topical application of curcumin inhibits chemically induced carcinogenesis on mouse skin, and oral administration of curcumin inhibits chemically induced **oral, forestomach, duodenal, and colon carcinogenesis**. Although curcumin alone had little or no effect on cellular differentiation in the human promyelocytic HL-60 **leukemia** cell model system, when it was combined with all-trans retinolic acid or 1alpha,25-dihydroxyvitamin D3 a synergistic effect was observed. It is possible that many dietary chemicals in fruits, vegetables, and other edible plants can prevent cancer by synergizing with endogenously produced stimulators of differentiation."

Liver

*Synergistic effects of beta-aescin and 5-fluorouracil in human **hepatocellular carcinoma** SMMC-7721 cells.* Ming ZJ, Hu Y, Qiu YH, Cao L, Zhang XG. Phytomedicine. 2010 Jul;17(8-9):575-80. **Key Finding**: "Mixtures of beta-aescin and 5-FU showed a synergistic effect on the 50% inhibitory effect when their ration was 4:1 when compared with either agent alone. The mechanism of action could be through the synergistic arrest of the cell cycle, induction of apoptosis, activation of caspases-3, 8 and 9, and down-regulation Bci-2 expression. The results suggest that mixtures of these two agents had a synergistic inhibitory effect on SMMC-7721 cells, an observation which might be useful for the further development of anti-cancer drugs."

Melanoma/skin

Synergistic effects of combined phytochemicals and **skin cancer** *prevention in SEN-CAR mice.* Kowalczyk MC, Kowalczyk P, Tolstykh, O, et al.Cancer Prev Res. 2010 Feb;3(2):170-8. **Key Finding**: "All combinations of combined phytochemicals showed either additive or synergistic effects. Especially, resveratrol combinations with ellagic acid, grape seed extract, and other phytochemicals are very potent inhibitors of skin tumorgenesis, based on the suppression of epidermal hyperplasia as well as on the modulation of intermediate biomarkers of cell proliferation, cell survival, inflammation, oncogene mutation, and apoptosis."

Differential effects of several phytochemicals and their derivatives on murine keratinocytes in vitro and in vivo: implications for **skin cancer** *prevention.* Kowalczyk MC, Walaszek Z, Kowalczyk P, et al. Carcinogenesis. 2009 Jun;30(6):1008-15. **Key Finding:** "Differential effects of tested phytochemicals on events and processes critical for the growth inhibition of keratinocytes in vitro and in vivo indicate that combinations of tested compounds may, in the future, better counteract both tumor initiation and tumor promotion/progression."

Suppression of growth and hepatic metastasis of murine B16FO melanoma cells by a novel nutrient mixture. Roomi MW, Kalinovsky T, Roomi NW, et al. Oncol Rep. 2008 Oct;20(4):809-17. **Key Finding:** A nutrient mixture extended the survival time of mice and induced extensive apoptosis in **melanoma** cells at 1000 microg/ml concentration.

In vivo and vitro antitumor effect of ascorbic acid, lysine, proline, and green tea extract on human **melanoma** *cell line A2058.* Roomi MW, Ivanov V, Netke S, In Vivo. 2006 Jan-Feb;20(1):25-32. **Key Finding:** "These results suggest that the nutrient mixture may have a therapeutic potential in melanoma."

Multiple myeloma

Synergistic apoptotic effect of arabinoxylan rice bran (MGN-3/Biobran) and curcumin (turmeric) on human multiple myeloma cell line U266 in vitro. Ghoneum M, Gollapudi S. Neoplasma. 2011;58(2):118-23. **Key Finding**: "We conclude that MGN-3 and curcumin synergize in the induction of U266 cell apoptosis. This data may establish the foundation for in vivo studies that could have therapeutic implications."

Oral

*Total cranberry extract versus its phytochemical constituents: antiproliferative and synergistic effects against human **tumor cell** lines.* Seeram NP, Adams LS, Hardy ML, Heber D. J Agric Food Chem. 2004 May 5;52(9):2512-7. **Key Finding:** "All cranberry fractions were evaluated against human **oral, colon, and prostate cancer** cell lines. The total polyphenol fraction was the most effective against all cell lines with 96.1% and 95% inhibition of KB and CAL27 oral cancer cells, respectively. For the colon cancer cells, the antiproliferative activity of this fraction was greater against HCT116 (92.1%) than against HT-29 (61.1%), SW480 (60%) and SW620 (63%). The enhanced antiproliferative activity of total polyphenols compared to total cranberry extract and its individual phytochemicals suggests synergistic or additive antiproliferative interactions of the anthoycyanins, proanthocyanidins, and flavonol glycosides within the cranberry extract."

Some perspectives on dietary inhibition of carcinogenesis: studies with curcumin and tea. Conney AH, Lou YR, Xie JG, et al. Proc Soc Exp Biol Med. 1997 Nov;216(2):234-45. **Key Finding:** "Topical application of curcumin inhibits chemically induced carcinogenesis on mouse skin, and oral administration of curcumin inhibits chemically induced **oral, forestomach, duodenal, and colon carcinogenesis**. Although curcumin alone had little or no effect on cellular differentiation in the human promyelocytic HL-60 **leukemia** cell model system, when it was combined with all-trans retinolic acid or 1alpha,25-dihydroxyvitamin D3, a synergistic effect was observed. It is possible that many dietary chemicals in fruits, vegetables, and other edible plants can prevent cancer by synergizing with endogenously produced stimulators of differentiation."

*Quantitation of chemopreventive synergism between (-)-epigallocatechin-3-gallate and curcumin in normal, premalignant and malignant human **oral epithelial cells**.* Khafif A, Schantz SP, Chou TC, Edelstein D, Sacks PG. Carcinogenesis. 1998; 19(3):419-24. **Key Finding:** "An in vitro model for oral cancer was used to examine the growth inhibitory effects of chemopreventive agents when used singly and in combination. EGCG from green tea was less effective with cell progression. In contrast, curcumin was equally effective regardless of the cell type tested. The combination of both agents showed synergistic interactions in growth inhibition and increased sigmoidicity (steepness) of the dose-effect curves, a response that was dose and cell type dependent."

Osteosarcoma

*Antitumor effect of nutrient synergy on human **osteosarcoma** cells U-20S, MNNG-HOS and Ewing's sarcoma SK-ES.1.* Roomi MW, Ivanov V, Kalinovsky T, Niedzwiecki A, Rath M. Oncol Rep. 2005 Feb;13(2):253-7. **Key Finding:** "Our results suggest the nutrient mixture containing lysine, proline, arginine, ascorbic acid and epigallocatechin gallate is an excellent candidate for therapeutic use in the treatment of osteosarcoma by inhibiting cancer cell invasion, and secretion of MMPs and VEGF, all critical parameters for cancer control and prevention."

Pancreatic

*Synergistic effects of multiple natural products in **pancreatic cancer** cells.* Wang Z, Desmoulin S, Banerjee S, et al. Life Sci. 2008 Aug 15;83(7-8):293-300. **Key Finding:** "Here we examined whether isoflavone together with curcumin could elicit a greater inhibition of growth of pancreatic cancer cells than either agent alone. We found that the inhibition of cell growth and induction of apoptosis was significantly greater in the combination group than what could be achieved by either agent alone. Moreover, we found that the combination of four natural agents at lower concentration was much more effective. Our results suggest that diets containing multiple natural products should be preferable over single agents for the prevention and/or treatment of pancreatic cancer. The superior effects of the combinatorial treatment could partly be attributed to the inhibition of constitutive activation of Notch-1 and NF-kappaB signaling pathways."

*Antitumor effect of a combination of lysine, proline, arginine, ascorbic acid, and green tea extract on **pancreatic cancer** cell line MIA PaCa-2.* Roomi MW, Ivanov V, Kalinovsky T, Niedzwiecki A, Rath M. Int J Gastrointest Cancer.

2005;35(2):97-102. **Key Finding:** "Our results suggest that the formulation of green tea extract, lysine, proline, and ascorbic acid, tested as a promising adjunct to standard treatment of pancreatic cancer by inhibiting MMP expression and invasion without toxic effects, important parameters in cancer metastasis."

*Inhibitory effects of rosmarinic acid extracts on porcine **pancreatic** amylase in vitro.* McCue PP, Shetty K. Asia Pac J Clin Nutr. 2004;13(1):101-6. **Key Finding:** "The extent of amylase inhibition correlated with increased concentration of rosmarinic acid. RA-containing oregano extracts yielded higher than expected amylase inhibition than similar amount of purified RA, suggesting that other phenolic compounds or phenolic synergies may contribute to additional amylase inhibitory activity. The significance of food-grade, plant-based amylase inhibitors for modulation of diabetes mellitus and other oxidation-linked diseases is hypothesized and discussed."

Prostate

*Genistein-selenium combination induces growth arrest in **prostate cancer** cells.* Kumi-Diaka J, Merchant K, Haces A, Hormann V, Johnson M. J Med Food. 2010 Aug;13(4):842-50. **Key Finding**: "Several in vitro studies together with animal models and epidemiological studies have indicated that phytochemicals can be antitumorigenic and may be protective against human cancers. In this study we investigated the effects of genistein-selenium combination on prostate cancer cells. This combination induced significant growth inhibition in both MMP-2 and LNCaP cell lines. The data obtained from the present study indicate that Gn-Se combination may have chemopreventive value for prostate tumors independent of hormonal status."

*Synergistic chemoprotective mechanisms of dietary phytoestrogens in a select combination against **prostate cancer**.* Kumar R, Verma V, Jain A, Jain RK. J Nutr Biochem. 2010 Nov 8. [epub ahead of print] **Key Finding:** "Our findings suggest that selectively combining anticancer phytoestrogens could significantly increase the efficacy of individual components resulting in improved efficacy at physiologically achievable concentrations. The combination mechanism of multiple anticancer phytochemicals may be indicative of the potential of some vegetarian diet components to elicit chemopreventive effects against prostate cancer at their physiologically achievable concentrations in vivo."

Targeting CWR22Rv1 **prostate cancer** *cell proliferation and gene expression by combinations of the phytochemicals EGCG, genistein and quercetin.* Hsieh TC, Wu JM. Anticancer Res. 2009 Oct;29(10):4025-32. **Key Finding**: "These results demonstrate the feasibility of developing a diet-based combinatorial approach for prostate cancer prevention and treatment and raises the possibility that serum added to culture medium might affect uptake, bioavailability and biological efficacy of dietary phytochemicals."

Genistein and resveratrol, alone and in combination, suppress **prostate cancer** *in SV-40 tag rats.* Harper CE, Cook LM, Patel BB, et al. Prostate. 2009 Nov 1;69(15):1668-82. **Key Finding:** "Genistein and resveratrol, alone and in combination, suppress prostate cancer development in the SV-40 Tag (rat) model. Regulation of SRC-3 and growth factor signaling proteins are consistent with these nutritional polyphenols reducing cell proliferation and increasing apoptosis in the prostate."

Murine **prostate cancer** *inhibition by dietary phytochemicals – curcumin and phenyethylisothiocyanate.* Barve A, Khor TO, Hay X, et al. Pharm Res. 2008 Sept;25(9):2181-9. **Key Finding:** "Our data lucidly evidence the chemopreventive merits of dietary phytochemicals curcumin and PEITC in suppressing prostate adenocarcinoma."

Interaction of tomato lycopene and ketosamine against rat **prostate tumorigenesis**. Mossine VV, Chopra P, Mawhinney TP. Cancer Res. 2008 Jun 1;68(11):4384-91. **Key Finding**: "We investigated whether ketosamines, a group of carbohydrate derivatives present in dehydrated tomato products, may interact with lycopene against prostate tumorigenesis. One ketomsamine, FruHis, strongly synergized with lycopene against proliferation of the highly metastatic rat prostate adenocarcinoma MAT-LyLu cell line in vitro. The FruHis/lycopene combination significantly inhibited in vivo tumor formation by MAT-LyLu cells in syngeneic Copenhagen rats. FruHis, therefore, may exert tumor preventive effect through its antioxidant activity and interaction with lycopene."

Combinations of tomato and broccoli enhance **antitumor** *activity in dunning r3327-h* **prostate** *adenocarcinomas.* Canene-Adams K, Lindshield BL, Wang S, et al. Cancer Res. 2007 Jan 15;67(2):836-43. **Key Finding:** "The combination of tomato and broccoli was more effective at slowing tumor growth than either tomato or broccoli alone and supports the public health recommendations to increase the intake of a variety of plant components."

Compounds from Wedelia chinensis synergistically suppress androgen activity and growth in **prostate cancer** *cells.* Lin FM, Chen LR, Lin Eh, et al. Carcinogenesis. 2007: 28(12):2521-29. **Key Finding:** Chronic inflammation can augment tumor development in various types of cancers, including prostate cancer. Four anti-proliferative phytocompounds—indole-3-carboxylaldehyde, wedelolactone, luteolin and apigenin—in Wedelia chinensis, an oriental herbal medicine, were tested. These active compounds specifically inhibited the growth of AR-dependent PCa cells and as a combination formula they also synergistically suppressed growth in AR-dependent PCa cells.

Combined lycopene and vitamin E treatment suppresses the growth of PC-346C **prostate cancer** *cells in nude mice.* Limpens J, Schroder FH, De Ridder CM, et al. J Nutr. 2006 May;136(5):1287-93. **Key Finding:** "Our data provide evidence that lycopene combined with vitamin E may inhibit the growth of prostate cancer and that PSA can serve as a biomarker of tumor response for this treatment regimen."

Inhibition of EGFR signaling in human **prostate cancer** *PC-3 cells by combination treatment with beta-phenylethyl isothiocyanate and curcumin.* Kim JH, Xu C, Keum YS, et al. Carcinogenesis. 2006 Mar;27(3): 475-82. **Key Finding:** "We conclude that the simultaneous targeting of EGFR, AKt and Nf-Kappab signaling pathways by PEITC and curcumin could be the molecular targets by which PEITC and curcumin exert their additive inhibitory effects on cell proliferation and ultimately lead to programmed cell death of tumor cells."

Combined inhibitory effects of curcumin and phenethyl isothiocyanate on the growth of human PC-3 **prostate xenografts** *in immunodeficient mice.* Khor TO, Keum YS, Lin W, et al.Cancer Res. 2006 Jan 15;66(2):613-21. **Key Finding:** "Our results show that PEITC and curcumin alone or in combination possess significant cancer-preventive activities in the PC-3 prostate tumor xenografts. Furthermore, we found that combination of PEITC and curcumin could be effective in the cancer-therapeutic treatment of prostate cancers."

*Inhibition of **prostate cancer** cell growth by an avocado extract: role of lipid-soluble bioactive substances.* Lu OY, Arteaga JR, Zhang Q, et al. J Nutr Biochem. 2005 Jan;16(1):23-30. **Key Finding:** "An acetone extract of avocado containing these carotenoids (zeaxanthin, alpha-carotene and beta carotene) and tocopherols was shown to inhibit the growth of both androgen-dependent and androgen-independent prostate cancer cell lines in vitro. Because the avocado also contains a significant amount of mono-saturated fat, these bioactive carotenoids are likely to be absorbed into the bloodstream, where in combination with other diet-derived phytochemicals they may contribute to the significant cancer risk reduction."

Anti-tumor effect of ascorbic acid, lysine, proline, arginine, and epigallocatechin gallate on prostate cancer cell lines PC-3, LNaP, and DU145. Roomi MW, Ivanov V, Kalinovsky T, Niedzwiecki A, Rath M. Res Commun Mol Pathol Pharmacol. 2004;115-116:251-64. **Key Finding:** "Inhibition of MMP expression and invasion suggests the mixture of nutrients studied is a potent, natural anticancer agent for the treatment of **prostate cancer**."

*Potential mechanism of phytochemical-induced apoptosis in human **prostate adenocarcinoma** cells: therapeutic synergy in genistein and B-lapachone combination treatment.* Kumi-Diaka J. Saddler-Shawnette S. Aller A. Brown J. Cancer Cell Int. 2004 Aug 17;4(1):5. **Key Finding:** "The demonstrated synergism between genistein and bLap justifies consideration of these phytochemicals in chemotherapeutic strategic planning."

*Total cranberry extract versus its phytochemical constituents: antiproliferative and synergistic effects against human **tumor cell** lines.* Seeram NP, Adams LS, Hardy ML, Heber D. J Agric Food Chem. 2004 May 5;52(9):2512-7. **Key Finding:** "All cranberry fractions were evaluated against human **oral, colon, and prostate cancer** cell lines. The total polyphenol fraction was the most effective against all cell lines with 96.1% and 95% inhibition of KB and CAL27 oral cancer cells, respectively. For the colon cancer cells, the antiproliferative activity of this fraction was greater against HCT116 (92.1%) than against HT-29 (61.1%), SW480 (60%) and SW620 (63%). The enhanced antiproliferative activity of total polyphenols compared to total cranberry extract and its individual phytochemicals suggests synergistic or additive antiproliferative interactions of the anthoycyanins, proanthocyanidins, and flavonol glycosides within the cranberry extract."

Soy phytochemicals and tea bioactive components synergistically inhibit androgensensitive human **prostate tumor** *in mice.* Zhou JR, Yu L, Zhong Y, Blackburn G. J Nutr. 2003 Feb;133(2):516-21. **Key Finding:** The combination of soy phytochemical concentrate and green tea synergistically inhibited final tumor weight and metastasis and significantly reduced serum concentrations of both testosterone and DHT in vivo.

Tomatoes, lycopene, and **prostate cancer:** *progress and promise.* Hadley CW, Miller EC, Schwartz SJ, Clinton SK. Exp Biol Med. 2002 Nov;227(10):869-80. **Key Finding:** "In contrast to the pharmacologic approach with pure lycopene, many nutritional scientists direct their attention upon the diverse array of tomato products as a complex mixture of biologically active phytochemicals that together may have anti-prostate cancer benefits beyond those of any single constitutent."

Synergistic effects of thearubigin and genistein on human **prostate tumor** *cell (PC-3) growth via cell cycle arrest.* Sakamoto K. Cancer Lett. 2000 Apr 3;151(1):103-9. **Key Finding:** "There is evidence that habitual consumption of green tea by Japanese men is correlated with a reduction in cancers, including prostate; soybean isoflavones are also associated with increased protection. The present study compared the anti-proliferative effect of black tea polyphenol, thearubigin, alone or combined, with the isoflavone genistein, on human prostate PC-3 carcinoma cells. Thearubigin administered alone did not result in any alteration of cell growth. When combined with genistein, however, it significantly inhibited cell growth and induced a G2/M phase cell cycle arrest in a dose dependent manner. These findings indicate the potential use of combined phytochemicals to provide protection against prostate cancer."

Renal

Anticancer effect of lysine, proline, arginine, ascorbic acid and green tea extract on human renal adenocarcinoma line 786-0. Roomi MW, Ivanov V, Kalinovsky T, Niedzwiecki A, Rath M. Oncol Rep. 2006 Nov;16(5):943-7. **Key Finding:** "Our results support a potential role for the nutrient mixture tested in the treatment of **renal cell carcinoma**, by inhibition of MMP-2 and MMP-9 secretion and invasion."

Testicular

*Inhibitory effects of a nutrient mixture on human **testicular cancer** cell line NT 2/DT matrigel invasion and MMP activity.* Roomi MW, Ivanov V, Kalinovsky T, Niedzwiecki A, Rath M. Med Oncol. 2007;24(2):193-8. **Key Finding:** A nutrient mixture containing lysine, proline, arginine, ascorbic acid, and green tea extract significantly inhibited MMP secretion and matrix invasion in testicular cancer cells without toxic effect, indicating potential as an anticancer agent.

Candida

Synergistic antiyeast activity of garlic oil and allyl alcohol derived from alliin in garlic. Chung I, Kwon SH, Shim ST, Kyung KH. J Food Sci. 2007 Nov;72(9):M437-40. **Key Finding:** "Combinations of AA and GO at 1 and 9 ppm, 5 and 5 ppm, and 6 and 3 ppm, respectively, inhibited *C. utilis* **(Candida)** completely. The sum of the fractional inhibitory concentrations (FICs) in the 2-component (GO and AA) combination was as low as 0.37 for *C. utilis*, indicating strong synergism."

Cardioprotection

Co-ordinated autophagy with resveratrol and y-tocotrienol confers synergetic cardioprotection. Lekli I, Ray D, Mukherjee S, et al. J Cell Mol Med. 2010 Oct;14(10):2506-18. **Key Finding:** "This study compared two dietary phytochemicals, grape-derived resveratrol and palm oil-derived y-tocotrienol, either alone or in combination, on the contribution of autophagy in cardioprotection during ischaemia and reperfusion. Reservatrol and y-tocotrienol acted synergistically, providing [a] greater degree of cardioprotection [while] simultaneously generating [a] greater amount of survival signal through the activation of Akt-Bcl-2 survival pathway."

Cardiovascular disease

*Co-ordinated autophagy with resveratrol and y-tocotrienol confers a synergetic **cardioprotection***. Lekli I, Ray D, Mukherjee S, et al. J Cell Mol Med. 2010 Oct;14(10):2506-18. **Key Finding:** "Palm oil-derived gamma-tocotrienol and resveratrol from grapes acted synergistically, providing [a] greater degree of cardioprotection [while] simultaneously generating [a] greater amount of survival signal through the activation of Akt-Bcl-2 survival pathway. It is tempting to speculate that during ischemia and reperfusion autophagy along with enhanced survival signals helps to recover the (rat heart) cells from injury."

Cranberries inhibit LDL oxidation and induce LDL receptor expression in hepatocytes. Chu YF, Liu RH. Life Sci. 2005 Aug 26;77(15):1892-1901. **Key Finding:** "Cranberries were evaluated for their potential roles in dietary prevention of **cardiovascular disease**. Cranberry extracts were found to have potent antioxidant capacity preventing in vitro LDL oxidation with increasing delay and suppression of LDL oxidation in a dose dependent manner. We propose that additive or synergistic effects of phytochemicals in cranberries are responsible for the inhibition of LDL oxidation, the induced expression of LDL receptors, and the increased uptake of cholesterol in hepatocytes."

Cataracts

Dietary carotenoids, vitamins C and E, and risk of cataract in women: a prospective study. Christen WG, Liu S, Glynn RJ, Gaziano JM, Buring JE. Arch Ophthalmol. 2008 Nov;126(11):1606-7. **Key Finding:** "In these prospective observational data from a large cohort of female health professionals, higher dietary intakes of lutein/zeaxanthin and vitamin E from food and supplements were associated with significantly decreased risks of **cataracts**."

Cholesterol

Avenanthramides and phenolic acids from oats are bioavailable and act synergistically with vitamin C to enhance hamster and human LDL resistance to oxidation. Chen CY, Milbury P, Kwak HK, et al. J Nutri. 2004; 134:1459-66. **Key Finding:** "Combining the oat phenolics with 5 umol/L ascorbic acid extended the lag time in a synergistic fashion. Thus, oat phenolics, including avenanthramides, are bioavailable in hamsters and interact synergistically with vitamin C to protect **LDL** during oxidation."

Synergistic inhibition of low-density lipoprotein oxidation by rutin, y-terpinene, and ascorbic acid. Mildea J, Elstnera EP, Grabmann J. Phytomedicine. 2004;11(2):105-13. **Key Finding:** "Low-density lipoprotein LDL oxidation may play a significant role in **atherogenesis**. We investigated the combination of rutin with a hydrophilic (ascorbate) and a lipophilic antioxidant (y-terpinene) in copper-mediate LDL oxidation. In both cases we found a synergistic effect on lag phase prolongation."

Soy and alfalfa phytoestrogen extracts become potent low-density lipoprotein antioxidants in the presence of acerola cherry extract. Hwang J, Hodis HN, Sevanian A. J Agric Food Chem. 2001;49(1):308-14. **Key Finding:** Antioxidant activity of phytoestrogen extracts from soy and alfalfa was enhanced by the presence of acerola cherry extract, which is rich in ascorbic acid. "This synergy is complemented by a mechanism in which phytoestrogens stabilize the LDL, structure and suppress the propagation of radical chain reactions. The combination of these extracts markedly lowers the concentrations of phytoestrogens required to achieve significant antioxidant activity toward **LDL**."

Colitis

*Suppression of dextran sodium sulfate-induced **colitis** in mice by zerumbone, a subtropical ginger sesquiterpene, and nimesulide, separately and in combination.* Murakami A, Hayashi R, Tanaka T, et al. Biochem Pharmacol. 2003 Oct 1;66(7):1253-61. **Key Finding:** "Ulcerative colitis and Crohn's disease are inflammatory disorders of unknown cause and difficult to treat. The present study was undertaken to explore the suppressive efficacy of zerumbone, a sesquiterpenoid used as a condiment in Southeast Asian countries. Our results suggest that zerumbone is a novel food factor for mitigating experimental ulcerative colitis and that use of a combination of agents, with different modes of action, may be an effective anti-inflammatory strategy."

Coronary artery disease

Grape seed and grape skin extracts elicit a greater antiplatelet effect when used in combination than when used individually in dogs and humans. Shanmuganayagam D, Beahm MR, Osman HE, et al. J Nutr. 2002 Dec;132(12):3592-8. **Key Finding:** Grape products, rich in polyphenolics, inhibit platelet aggregation, a risk factor for **coronary artery disease**. The components when present in combination exhibit a greater antiplatelet effect than when present individually.

Diabetes

Effect of genistein with carnitine administration on lipid parameters and obesity in C57Bl/6J mice fed a high-fat diet. Yang JY, Lee SJ, Park HW, Cha YS. J Med Food. 2006;9(4):459-67. **Key Finding:** "We investigated the effect of dietary genistein (the principal soy isoflavone) alone and combined with L-carnitine to evaluate possible synergistic effects on the intentionally induced **prediabetic** state characterized by insulin resistance and obesity. Especially in liver, the results showed that genistein with carnitine transcriptionally up-regulated expressions of acyl-coenzyme A synthetase (ACS) and carnitine palmitoyltransferase-I (CPT-I) by approximately 50% and 40%, respectively, compared with genistein alone."

*Potential of cranberry-based herbal synergies for **diabetes** and **hypertension** management.* Apostolidis E, Kwon YI, Shetty K. Asia Pac J Clin Nutr. 2006;15(3):433-41. **Key Finding:** "Water soluble cranberry-based phytochemical combinations with oregano, rosemary, and Rhodiola rosea were evaluated for total phenolic content, related antioxidant activity and inhibition of diabetes management-related alpha-glucosidase, pancreatic alpha-amylase inhibition, and hypertension-related ACE-I inhibitory activities. The 75% cranberry and 25% oregano combinations had the highest penolics among all combinations tested; that same combination also had the highest DPPH radical inhibition activity, and the highest ACE-I inhibitory activity. By bringing together synergistic combinations to cranberry, health beneficial functionality was enhanced. This enhanced functionality in terms of high alpha-glucosidase and alpha-amylase inhibitory activities indicate the potential for diabetes management, and high ACE-I inhibitory activity indicates the potential for hyptension management."

Potential of cranberry-based phytochemical synergies for **diabetes** *and* **hypertension** *management.* Kwon YI, Lin YT, Shetty K. Department of Food Science, University of Massachusetts. Available at http://ift.confex.com/direct/ift/2005/techprogram/paper_29028.htm. Accessed on May 20, 2011. **Key Finding:** "There is a synergistic inhibitory effect of various phytochemical combinations on above enzyme activities. These findings indicate that cranberry-based phytochemical synergies have potential as functional ingredients in the dietary management of diabetes and hypertension."

Health benefits (in general)

Food synergy—an operational concept for understanding nutrition. Jacobs DR Jr., Gross MD, Tapsell LC. Am J Clin Nutr. 2009 May; 89(5):1543-48S. **Key Finding**: "The evidence for health benefit appears stronger when put together in a synergistic dietary pattern than for individual foods or food constituents…Many examples are provided of superior effects of whole foods over their isolated constituents."

Bioactivity of grape chemicals for human health. Iriti M, Faoro F, Nat Prod Commun. 2009 May;4(5):611-34. **Key Finding:** "The health benefits arising from grape product intake can be ascribed to the potpourri of biologically active chemicals occurring in grapes. Among them, the recently discovered presence of melatonin adds a new element to the already complex grape chemistry. Melatonin, and its possible synergistic action with the great variety of polyphenols, contributes to further explaining the observed health benefits associated with regular grape product consumption."

Diet synergies and mortality—a population-based case-control study of 32,462 Hong Kong Chinese older adults. Schooling CM, Ho SY, Leung GM, et al. Int J

Epidemiol. 2006;35(2):418-26. **Key Finding:** "There was a significant trend of increasing all-cause mortality risk with decreasing healthy food consumption. Intake of some dietary items may modify the effect of others. An analysis framework explicitly recognizing complementary and potentially synergistic effects of food, drinks, and smoking could enhance our understanding of dietary epidemiology."

Nutraceuticals synergistically promote proliferation of human stem cells. Bickford PC, Tan J, Shytle RD, et al. Stem Cells Dev. 2006 Feb;15(1):118-23. **Key Finding:** "We report here the effects of several natural compounds on the proliferation of human bone marrow and human CD34(+) and CD133(+) cells. A dose-related effect of blueberry, green tea, catechin, carnosine and vitamin D(3) was observed on proliferation with human bone marrow. We further show that combinations of nutrients produce a synergistic effect to promote proliferation of human hematopoietic progenitors. This demonstrates that nutrients can act to promote **healing** via an interaction with stem cell populations."

Mediterranean diet health benefits may be due to a synergistic combination of phytochemicals and fatty-acids. Fortes C, Forastiere F, Farchi S, Mailone S. BMJ. 2005 July 9;331:E366. **Key Finding:** Two different epidemiological studies of the Mediterranean diet found the health benefits came from a combination of high intake of fruits and vegetables, the use of olive oil, the use of fresh aromatic herbs such as sage and rosemary, and the intake of omega-3 fatty acids.

Health benefits of fruit and vegetables are from additive and synergistic combinations of phytochemicals. Liu RH. Am J Clin Nutr. 2003 Sep;78(3 Suppl): 517-20S. **Key Finding:** "We propose that the additive and synergistic effects of phytochemicals in fruit and vegetables are responsible for their potent antioxidant and anticancer activities, and that the benefit of a diet rich in fruit and vegetables is attributed to the complex mixture of phytochemicals present in whole foods."

Nutrients, foods, and dietary patterns as exposures in research: a framework for food synergy. Jacobs D, Steffen LM. Am J Clin Nutr. 2003 Sep;78(3):508-13S. **Key Finding:** Foods and food patterns act synergistically to influence the risk of several chronic diseases. Benefit accrues when all edible parts of the plant are included. Phytochemicals located in the fiber matrix, in addition to or instead of the fiber itself, are responsible for the reduced risk of diseases.

Carotenoids in staple foods: their potential to improve human nutrition. Graham R, Rosser J. Food Nutr Bull. 2000;21(4): 404-9. **Key Finding:** Among three micronutrients–iron, zinc and carotenoids—there are important synergies in absorption, transport, and function that strongly indicate substantial benefits to enhancing all three nutrients together.

HIV infection

*Anti-stress, anti-**HIV** and vitamin C-synergized radical scavenging activity of mulberry juice fractions.* Sakagami H, Asano K, Satoh K, et al. In Vivo. 2007 May-Jun;21(3):499-505. **Key Finding:** "Anti-stress and anti-HIV activity of mulberry juice were separated by centrifugation. The kinetic study revealed that the anti-stress activity was maintained for 4 hours after cessation of the administration of mulberry juice. The lignin fraction in the precipitate fraction scavenged superoxide and hydroxyl radicals more efficiently than other fractions, in a synergistic fashion with sodium ascorbate. Anti-HIV activity of mulberry juice was concentrated in the lignin fraction, whereas blueberry juice, which has no precipitating fibrous materials, did not show anti-HIV activity. The present study suggests the functionality of mulberry juice as an alternative medicine."

Hypercholesterolemia

*Assessment of the longer-term effects of a dietary portfolio of cholesterol-lowering foods in **hypercholesterolemia**.* Jenkins DJ, Kendall CW, Faulkner DA, et al. Am J Clin Nutr. 2006 Mar;83(3):582-91. **Key Finding:** "Cholesterol-lowering foods may be more effective when consumed as combinations rather than as single foods. Our aims were to determine the effectiveness of consuming a combination of cholesterol-lowering foods (plant sterols, viscous fibers, almonds) under real-world conditions and compare the results to the effects of a statin. More than 30% of motivated participants who ate the dietary portfolio of cholesterol-lowering foods were able to lower LDL-cholesterol concentrations >20%, which was not significantly different from their response to a first-generation statin."

Hypertension

*Potential of cranberry-based herbal synergies for **diabetes** and **hypertension** management.* Apostolidis E, Kwon YI, Shetty K. Asia Pac J Clin Nutr. 2006;15(3):433-41. **Key Finding:** "Water soluble cranberry-based phytochemical combinations with oregano, rosemary, and Rhodiola rosea were evaluated for total phenolic content, related antioxidant activity and inhibition of diabetes management-related alpha-glucosidase, pancreatic alpha-amylase inhibition, and hypertension-related ACE-I inhibitory activities. The 75% cranberry and 25% oregano combinations had the highest penolics among all combinations tested; that same combination also had the highest DPPH radical inhibition activity, and the highest ACE-I inhibitory activity. By bringing together synergistic combinations to cranberry, health-beneficial functionality was enhanced. This enhanced functionality in terms of high alpha-glucosidase and alpha-amylase inhibitory activities indicate the potential for diabetes management, and high ACE-I inhibitory activity indicates the potential for hypertension management."

*Potential of cranberry-based phytochemical synergies for **diabetes** and **hypertension** management.* Kwon YI, Lin YT, Shetty K. Department of Food Science, University of Massachusetts. Available at http://ift.confex.com/direct/ift/2005/techprogram/paper_29028.htm. Accessed on May 20, 2011. **Key Finding:** "There is a synergistic inhibitory effect of various phytochemical combinations on above enzyme activities. These findings indicate that cranberry-based phytochemical synergies have potential as functional ingredients in the dietary management of diabetes and hypertension."

Hypoglycemia

*Synergistic effect of phytochemicals in combination with **hypoglycemic** drugs on glucose uptake in myotubes.* Prabhakar PK, Doble M. Phytomedicine. 2009 Dec;16(12):1119-26. **Key Finding:** "The present study analyzes the effect of two plant phenolic compounds, chlorogenic acid and ferulic acid, in combination with two commercial oral phyotglycemic drugs. A combination of different concentrations of chlorogenic acid and metformin or THZ, has a synergistic effect in the uptake of 2DG with a maximum of 5.0 and 5.3-time respectively, with reference to the base value (without the drugs or the natural products.) Ferulic acid in combination with metformin has also shown a synergistic effect and the 2DG uptake increases by 4.98 and 5.11-fold when compared to the control respectively. The current findings suggest that the phytochemicals can replace the commercial drugs in part, which could lead to a reduction in toxicity and side effects of the latter."

Inflammation

Synergistic effect of combination of phenethyl isothiocyanate and sulforaphane or curcumin and sulforaphane in the inhibition of **inflammation***.* Cheung KL, Khor TO, Kong AN. Pharm Res. 2009 Jan;26(1):224-31. **Key Finding:** "Our data suggest that CUR (curcumin) **+** SFN (sulforaphane) and PEITC (phenethyl isothiocyanate) **+** SFN combinations could be more effective than used alone in preventing inflammation and possibly its associated diseases including cancer."

Synergistic effect of Kalpaamruthaa on antiarthritic and anti-inflammatory properties—its mechanism of action. Mythilypriya R, Shanthi P, Sachdanandam P. Inflammation. 2008 Dec;31(6):391-8. **Key Finding:** The nut milk extract combined with honey and Emblica officinalis, Kalpaamruthaa (KA), "exhibited enhanced effect on **anti-inflammatory** and **anti-arthritic** properties than sole nut milk extract treatment, and the collective effect might be due to the combined interactions of the phytochemicals such as flavonoids, tannins, and other compounds such as vitamin C present in KA."

Grape seed and skin extracts inhibit platelet function and release of reactive oxygen intermediates. Vitseva O, Varghese S, Chakrabarti S, Folts JD, Freedman JE. J Cardiovasc Pharmacol. 2005 Oct;46(4):445-51. **Key Finding:** "coincubation with seeds and skins led to additive inhibition of platelet aggregation, enhanced NO release, and prevented superoxide production. Thus, the extracts from purple grape skins and seeds inhibit platelet function and platelet-dependent **inflammatory** responses at pharmacologically relevant concentrations."

*Hydrolyzed olive vegetation water in mice has **anti-inflammatory** activity.* Bitler CM, Viale TM, Damaj B, Crea R. J. Nutr. 2005 June;135:1475-79. **Key Finding:** Olive vegetation water when combined with glucosamine "acted synergistically to reduce serum TNF levels in LPS-treated mice," which means this combination "may be an effective therapy for a variety of inflammatory processes, including **rheumatoid** and **osteoarthritis**."

Liver damage

Protective effects of garlic and silymarin on NDEA-induced rats hepatoxicity. Shaarawy SM, Tohamy AA, Elgendy SM, et al. Int J Biol Sci. 2009 Aug 11;5(6):549-57. **Key Finding:** "These novel findings suggest that silymarin and garlic have a synergistic effect, and could be used as hepatoprotective agents against **hepatotoxicity** (chemical-driven liver damage)."

Osteoarthritis

Synergistic chondroprotective effects of curcumin and resveratrol in human articular chondrocytes: inhibition of IL-1beta-induced NF-kappaB-mediated inflammation and apoptosis. Csaki C, Mobasheri A, Shakibaei M. Arthritis Res Ther. 2009 Nov 4;11(6):R165. **Key Finding:** "Currently available treatments for **osteoarthritis** are restricted to nonsteroidal anti-inflammatory drugs, which exhibit numerous side effects and are only temporarily effective. Naturally occurring polyphenolic compounds, such as curcumin and resveratrol, are potent agents for modulating inflammation. The aim of this study was to investigate the potential synergistic effects of curcumin and resveratrol on IL-1beta-stimulated human chondrocytes in vitro. Treatment with curcumin and resveratrol suppressed NF-kappaB-regulated gene products involved in inflammation. We propose that combining these natural compounds may be a useful strategy in osteoarthritis therapy as compared with separate treatment with each individual compound."

*Hydrolyzed olive vegetation water in mice has **anti-inflammatory** activity.* Bitler CM, Viale TM, Damaj B, Crea R. J Nutr. 2005 June;135:1475-79. **Key**

Finding: Olive vegetation water when combined with glucosamine "acted synergistically to reduce serum TNF levels in LPS-treated mice," which means this combination "may be an effective therapy for a variety of inflammatory processes, including **rheumatoid** and **osteoarthritis**."

Prostate health

*Role of lycopene and tomato products in **prostate** health.* Stacewicz-Sapuntzakis M, Bowen PE. Biochem Biophys Acta. 2005 May 30;1740(2):202-5. **Key Finding:** "We conducted a small intervention trial among patients diagnosed with prostate adenocarcinoma. Tomato sauce pasta was consumed daily for 3 weeks. Oxidative DNA damage in leukocytes and prostate tissues was significantly diminished, the latter mainly in the tumor cell nuclei, possibly due to the antioxidant properties of lycopene. Quite surprising was the decrease in blood prostate-specific antigen, which was explained by the increase in apoptotic death of prostate cells, especially in carcinoma regions. Other phytochemicals in tomato may act in synergy with lycopene to potentiate protective effects and to help in the maintenance of prostate health."

Ulcers

Inhibition of Helicobacter pylori and associated urease by oregano and cranberry phytochemical synergies. Lin YT, Kwon YI., Labbe RG, Shetty K. Appl Environ Microbiol. Dec 2005;71(12):8558-64. **Key Finding:** "The results indicated that the antimicrobial activity was greater in extract mixtures than in individual extracts of each species. The results also indicate that the synergistic contribution of oregano and cranberry phenolics may be more important for inhibition than any species-specific phenolic concentration." (H. pylori is linked to a majority of **peptic ulcers**.)

CHAPTER THREE

The Effects of Caloric Restriction and Intermittent Fasting on Human Health and Lifespan

SOME YEARS AGO, A SWISS PUBLISHER approached me to write a book on longevity. As I began my research on the central cause for long life, it became evident that nutrition and the way we utilize it was fundamental.

For most of the time people have walked the earth, we were nomadic, moving from place to place following the food sources. This put us in a position where we would not only eat simply, but also rarely. This is how the human anatomy was designed and how it operated until recent generations.

Today, we consumers confront a format placed before us of breakfast, lunch, and dinner, mostly relying on processed foods. Additionally we are told that if we do not consistently consume, we will be malnourished, which is ironic since most "food choices" have little to do with true nutrition.

Cornell University scientists made the initial discovery in 1935 that a very low-calorie diet could extend the lives of rats by 33 percent and bestow other health benefits. Since then, other researchers have documented how caloric restriction slows the aging process in a wide range of life forms. In 2009, after a two-decade-long experiment with rhesus monkeys, University of Wisconsin researchers concluded that monkeys who had eaten a third fewer calories than a control group of monkeys aged more slowly and had a lower incidence of cancer, cardiovascular disease, and muscle and brain deterioration.

For the hundreds of thousands of people who have attended the Hippocrates Health Institute, a minimum of a one-day fast per week has been a core principle of our program. We have documented many health benefits, including this example from the realm of obesity and eating disorders.

Arnie Weintraub weighed more than 320 pounds in the three years before he changed his diet. He worked as the food services director for a community hospital. When I met him, Arnie described himself this way: "My body was a mess. I suffered an array of ailments from arthritis, bursitis, sleep apnea, heal spurs and bad knees. I was also pre-diabetic, had high blood pressure, allergies and constant headaches."

Arnie began a raw organic diet for health reasons. The caloric restriction of periodic 24-hour fasting combined with nutrient-dense vegan food paid off. He experienced the benefits almost immediately. "The weight began to drop off quickly. I lost about 25 pounds a month for the first four months. The program didn't even focus on weight. It focused on health. The rest of the weight continued to melt away over the next six months until I had lost 175 pounds. Today, I'm a much happier and healthier person."

Here's another example:

At the age of 42, Fiona Burns was diagnosed with ovarian cancer. This native of Britain came to us and shared the circumstances of her condition: "My oncologist told me I needed to have a full hysterectomy and have my appendix and omentum removed, and follow up with chemo and radiotherapy. He said that if I followed his recommendations, I had a 20 to 30 percent chance of being alive in five years and a 10 percent chance of being alive in ten-years' time."

Further blood testing revealed that Fiona had a cervical adenocarcinoma, a tumor on her cervix, that had metastasized to her ovaries. Her stomach swelled up, making her look pregnant, and fluid began to fill her lungs, making breathing difficult. Facing a dire prognosis, she decided to walk away from orthodox medicine and try alternative therapies. "I am not going to be ill for a long time," she told herself and others. "Either I am going to get better fast, or I will die."

Fiona's journey back to health is a complicated one, involving experimentation with combinations of herbs and positive thinking. But a key component for her was raw food, sprouts, and periodic fasting. Subsequently after adopting this regimen, each scan and blood test showed a shrinkage in the tumors until the cervical adenocarcinoma completely disappeared nine months after it was first diagnosed. "As for my ovaries," Fiona relates, "there is some scarring, but I no longer have any cancer in my body. I have my energy and my lust for life back and I actually feel as good now as I did when I was in my 20s. Nobody can believe that I am 43-years old."

Arnie's and Fiona's experiences are typical of the case studies we have chronicled. We believe that one-fifth to one-quarter of your biological health is attained by the absence of food, not its ingestion. Every legitimate study focusing on this scientific premise has shown the same results: People who consume small amounts of high-quality food, which generally contain lower amounts of calories, suffer less disease and experience longer life spans.

From the following medical studies you will find more evidence for this profound truth.

Aging

Caloric restriction: from soup to nuts. Spindler SR. Ageing Res Rev. 2010 Jul;9(3):324-53. **Key Finding**: "Caloric restriction, reduced protein, methionine, or tryptophan diets, and reduced insulin and/or IGFI intracellular signaling can extend mean and/or **maximum lifespan** and delay deleterious age-related physiological changes in animals. Many health benefits are induced by even brief periods of caloric restriction. In primates, caloric restriction provides protection from type 2 diabetes, cardiovascular and cerebral vascular diseases, immunological decline, malignancy, hepatotoxicity, liver fibrosis and failure, sarcopenia, inflammation, and DNA damages. It also enhances muscle mitochrondrial biogenesis, affords neuroprotection, and extends mean and maximum lifespan."

*Curcumin, inflammation, **ageing and age-related diseases**.* Sikora E, Scapagnini G, Barbagallo M. Immun Ageing. 2010 Jan 17;7(1):1. **Key Finding**: "Ageing is manifested by the decreasing health status and increasing probability to acquired age-related disease such as cancer, Alzheimer's disease, atherosclerosis, metabolic disorders and others. They are likely caused by low-grade inflammation driven by oxygen stress and manifested by the increased level of pro-inflammatory cytokines. It is believed that ageing is plastic and can be slowed down by **caloric restriction** as well as by some nutraceuticals. Accordingly, slowing down ageing and postponing the onset of age-related diseases might be achieved by blocking the NF-kappaB-dependent inflammation. In this review we consider the possibility of the spice curcumin, a powerful antioxidant and anti-inflammatory agent possibly capable of improving the health status of the elderly."

Calorie restriction: what recent results suggest for the future of **ageing** *research.* Smith DL, Nagy TR, Allison DB. Eur J Clin Invest. 2010 May;40(5):440-50. **Key Finding**: "The first results from a long-term, randomized, controlled caloric restriction study in nonhuman primates showing statistically significant benefits on longevity have now been reported. Whether current positive results will translate into longevity for humans remains an open question. However, the apparent health benefits that have been observed with caloric restriction suggest that regardless of longevity gains, the promotion of healthy ageing and disease prevention may be attainable."

Sirt3 mediates reduction of oxidative damage and prevention of age-related **hearing loss** *under caloric restriction.* Someya S, Yu W, Hallows WC, et al. Cell. 2010 Nov 24;143(5):802-12. **Key Finding**: "Our findings identify Sirt3 as an essential player in enhancing the mitochondrial glutathione antioxidant defense system during caloric restriction and suggest that Sirt3 dependent mitochdonrial adaptations may be a central mechanism of aging retardation in mammals."

Caloric restriction attenuates **age-related changes** *of DNA methyltransferase 3a in mouse hippocampus.* Chouliaras L, van den Hove DL, Kenis G, et al. Brain Behav Immun. 2011 May;25(4):616-23. **Key Finding**: "Recent studies have suggested that DNA methlation is implicated in age-related changes in gene expression as well as in cognition. Because caloric restriction and upregulation of antioxidants have been suggested as strategies to attenuate age-related alterations in the brain, we hypothesized that both a diet restricted in calories and transgenic overexpression of normal human Cu/Zn superoxide dismutase 1 attenuate age-related changes in Dnmt3a in the aging mouse hippocampus. We performed qualitative and quantitative analyses in Dnmt3a in the aging mouse hippocampus. Changes in Dnmt3a levels in the mouse hippocampus may have a significant impact on gene expression and associated cognitive functioning."

*Adult-onset, short-term dietary restriction reduces **cell senescence** in mice.* Wang C, Maddick M, Miwa S, et al. Aging. 2010 Sep;2(9):555-66. **Key Finding**: "Dietary restriction (DR) extends the lifespan of a wide variety of species and reduces the incidence of major age-related diseases. Cell senescence has been proposed as one causal mechanism for tissue and organism ageing. We show for the first time that adult-onset, short-term DR reduced frequencies of senescent cells in the small intestinal epithelium and liver of mice, which are tissues known to accumulate increased numbers of senescent cells with advancing age."

*Lifelong calorie restriction alleviates **age-related oxidative damage** in peripheral nerves.* Opalach K, Rangaraju S, Madorsky I, Leeuwenburgh C, Notterpek L. Rejuvenation Res. 2010 Feb;13(1):65-74. **Key Finding**: "These results show that dietary restriction is an efficient means of defying age-related oxidative damage and maintaining a younger state in peripheral nerves."

*Effects of caloric restriction on **age-related hearing loss** in rodents and rhesus monkeys.* Someya S, Tanokura M, Weindruch R, Prolla TA, Yamasoba, T. Curr Aging Sci. 2010 Feb;3(1):20-5. **Key Finding:** "Caloric restriction extends the lifespan of most mammalian species, delays the onset of multiple age-related diseases, and attenuates both the degree of oxidative damage and the associated decline in physiological function. Here we review studies on caloric restriction's ability to prevent cochlear pathology and age-related hearing loss in laboratory animals and discuss potential molecular mechanisms of CR's actions."

*Caloric restriction counteracts **age-related** changes in the activities of sorbitol metabolizing enzymes from mouse liver.* Hagopian K, Ramsey JJ, Weindruch R. Biogerontology. 2009 Aug;10(4): 471-9. **Key Finding:** "The results indicate that decreased glucose levels under caloric restriction conditions lead to decreased sorbitol pathway enzyme activities and metabolite levels, and could contribute to the beneficial effects of long-term CR through decreased sorbitol levels and NADPH sparing."

*Caloric restriction and **aging**: studies in mice and monkeys.* Anderson RM, Shanmuganayagam D, Weindruch R. Toxicol Pathol. 2009; 37(1): 47-51. **Key Find-**

ing: "It is widely accepted that caloric restriction (CR) without malnutrition delays the onset of aging and extends lifespan in diverse animal models." CR in rhesus monkeys reduces the rate of age-associated muscle loss.

Metabolic shifts due to long-term caloric restriction revealed in nonhuman primates. Rezzi S, Marin FP, Shanmuganayagam D, et al. Exp. Gerontol. 2009 May; 44(5): 356-62. **Key Finding:** "We report new metabolic insights into long-term CR (caloric restriction) in nonhuman primates revealed by the holistic inspection of plasma (1)H NMR spectroscopic metabolic and lipoprotein profiles. The results revealed attenuation of **aging-dependent alterations** of lipoprotein and energy metabolism by CR."

Optimal window of caloric restriction onset limits its beneficial impact on T-cell senescence in primates. Messaoudi I, Fischer M, Warner J, et al. Aging Cell. 2008 Dec; 7(6): 908-19. **Key Finding:** "Our data demonstrate that the beneficial effects of adult-onset caloric restriction on **T-cell aging** were lost by both early and late CR onset. This suggests that there may be an optimal window during adulthood where CR can delay immune senescence and improve correlates of immunity in primates."

*Human caloric restriction for retardation of **aging**: current approaches and preliminary data.* Roberts SB, Schoeller DA. J Nutr. 2007 Apr 1;137(4):1076-77. **Key Finding:** Evidence from animal studies suggest "the potential for significant beneficial effects of CR in humans consistent with the effects that are emerging in the nonhuman primate studies."

Calorie restriction in nonhuman primates: assessing effects on brain and behavioral aging. Ingram DK, Young J, Mattison JA. Neuroscience. 2007 Apr 14;145(4):1359-64. **Key Finding:** "Recent results emerging from ongoing studies of caloric restriction in human and nonhuman primates suggest that many of the same anti-disease and anti-aging benefits observed in rodent studies may be applicable to long-lived species. The current review discusses approaches taken in studies of rhesus monkeys to analyze **age-related changes** in brain and behavioral function and the impact of CR on these changes."

*Caloric restriction, the traditional Okinawan diet, and healthy **aging**: the diet of the world's longest-lived people and its potential impact on morbidity and life span.*

Willcox BJ, Willcox DC, Todoriki H, et al. Ann NY Acad Sci. 2007 Oct; 1114: 434-55. **Key Finding:** Six decades of archived population data on the elderly in Okinawa was investigated. "This study lends epidemiological support for phenotypic benefits of CR in humans and is consistent with the well-known literature on animals with regard to CR phenotypes and healthy aging."

*Overview of caloric restriction and **ageing**.* Masoro EJ. Mech Ageing Dev. 2005 Sep;126(9):913-22. **Key Finding:** "It is proposed that low-intensity stressors, such as CR, activate ancient hermetic defense mechanisms in organisms ranging from yeast to mammals, defending them against a variety of adversities and, when long-term, retarding senescent processes."

*The impact of alpha-lipoic acid, coenzyme Q10 and caloric restriction on **life span** and gene expression patterns in mice.* Lee CK, Pugh TD, Klopp RG, et al. Free Radic Biol Med. 2004 Apr 15;36(8):1043-57. **Key Finding:** "Our observations suggest that supplementation with LA or CQ results in transcriptional alterations consistent with a state of reduced oxidative stress in the heart, but that these dietary interventions are not as effective as CR in inhibiting the **aging process** in the heart."

*Caloric restriction and **aging**: review of the literature and implications for studies in humans.* Heilbronn LK, Ravussin E. Am J Clin Nutr. 2003 Sep;78(3): 361-9. **Key Finding:** "The absence of adequate information on the effects of good quality, caloric-restricted diets in nonobese humans reflects the difficulties involved in conducting long-term studies in an environment so conducive to overfeeding."

*Caloric restriction, **aging**, and **cancer** prevention: mechanisms of action and applicability to humans.* Hursting SD, Lavigne JA, Berrigan D, Perkins SN, Barrett JC. Annu Rev Med. 2003 Feb;54:131-52. **Key Finding:** "Calorie restriction (CR) is the most effective and reproducible intervention for increasing lifespan in a variety of animal species, including mammals. CR is also the most potent, broadly acting cancer-prevention regimen in experimental carcinogenesis models."

*Caloric restriction and **aging** in primates: relevance to humans and possible CR mimetics.* Lane MA, Maittson J, Ingram DK, Roth GS. Microsc Res Tech.

2002 Nov 15;59(4):335-8. **Key Finding:** "Even if CR can be shown to impact upon human aging, it is unlikely that most people will be able to maintain the strict dietary control required for this regimen. Thus, elucidation of the biological mechanisms of CR and development of alternative strategies to yield similar benefits is of primary importance. CR mimetics, or interventions that 'mimic' certain protective effects of CR, may represent one such alternative strategy."

Caloric restriction in primates. Lane MA, Black A, Handy A, et al. Ann NY Acad Sci. 2001 Apr;928:287-95. **Key Finding:** "The emerging data from the ongoing primate studies strengthens the possibility that the diverse beneficial effects of CR on **aging** in rodents will also apply to non-human primates and perhaps ultimately to humans."

*Caloric restriction and **aging**: an update.* Masoro EJ. Exp Gerontol. 2000 May;35(3): 299-305. **Key Finding:** Three mechanisms for the observed antiaging action of caloric restriction are considered: 1) attenuation of **oxidative damage**; 2) modulation of **glycemia** and insulinemia; 3) hormesis. A scenario unifying the mechanisms is presented.

Caloric intake and aging. Weindruch R, Sohal RS. N Engl J Med. 1997 Oct 2;337:986-994. **Key Finding:** "Several lines of evidence suggest that caloric intake influences the rate of **aging** and the onset of associated diseases in animals and possibly, humans."

*The retardation of **aging** by caloric restriction: studies in rodents and primates.* Weindruch R. Toxicol Pathol. 1996 Nov-Dec; 24(6):742-5. **Key Finding:** "There is evidence to suggest that age-associated increases in oxidative damage may represent a primary aging process that is attenuated by CR."

*Protein oxidation associated with **aging** is reduced by dietary restriction of protein or calories.* Youngman LD, Park JY, Ames BN. Proc Natl Acad Sci. 1992 Oct 1; 89(19): 9112-6. **Key Finding:** Rats were fed diets restricted in either protein, calories, or total diet. Either protein or caloric restriction markedly inhibited the accumulation of **oxidatively damaged** proteins.

Alzheimer's disease

Dietary manipulation and caloric restriction in the development of mouse models relevant to neurological diseases. Schroeder JE, Richardson JC, Virley DJ. Biochem Biophys Acta. 2010 Oct;1802(10):840-6. **Key Finding**: "Reduced calorie consumption appears to increase the resistance of neurons to intracellular and extracellular stress and consequently improves the behavioural phenotype in animal models of neurological diseases such as **Alzheimer's disease.**"

*Intermittent fasting and caloric restriction ameliorate age-related behavioral deficits in the triple-transgenic mouse model of **Alzheimer's** disease.* Halagappa VK, Guo Z, Pearson M, et al. Neurobiol Dis. 2007 Apr; 26(1):212-20. **Key Finding:** "We conclude that CR and IF dietary regimens can ameliorate age-related deficits in cognitive function by mechanisms that may or may not be related to Abeta and tau pathologies."

*Calorie restriction attenuates **Alzheimer's disease** type brain amyloidosis in squirrel monkeys (Saimiri sciureus).* Qin W, Chachich M, Lane M, et al. J Alzheimers Dis. 2006 Dec;10(4):417-22. **Key Finding:** "Collectively, the study suggests that investigation of the role of CR in non-human primates may provide a valuable approach for further clarifying the role of CR in AD."

*Caloric intake and the risk of **Alzheimer's** disease.* Luchsinger JA, Tang MX, Shea S, Mayeux R. Arch Neurol. 2002;59:1258-63. **Key Finding:** "Higher intake of calories and fats may be associated with higher risk of AD in individuals carrying the apolipoprotein E 4allele."

Antioxidation

***Anti-oxidative** and **anti-inflammatory** vasoprotective effects of caloric restriction in **aging**: role of circulating factors and SIRT1.* Csiszar A, Labinskyy N, Jimenez R, et al. Mech Ageing Dev. 2009 Aug;130(8):518-27. **Key Finding:** "Endothelial dysfunction, oxidative stress and inflammation are associated with vascular aging and promote the development of cardiovascular disease. Caloric restriction mitigates conditions associated with aging. Caloric restriction exerts anti-oxidant and anti-inflammatory vascular effects."

Chronic calorie restriction attenuates experimental autoimmune encephalomyelitis. Piccio L, Stark JL, Cross AH. J Leukoc Biol. 2008;84:940-48. **Key Finding:** "CR induces multiple metabolic and physiologic modifications, including **anti-inflammatory, antioxidant, and neuroprotective effects** that may be beneficial in **multiple sclerosis**. The CR-induced hormonal, metabolic and cytokine changes observed in our studies suggest a combined anti-inflammatory and neuroprotective effect. CR with adequate nutrition and careful medical monitoring should be explored as a potential treatment for MS."

Cellular stress responses: a novel target for chemoprevention and nutritional neuroprotection in aging, neurodegenerative disorders and longevity. Calabrese V, Cornelius C, Mancuso C, et al. Neurochem Res. 2008 Dec; 33(12):2444-71. **Key Finding:** "In this review the importance of vitagenes in the cellular stress response and the potential use of dietary **antioxidants** in the prevention and treatment of **neurodegenerative disorders** is discussed."

Minireview: the role of **oxidative stress** *in relation to caloric restriction and longevity.* Gredilla R, Barja G. Endocrinology. 2005;146(9):3713-17. **Key Finding:** Investigations have reported reductions in steady-state oxidative damage to proteins, lipids, and DNA in animals subjected to restricted caloric intake. Several investigations have reported that decreases in oxidative damage are related to a lowering of mitochondrial free radical generation. A decrease in mitochondrial free radical generation has been suggested to be one of the main determinants of the extended **life span** observed in caloric restricted animals.

Caloric restriction and **aging**: *an update.* Masoro EJ. Exp Gerontol. 2000 May; 35(3):299-305. **Key Finding:** Three mechanisms for the observed antiaging action of caloric restriction are considered: 1) attenuation of **oxidative damage**; 2) modulation of **glycemia** and insulinemia; 3) hormesis. A scenario unifying the mechanisms is presented.

Oxidative stress, caloric restriction, and aging. Sohal RS, Weindruch R. Science. 1996 July 5;273(5271):59-63. **Key Finding:** "Restriction of caloric intake lowers steady-state levels of **oxidative stress** and damage, retards age-associated changes, and extends the maximum **life-span** in mammals."

*Protein oxidation associated with **aging** is reduced by dietary restriction of protein or calories.* Youngman LD, Park JY, Ames BN. Proc Natl Acad Sci. 1992 Oct 1; 89(19): 9112-6. **Key Finding:** Rats were fed diets restricted in either protein, calories, or total diet. Either protein or caloric restriction markedly inhibited the accumulation of **oxidatively damaged** proteins.

Arthritis (rheumatoid)

*Gluten-free vegan diet induces decreased LDL and oxidized LDL levels and raised atheroprotective natural antibodies against phosphorylcholine in patients with **rheumatoid arthritis**: a randomized study.* Elkan AC, Sjoberg B, Kolsrud B, et al. Arthritis Res Ther. 2008;10(2):R34. **Key Finding**: "A gluten-free vegan diet in rheumatoid arthritis patients induces changes that are potentially atheroprotective and anti-inflammatory, including decreased LDL."

*Effects of a very **low-fat vegan diet** in subjects with **rheumatoid arthritis**.* McDougall J, Bruce B, Spiller G, Westerdahl J, McDougall M. J Altern Complement Med. 2002 Feb;8(1):71-5. **Key Finding: "**This study showed that patients with moderate to severe rheumatoid arthritis, who switch to a very low-fat vegan diet, can experience significant reductions in RA symptoms."

*Fasting followed by vegetarian diet in patients with **rheumatoid arthritis**: a systematic review.* Muller H, de Toledo FW, Resch KL. Scand J Rheumatol. 2001;30(1):1-10. **Key Finding**: "We reviewed the available scientific evidence that fasting followed by vegetarian diet may help patients with rheumatoid arthritis (RA). Thirty-one reports of fasting studies in patients with RA were found. Only four controlled studies investigated the effects of fasting and subsequent diets for at least three months. The pooling of these studies showed a **statistically and clinically significant beneficial long-term effect**."

*Antioxidants in vegan diet and **rheumatic disorders**.* Hanninen O, Kaartinen K, Rauma AL, et al. Toxicology. 2000 Nov 30;155(1-3):45-

53. **Key Finding**: "Interventions and cross sectional studies on subjects consuming an **uncooked vegan diet called living food** have been carried out. The shift of **fibromyalgic** subjects to living foods resulted in a decrease of their joint stiffness and pain as well as an improvement of their self-experienced health. The rheumatoid arthritis patients eating the living foods diet also reported similar positive responses and the objective measures supported this finding."

Rheumatoid arthritis treated with vegetarian diets. Kjeldsen-Kragh J. Am J Clin Nutr. 1999 Sep;70(3 Suppl):594S-600S. **Key Finding**: "For all clinical variables and most laboratory variables measured, the 27 patients in the **fasting and vegetarian diet groups** improved significantly compared with the 26 patients in the control group who followed their usual omnivorous diet throughout the study period."

Faecal microbial flora and disease activity in **rheumatoid arthritis** *during a vegan diet.* Peltonen R, Nenonen M, Helve T, et al. Br J Rheumatol. 1997 Jan;36(1):64-8. **Key Finding**: "43 rheumatoid arthritis (RA) patients were randomized into two groups: the test group to receive living food, a form of **uncooked vegan diet** rich in lactobacilli, and the control group to continue their ordinary omnivorous diets. A significant, diet-induced change in the faecal flora was observed in the test group but not in the control group. We conclude that a vegan diet changes the faecal microbial flora in RA patients and changes in the faecal flora are associated with improvement in RA activity."

Effect of a strict vegan diet on energy and nutrient intakes by Finnish **rheumatoid patients**. Rauma AL, Nenonen M, Helve T, Hanninen O. Eur J Clin Nutr. 1993 Oct;47(10):747-9. **Key Finding**: "Dietary intake data of 43 Finnish rheumatoid arthritis patients were collected using 7-day food records. The subjects were randomized into a control and a vegan diet group. Shifting to the **uncooked vegan diet** significantly increased the intakes of energy and many nutrients. In spite of the increased energy intake, the group on the vegan diet lost 9% of their **body weight** during the intervention period."

*Controlled trial of fasting and one-year vegetarian diet in **rheumatoid arthritis**.* Kjeldsen-Kragh J, Haugen M, Borchgrevink CF, et al. Lancet. 1991 Oct 12;338(8772):899-902. **Key Finding:** "After four weeks at the health farm the **diet group showed a significant improvement** in number of tender joints, Ritchie's articular index, number of swollen joints, pain score, duration of morning stiffness, grip strength, erythrocyte sedimentation rate, C-reactive protein, white blood cell counts, and a health assessment questionnaire score. The benefits in the diet group were still present after one year."

Atherosclerosis

Long-term calorie restriction is highly effective in reducing the risk for atherosclerosis in humans. Fontana L, Meyer TE, Klein S, Holloszy JQ. Proc Natl Acad Sci. 2004 Apr 27;101(17):6659-63. **Key Finding:** The effect of CR on risk for **atherosclerosis** was studied in 18 individuals who had been on CR for an average of six years compared with 18 age-matched individuals on typical American diets. "Cartoid artery IMT was approximately 40% less in the CR group than in the comparison group. Based on a range of risk factors, it appears that long-term CR has a powerful protective effect against atherosclerosis."

Attention deficit hyperactivity disorder

Caloric restriction alters seizure disposition and behavioral profiles in seizure-prone (fast) versus seizure-prone (slow) rats. Azarbar A, McIntyre DC, Gilby KL. Behav Neurosci. 2010 Feb;124(1):106-14. **Key Finding**: "These results clearly endorse further investigation into the potential benefits of caloric restriction for both **epilepsy** and **attention-deficit hyperactivity disorder** (ADHD)."

Cancer (breast, chemotherapy side effects, lymphoma, prostate)

*Effect of chronic and intermittent caloric restriction on serum adiponectin and leptin and **mammary tumorigenesis**.* Rogozina OP, Bonorden MJ, Seppanen

CM, Grande JP, Cleary MP. Cancer Prev Res. 2011 Jan 21 [Epub ahead of print]. **Key Finding**: "Mammary tumor incidence in mice was 71% for the control group, 35.4% for the chronic caloric restriction group, and 9.1% for the intermittent caloric restriction group. Although we did not demonstrate an association of either adiponectin or leptin with individual mice in relation to mammary tumorigenesis, we did find that reduced serum leptin and elevated adiponectin leptin ratio were associated with the protective effect of intermittent calorie restriction."

*Calorie restriction and **cancer prevention**: metabolic and molecular mechanisms.* Longo VD, Fontana L. Trends Pharmacol Sci. 2010 Feb;31(2):89-98. **Key Finding**: "Calorie restriction without malnutrition has been shown to be broadly effective in cancer prevention in laboratory strains of rodents. Adult-onset moderate caloric restriction also reduces cancer incidence by 50% in monkeys. Here we discuss the link between nutritional interventions and cancer prevention with focus on the mechanisms that might be responsible."

*Fasting and differential **chemotherapy protection** in patients.* Raffaghello L, Safdie F, Bianchi G, et al. Cell Cycle. 2010 Nov 15;9(22):4474-6. **Key Finding**: "Chronic calorie restriction has been known for decades to prevent or retard cancer growth, but its weight-loss effect and the potential problems associated with combining it with chemotherapy have prevented its clinical application. Based on the discovery in model organisms that short term starvation (STS or fasting) causes a rapid switch of cells to a protected mode, we described a fasting-based intervention that causes remarkable changes in the levels of glucose, IGF-I and many other proteins and molecules and is capable of protecting mammalian cells and mice from various toxins, including chemotherapy. Because oncogenes prevent the cellular switch to this stress resistance mode, starvation for 48 hours or longer protects normal yeast and mammalian cells but not cancer cells from chemotherapy. Ten patients who fasted in combination with chemotherapy reported that fasting was not only feasible and safe but caused a reduction in a wide range of side effects accompanied by an apparently normal and possibly augmented chemotherapy efficacy. Together with the remarkable results observed in animals, these data provide preliminary evidence in support of the human application of this fundamental biogerontology finding, particularly for terminal patients receiving chemotherapy."

*Glucose restriction can extend normal cell **lifespan** and impair **precancerous cell** growth through epigenetic control of hTERT and p16 expression.* Li Y, Liu L, Tollefsbol TO. FASEB J. 2009 Dec 17 [Epub ahead of print]. **Key Finding:** Restricted calorie diets—specifically in the form of restricted glucose—help human cells live longer. "Cancer cells metabolize glucose at elevated rates and have a higher sensitivity to glucose reduction. We analyzed normal WI-38 and immortalized WI-38/S fetal lung fibroblasts and found that glucose restriction resulted in growth inhibition and apoptosis in WI-38/S cells, whereas it induced lifespan extension in WI-38 cells. Glucose restriction can extend normal cell lifespan and impair precancerous cell growth through epigenetic control of hTERT and p16 expression."

*Starvation-dependent differential stress resistance protects normal but not **cancer** cells against high-dose chemotherapy.* Raffaghello L, Lee C, Safdie FM, et al. Proc Natl Acad Sci. 2008 June 17; 105(24): 8215-20. **Key Finding:** "These studies describe a starvation-based differential stress resistance strategy to enhance the efficacy of chemotherapy and suggest that specific agents among those that promote oxidative stress and DNA damage have the potential to maximize the differential toxicity to normal and cancer cells." This experiment in mice confirmed the protective effects of fasting. Healthy cells can be protected from the side effects of chemotherapy.

Modified alternate-day fasting regimens reduce cell proliferation rates to a similar extent as daily calorie restriction in mice. Varady KA, Roohk DJ, McEvoy-Hein BK, et al. FASEB J. 2008;22:2090-6. **Key Finding:** "Calorie restriction CR and alternate-day fasting ADF reduce **cancer risk** and reduce cell proliferation rates." Cell proliferation rates in mice were measured using ADF, modified ADF, and daily CR. "In summary, modified ADF, allowing the consumption of 15% of energy needs on the restricted intake day, decreases global cell proliferation similarly as true ADF and daily CR without reducing body weight."

Prevention of **mammary tumorigenesis** *by intermittent caloric restriction: does caloric intake during refeeding modulate the response?* Cleary MP, Hu X, Grossmann ME, et al. Exp Biol Med. 2007;232:70-80. **Key Finding:** "These results confirm that intermittent caloric restriction prevents development of mammary tumors to a greater extent than does chronic caloric restriction, although 'overeating' during refeeding may compromise this protection."

Alternate-day fasting and chronic disease prevention: a review of human and animal trials. Varady KA, Hellerstein MK. Am J Clin Nutr. 2007 Jul; 86(1):7-13. **Key Finding**: Animal studies of alternate day fasting (ADF) find lower **diabetes** incidence and lower fasting glucose and insulin concentrations, effects that are comparable to those of caloric restriction (CR). Human trials to date report greater insulin-mediated glucose uptake but no effect on fasting glucose or insulin concentrations. Animal ADF data on cardiovascular disease show lower total cholesterol and triacylglycerol concentrations, a lower heart rate and lower blood pressure. Limited human evidence suggests higher HDL-cholesterol concentrations and lower triacylglycerol concentrations but no effect on blood pressure. There is no human evidence to date on **cancer** risk, but animal studies have found decreases in **lymphoma** incidence, longer survival after tumor inoculation, and lower rates of proliferation of several cell types. The findings in animals suggest that ADF may effectively modulate several risk factors, thereby preventing chronic disease, and that ADF may modulate disease risk to an extent similar to that of CR.

Dose effects of modified alternate-day fasting regimens on in vivo cell proliferation and plasma insulin-like growth factor-1 in mice. Varady KA, Roohk DJ, Hellerstein MK. J Appl Physiol. 2007 Aug;103(2):547-51. **Key Finding:** This four-week study with mice confirmed the beneficial effects of alternate-day fasting (100% caloric restriction on fast day) on **cancer risk** by decreasing cell proliferation and IGF-1 levels and suggest that modified alternate-day fasting regimens comprising 25%-50% caloric restriction on the fast day do not replicate these effects.

Long-term low-protein, **low-calorie** *diet and endurance exercise modulate metabolic factors associated with* **cancer** *risk.* Fontana L, Klein S, Holloszy JO. Am J

Clin Nutr. 2006 Dec;84(6):1456-62. **Key Finding**: "Exercise training, decreased adiposity, and long-term consumption of a low-protein, low-calorie diet are associated with low plasma growth factors and hormones that are linked to an increased risk of cancer. Low protein intake may have additional protective effects because it is associated with a decrease in circulating IGF-I independent of body fat mass."

*Caloric restriction, **aging**, and **cancer** prevention: mechanisms of action and applicability to humans.* Hursting SD, Lavigne JA, Berrigan D, Perkins SN, Barrett JC. Annu Rev Med. 2003 Feb;54:131-52. **Key Finding:** "Calorie restriction (CR) is the most effective and reproducible intervention for increasing lifespan in a variety of animal species, including mammals. CR is also the most potent, broadly acting cancer-prevention regimen in experimental carcinogenesis models."

Prostate carcinogenesis in N-methyl-N-nitrosourea (NMU)-testosterone-treated rats fed tomato powder, lycopene, or energy-restricted diets. Boileau TW, Liao Z, Kim S, et al. J Natl Cancer Inst. 2003 Nov 5;95(21):1578-86. **Key Finding:** "Consumption of tomato powder but not lycopene inhibited prostate carcinogenesis, suggesting that tomato products contain compounds in addition to lycopene that modify prostate carcinogenesis. Diet restriction also reduced the risk of **prostate cancer**. Tomato phytochemicals and diet restriction may act by independent mechanisms."

*Adult-onset calorie restriction and fasting delay spontaneous **tumorigenesis** in p53-deficient mice.* Berrigan D, Perkins SN, Haines DC, Hursting SD. Carcinogenesis. 2002 May;23(5):817-22. **Key Finding:** "Our findings that CR or a 1 day/week fast suppressed carcinogenesis–even when started late in life in mice predestined to develop tumors due to decreased p53 gene dosage–support efforts to identify suitable interventions influencing energy balance in humans as a tool for cancer prevention."

Caloric restriction as a mechanism mediating resistance to environmental disease. Frame LT, Hart RW, Leakey JE. Environ Health Perspect. 1998 Feb;106 (suppl 1): 313-24. **Key Finding:** Caloric restriction may confer added protection against environmental stress, such as chemically induced **cancers.**

Five-year survival rates of **melanoma** *patients treated by diet therapy after the manner of Gerson: a retrospective review.* Hildenbrand GL, Hildenbrand LC, Bradford K, Cavin SW. Altern Ther Health Med. 1995 Sep;1(4):29-37. **Key Finding**: "**Gerson's diet therapy**: **lactovegetarian,** low sodium, low fat and (temporarily) protein, high potassium, fluid, and nutrients (hourly **raw vegetable**/fruit juices). Calorie supply limited to 2600-3200 calories per day. Of 14 patients with stages I and II (localized) melanoma, 100% survived for 5 years. Of 17 with stage IIIA (regionally metastasized melanoma) 82% were alive at 5 years. The 5-year survival rates reported here are considerably higher than those reported elsewhere."

Cardiovascular protection

Cardiovascular protection afforded by caloric restriction: essential role of nitric oxide synthase. Shinmura K. Geriatr Gerontol Int. 2011 Apr;11(2):143-56. **Key Finding**: "It is possible that long-term caloric restriction partially retards cardiac senescence by attenuating oxidative damage in the aged heart. Overall, we strongly believe that caloric restriction could reduce morbidity and mortality of cardiovascular events in humans."

Caloric restriction and heart function: is there a sensible link? Han X, Ren J. Acta Pharmacol Sin. 2010 Sep;31(9):1111-7. **Key Finding**: "Ample clinical and experimental evidence has demonstrated that caloric restriction is capable of retarding the aging process and the development of **cardiovascular disease**. Despite the apparent beneficial cardiovascular effects of caloric restriction, implementation of CR in the health care management is still hampered by apparent applicability issues and health concerns."

Effect of a 21-day Daniel Fast on metabolic and **cardiovascular disease** *risk factors in men and women.* Bloomer RJ, Kabir MM, Canale RE, et al. Lipids Health Dis. 2010 Sep 3;9:94. **Key Finding**: "A 21-day period of modified dietary intake in accordance with the Daniel Fast improves several risk factors for metabolic and cardiovascular disease."

Cholesterol

Caloric restriction and aging as viewed from Biosphere 2. Walford RL, Weber L, Panov S. Receptor. 1995 Spring;5(1):29-33. **Key Finding:** Over the two year period of caloric restriction the eight persons sealed inside the closed ecological space known as Biosphere 2 demonstrated a "substantial **weight loss,** remarkable fall in blood **cholesterol, blood pressure, fasting blood sugar,** and low white blood cell counts – exactly as seen in rodents on such a regimen."

*The calorically restricted low-fat, nutrient-dense diet in Biosphere 2 significantly lowers **blood glucose**, total leukocyte count, **cholesterol**, and **blood pressure** in humans.* Walford RL, Harris SB, Gunion MW. Proc Natl Acad Sci. 1992 Dec 1; 89(23): 11533-7. **Key Finding:** "We conclude that drastic reductions in cholesterol and blood pressure may be instituted in normal individuals in Western countries by application of a carefully chosen diet and that a low-calorie, nutrient-dense regime shows physiologic features in humans similar to those in other animal species."

Diet and serum lipids in vegan vegetarians: a model for risk reduction. Resnicow K, Barone J, Engle A, et al. J Am Diet Assoc. 1991 Apr;91(4):447-53. **Key Finding:** "The lipid levels and dietary habits of 31 Seventh-Day Adventist vegan vegetarians (aged 5 to 46 years) who consume no animal products were assessed. Mean serum total **cholesterol**, low-density-lipoprotein cholesterol and triglyceride levels were lower than expected values derived from the Lipid Research Clinics Population Studies prevalence data. The vegan diet was characterized by increased consumption of almonds, cashews, and their nut butters; dried fruits; citrus fruits; soy milk and greens. We conclude from the present study that a strict vegan diet, which is typically very low in saturated fat and dietary cholesterol and high in fiber, can help children and adults maintain or achieve desirable blood lipid levels."

Cognitive impairment

*Gene expression in the **hippocampus**: regionally specific effects of aging and caloric restriction.* Zeier Z, Madorsky I, Xu Y, et al. Mech Ageing Dev. 2011

Jan-Feb;132(1-2):8-19. **Key Finding**: "We measured changes in gene expression induced by aging and caloric restriction in three hippocampal subregions. When analysis included all regions, aging was associated with expression of genes linked to mitochondrial dysfunction, inflammation, and stress responses, and in some cases, expression was reversed by caloric restriction."

Caloric restriction attenuates age-related changes of DNA methyltransferase 3a in mouse **hippocampus**. Chouliaras L, van den Hove DL, Kenis G, et al. Brain Behav Immun. 2011 May;25(4):616-23. **Key Finding**: "Because caloric restriction and upregulation of antioxidants have been suggested as strategies to attenuate age-related alterations in the brain, we hypothesized that both a diet restricted in calories and transgenic overexpression of normal human Cu/Zn superoxide dismutase 1 attenuate age-related changes in Dnmt3a in the aging mouse hippocampus."

Caloric restriction improves **memory** *in elderly humans.* Witte AV, Fobker M, Gellner R, Knecht S, Floel A. Proc Natl Acad Sci. 2009 Jan 27;106(4): 1255-60. **Key Finding:** "We found a significant increase in verbal memory scores after caloric restriction (mean increased 20%; P<0.001) which was correlated with decreases in fasting plasma levels of insulin and high sensitive C-reactive protein, most pronounced in subjects with best adherence to the diet."

Mediterranean diet and mild **cognitive impairment**. Scarmeas N, Stern Y, Mayeux R, et al.Arch Neurol. 2009 Jul; 66(7):912-3. **Key Finding:** "Higher adherence to the Mediterranean diet is associated with a trend for reduced risk of developing mild cognitive impairment and with reduced risk of MCI conversion to Alzheimer disease."

Chronic calorie restriction attenuates experimental autoimmune encephalomyelitis. Piccio L, Stark JL, Cross AH. J Leukoc Biol. 2008;84:940-48. **Key Finding:** "CR induces multiple metabolic and physiologic modifications, including **anti-inflammatory, antioxidant, and neuroprotective effects** that may be beneficial in **multiple sclerosis**. The CR-induced hormonal, metabolic and cytokine changes observed in our studies suggest a combined anti-inflammatory and neuroprotective effect. CR with adequate nutrition and careful medical monitoring should be explored as a potential treatment for MS."

Caloric restriction increases learning consolidation and facilitates synaptic plasticity through mechanisms dependent on NR2B subunits of the NMDA receptor. Fontan-Lozano A, Saez-Cassanelli JL, Inda MC, et al. J Neurosci. 2007 Sep 19;27(38):10185-95. **Key Finding:** Mature mice on a long-term intermittent fasting diet enhanced their learning and consolidation processes. "These data provide a molecular and cellular mechanism by which long-term intermittent fasting may enhance **cognition,** amerliorating some aging-associated cognitive deficits."

Coronary artery disease

*Modified alternate-day fasting and **cardioprotection:** relation to adipose tissue dynamics and dietary fat intake.* Varady KA, Hudak CS, Hellerstein MK. Metabolism. 2009 Jun; 58(6):803-11. **Key Finding:** Alternate day fasting with a low-fat diet may protect against **coronary heart disease**. Alternate day fasting may also be protective even in the presence of high-fat diets.

*Usefulness of routine periodic fasting to lower risk of **coronary artery disease** in patients undergoing coronary angiography.* Horne BD, May HT, Anderson JL, et al. Am J Cardiol. 2008 Oct 1;102(7):814-19. **Key Finding:** Fasting once a month for 24 hours is associated with a lower risk for coronary artery disease. Fasters among 515 people studied were 40 percent less likely to be diagnosed with clogged arteries than those who did not regularly fast.

***Cardioprotection** by intermittent fasting in rats.* Ahmet I, Wan R, Mattson MP, Lakatta EG, Talan M. Circulation. 2005 Nov 15; 112(20):3115-21. **Key Finding:** Intermittent fasting "protects the heart from ischemic injury and attenuates post-MI cardiac remodeling, likely via antiapoptotic and anti-inflammatory mechanisms."

Diabetes

*Caloric restriction reverses hepatic **insulin resistance** and steatosis in rats with low aerobic capacity.* Bowman TA, Ramakrishnan SK, Kaw M, et al. Endocrinology. 2010 Nov;151(11):5157-64. **Key Finding**: "Rats selectively bred for low aerobic running capacity exhibit the metabolic syndrome, including hyperinsulnemia, insulin resistance, visceral obesity, and dyslipidemia. They also exhibit features of nonalcoholic steatohepatitis, including chicken-wire fibrosis, inflammation, andoxidative stress. Caloric restriction by 30% over a period of 2-3 months improved insulin clearance in parallel to inducing the protein content and activation of the carcinoembryonic antigen-related cell adhesion molecule 1, a main player in hepatic insulin extraction. It also reduced glucose and insulin intolerance and serum and tissue triglyceride levels. Additionally, caloric restriction reversed inflammation, oxidative stress, and fibrosis in liver."

*Beneficial effects of dietary restriction in **type 2 diabetic** rats: the role of adipokines on inflammation and insulin resistance.* Crisóstomo J, Rodrigues L, Matafome P, et al. Br J Nutr. 2010 Jul;104(1):76-82. **Key Finding**: "These results indicate that dietary restriction in type 2 diabetes enhances adipose tissue metabolism leading to an improved skeletal muscle insulin sensitivity."

*The influence of dietary restriction on the development of **diabetes and pancreatitis** in female WBN/Kob-fatty rats.* Akimoto T, Terada M, Shimizu A, Sawai N, Ozawa H. Exp Anim. 2010;59(5):623-30. **Key Finding**: "In female fatty rats of the restricted feeding group, pathological changes of the pancreas were milder than those of the free-feeding fatty group. Although dietary restriction could not completely prevent pancreatitis in female fatty rats, the development of diabetes was inhibited by its reduction of the severity of pancreatitis."

*Combined effects of short-term caloric restriction and exercise on **insulin action** in normal rats.* Jiang HY, Koike T, Li P, et al. Horm Metab Res. 2010 Dec;42(13):950-4. **Key Finding:** "Our findings indicate that the combination of exercise and caloric restriction may be effective in enhancing insulin sensitivity at the skeletal muscle in normal subjects."

Changes in nutrient intake and dietary quality among participants with **type 2 diabetes** *following a* **low-fat vegan diet** *or a conventional diabetes diet for 22 weeks.* Turner-McGrievy GM. Barnard ND, Cohen J, et al. J Am Diet Assoc. 2008 Oct;108(10):1636-45. **Key Finding**: "Vegan diets increase intakes of carbohydrate, fiber, and several micronutrients, in contrast with the American Diabetes Association recommended diet. The vegan group improved its Alternate Healthy Eating Index score whereas the American Diabetes Association recommended diet group's score remain unchanged."

Alternate-day fasting and chronic disease prevention: a review of human and animal trials. Varady KA, Hellerstein MK. Am J Clin Nutr. 2007 Jul;86(1):7-13. **Key Finding**: Animal studies of alternate day fasting (ADF) find lower **diabetes** incidence and lower fasting glucose and insulin concentrations, effects that are comparable to those of caloric restriction (CR). Human trials to date report greater insulin-mediated glucose uptake but no effect on fasting glucose or insulin concentrations. Animal ADF data on cardiovascular disease show lower total cholesterol and triacylglycerol concentrations, a lower heart rate and lower blood pressure. Limited human evidence suggests higher HDL-cholesterol concentrations and lower triacylglycerol concentrations but no effect on blood pressure. There is no human evidence to date on **cancer** risk, but animal studies have found decreases in **lymphoma** incidence, longer survival after tumor inoculation, and lower rates of proliferation of several cell types. The findings in animals suggest that ADF may effectively modulate several risk factors, thereby preventing chronic disease, and that ADF may modulate disease risk to an extent similar to that of CR.

Intermittent fasting dissociates beneficial effects of dietary restriction on **glucose metabolism** *and* **neuronal resistance** *to injury from calorie intake.* Anson RM, Guo Z, de Cabo R, et al. Proc Natl Acad Sci. 2003 May 13;100(10):6216-20. **Key Finding:** "Intermittent fasting (in mice) resulted in beneficial effects that met or exceeded those of caloric restriction including reduced serum glucose and insulin levels and increased resistance of neurons in the brain to excitotoxic stress."

*Caloric restriction and **aging**: an update.* Masoro EJ. Exp Gerontol. 2000 May;35(3):299-305. **Key Finding:** Three mechanisms for the observed antiaging action of caloric restriction are considered: 1) attenuation of **oxidative damage**; 2) modulation of **glycemia** and insulinemia; 3) hormesis. A scenario unifying the mechanisms is presented.

Caloric restriction and aging as viewed from Biosphere 2. Walford RL, Weber L, Panov S. Receptor. 1995 Spring;5(1):29-33. **Key Finding:** Over the two-year period of caloric restriction the eight persons sealed inside the closed ecological space known as Biosphere 2 demonstrated a "substantial **weight loss,** remarkable fall in blood **cholesterol, blood pressure**, **fasting blood sugar**, and low white blood cell counts—exactly as seen in rodents on such a regimen."

*The calorically restricted low-fat, nutrient-dense diet in Biosphere 2 significantly lowers **blood glucose**, total leukocyte count, **cholesterol,** and **blood pressure** in humans.* Walford RL, Harris SB, Gunion MW. Proc Natl Acad Sci. 1992 Dec 1;89(23):11533-7. **Key Finding:** "We conclude that drastic reductions in cholesterol and blood pressure may be instituted in normal individuals in Western countries by application of a carefully chosen diet and that a low-calorie, nutrient-dense regime shows physiologic features in humans similar to those in other animal species."

Endothelial function

Short-term caloric restriction reverses vascular endothelial dysfunction in old mice by increasing nitric oxide and reducing oxidative stress. Ripee C, Lesniewski L, Connell M, et al. Aging Cell. 2010 Jun;9(3):304-12. **Key Finding**: "Short-term caloric restriction initiatied in old age reverses age-associated vascular endothelial dysfunction by restoring nitric oxide bioavailability, reducing oxidative stress and upregulation of sirtuin-1."

Caloric restriction improves endothelial dysfunction during vascular aging: effects on nitric oxide synthase isoforms and oxidative stress in rat aorta. Zanetti M, Gortan Cappellari G, Burekovic I, et al. Exp Gerontol. 2010 Nov;45(11):848-55. **Key Finding**: "Short-term caloric restriction improves age-related endothelial dysfunction. Reversal of altered iNOS/eNOS ratio, reduced oxidative stress and increased SOD enzyme activity rather than enhanced nitric oxide production appear to be involved in this effect."

Caloric restriction reverses high-fat diet-induced **endothelial dysfunction** *and vascular superoxide production in C57Bl/6 mice.* Ketonen J, Pilvi T, Mervaaia E. Heart Vessels. 2010 May;25(3):254-62. **Key Finding**: "The present study suggests that caloric restriction reverses obesity induced endothelial dysfunction and vascular oxidative stress, and underscores the importance of uncoupled endothelial nitric oxide synthase in the pathogenesis."

Epilepsy

Caloric restriction alters seizure disposition and behavioral profiles in seizure-prone (fast) versus seizure-prone (slow) rats. Azarbar A, McIntyre DC, Gilby KL. Behav Neurosci. 2010 Feb;124(1):106-14. **Key Finding**: "These results clearly endorse further investigation into the potential benefits of caloric restriction for both **epilepsy** and **attention-deficit hyperactivity disorder** (ADHD)."

Fibromyalgia

Antioxidants in vegan diet and **rheumatic disorders**. Hanninen O, Kaartinen K, Rauma AL, et al. Toxicology. 2000 Nov 30;155(1-3):45-53. **Key Finding**: "Interventions and cross-sectional studies on subjects consuming **uncooked vegan diet called living food** have been carried out. The shift of **fibromyalgic** subjects to living foods resulted in a decrease of their joint stiffness and pain as well as an improvement of their self-experienced health. The rheumatoid arthritis patients eating the living foods diet also reported similar positive responses and the objective measures supported this finding."

Vegan diet alleviates **fibromyalgia** *symptoms.* Kaartinen K, Lammi K, Hypen M, et al. Scand J Rheumatol. 2000;29(5):308-13. **Key Finding**: "The effect of a strict, low-salt, **uncooked vegan diet** rich in lactobacteria on symptoms in 18 fibromyalgia patients during and after a 3-month intervention period in an open, non-randomized controlled study was evaluated. The majority of patients were overweight to some extent at the beginning of the study and shifting to a vegan food diet caused a significant reduction in body mass. Total serum cholesterol showed a statistically significant lowering. It can be concluded that vegan diet had beneficial effects on fibromyalgia symptoms."

Health (in general)

Beneficial effects of mild stress (hermetic effects): **dietary restriction** *and* **health**. Kouda K, Iki M. J Physiol Anthropol. 2010;29(4):127-32. **Key Finding**: "In experimental animals, mild dietary stress (dietary restriction) without malnutrition delays most age-related physiological changes, and extends maximum and average lifespan. Animal studies have also demonstrated that dietary restriction can prevent or lessen the severity of cancer, stroke, coronary heart disease, autoimmune disease, allergy, Parkinson's disease and Alzheimer's disease."

How much should we eat? The association between energy intake and mortality in a 36-year follow-up study of Japanese-American men. Willcox BJ, Yang K, Chen R, et al. J Gerontol A Biol Sci Med Sci. 2004 Aug; 59(8):789-95. **Key Finding:** Men who consumed 15% below the group mean were at the lowest risk for **all-cause mortality.**

Calorie restriction in biosphere 2: alterations in physiologic, hematologic, hormonal and biochemical parameters in humans restricted for a 2-year period. Walford RL, Mock D, Verdery R, Maccallum T. J Gerontol A Biol Sci Med Sci. 2002 Jun;57(6):8211-24. **Key Finding:** "We conclude that healthy non-obese humans on a low-calorie, nutrient-dense diet show physiologic, hematologic, hormonal, and biochemical changes resembling those of rodents and monkeys on such diets. With regard to the health of humans on such a diet, we observed that despite the selective restriction in calories and marked **weight loss**, all crew members remained in excellent **health** and sustained a high level of physical and mental activity throughout the entire 2 years."

Heart health

*Impact of long-term caloric restriction on **cardiac senescence**: caloric restriction ameliorates cardiac diastolic dysfunction associated with aging.* Shinmura K, Tamaki K, Sano M, et al. J Mol Cell Cardiol. 2011 Jan;50(1):117-27. **Key Finding**: "Caloric restriction improves diastolic function in the senescent myocardium by amelioration of the age-associated deterioration in intracellular ca(2+) handling."

*Life-long caloric restriction elicits pronounced protection of the **aged myocardium**: a role for AMPK.* Edwards AG, Donato AJ, Lesniewski LA, et al. Mech Ageing Dev. 2010 Nov-Dec;131(11-12):739-42. **Key Finding**: "These results indicate that life-long caloric restriction profoundly protects the aged heart against ischemia/reperfusion injury and suggest that AMP-activated protein kinase may play a role in that protection."

*Severe, short-term food restriction improves **cardiac function** following ischemia/reperfusion in perfused rat hearts.* Yamagishi T, Bessho M, Yanagida S, Nishizawa K, et al. Heart Vessels. 2010 Sep;25(5):417-25. **Key Finding**: "These results involving Male Wistar rats suggest that severe, short-term food restriction improves ischemic tolerance in rat hearts vita altered expression of functional proteins induced by low serum T3 levels, decreased coronary conductance, and change in metabolic flux."

Hypertension

The impact of religious fasting on human health. Trepanowski JF, Bloomer RJ. Nutr J. 2010 Nov 22;9:57. **Key Finding**: "The Biblical-based Daniel Fast prohibits the consumption of animal products, refined carbohydrates, food additives, preservatives, sweeteners, flavorings, caffeine, and alcohol. It is most commonly partaken for 21 days, although fasts of 10 and 40 days have been observed. Our initial investigation of the Daniel Fast noted favorable effects on several health-related outcomes, including **blood pressure, blood lipids, insulin sensitivity,** and biomarkers of oxidative stress."

*Calorie restriction prevents **hypertension** and cardiac hypertrophy in the spontaneously hypertensive rat.* Dolinsky VW, Morton JS, Oka T, et al. Hypertension. 2010 Sep;56(3):412-21. **Key Finding**: "Our findings provide compelling evidence that short-term caloric restriction exerts beneficial effects and may serve as an effective nonpharmacological treatment of hypertension."

*Effects of the dietary approaches to stop **hypertension** diet, exercise, and caloric restriction on neurocognition in overweight adults with high blood pressure.* Smith PJ. Blumenthal JA, Babyak MA, et al. Hypertension. 2010 Jun;55(6):1331-8. **Key Finding**: "Combining aerobic exercise with the DASH diet and caloric restriction improves neurocognitive function among sedentary and overweight/obese individuals with prehypertension and hypertension."

*Long-term **low-calorie low-protein vegan** diet and endurance exercise are associated with low cardiometabolic risk.* Fontana L, Meyer TE, Klein S, Holloszy JO. Rejuvenation Res. 2007 Jun;10(2):225-34. **Key Finding**: "Long-term consumption of a low-calorie, low-protein vegan diet or regular endurance exercise training is associated with low cardiometabolic risk. Moreover, our data suggest that specific components of a low-calorie, low-protein vegan diet provide additional beneficial effects on **blood pressure**."

*Medically supervised water-only fasting in the treatment of borderline **hypertension**.* Goldhamer AC, Lisle DJ, Sultana P, et al. J Altern Complement Med. 2002 Oct; 8(5):643-50. **Key Finding:** "Medically supervised water-only fasting appears to be a safe and effective means of normalizing BP and may assist in motivating health-promoting diet and lifestyle changes."

Caloric restriction and aging as viewed from Biosphere 2. Walford RL, Weber L, Panov S. Receptor. 1995 Spring;5(1):29-33. **Key Finding:** Over the two year period of caloric restriction the eight persons sealed inside the closed ecological space known as Biosphere 2 demonstrated a "substantial **weight loss**, remarkable fall in blood **cholesterol, blood pressure, fasting blood sugar**, and low white blood cell counts—exactly as seen in rodents on such a regimen."

The calorically restricted low-fat nutrient-dense diet in Biosphere 2 significantly lowers **blood glucose**, *total leukocyte count,* **cholesterol,** *and* **blood pressure** *in humans.* Walford RL, Harris SB, Gunion MW. Proc Natl Acad Sci. 1992 Dec 1; 89(23):11533-7. **Key Finding:** "We conclude that drastic reductions in cholesterol and blood pressure may be instituted in normal individuals in Western countries by application of a carefully chosen diet and that a low-calorie, nutrient-dense regime shows physiologic features in humans similar to those in other animal species."

Immune system

Calorie restriction enhances T-cell-mediated **immune response** *in adult overweight men and women.* Ahmed T, Das SK, Golden JK, et al. J Gerontol A Biol Sci Med Sci. 2009 Nov;64(11):1107-13. **Key Finding:** Forty-six overweight men and women were randomly assigned to 30% or 10% calorie restriction (CR) groups for six months. Only after 30% was statistical significance reached. "These results, for the first time, show that 6-month CR in humans improves T-cell function."

Optimal window of caloric restriction onset limits its beneficial impact on T-cell senescence in primates. Messaoudi I, Fischer M, Warner J, et al. Aging Cell. 2008 Dec; 7(6): 908-19. **Key Finding:** "Our data demonstrate that the beneficial effects of adult-onset caloric restriction on **T-cell aging** were lost by both early and late CR onset. This suggests that there may be an optimal window during adulthood where CR can delay immune senescence and improve correlates of immunity in primates."

Mice and flies and monkeys too: caloric restriction rejuvenates the aging immune system of non-human primates. Nikolich-Zugich J, Messaoudi I. Exp Gerontol. 2005 Nov; 40(11): 884-93. **Key Finding:** "We review published data describing the impact of CR on the aging **immune system** of mice and primates, and discuss our unpublished data that delineate similarities and differences in the effects of CR upon T-cell aging and homeostasis between these two models."

Inflammation

*Effects of exercise combined with caloric restriction on **inflammatory** cytokines.* Reed JL, De Souza MJ, Williams NI. Appl Physiol Nutr Metab. 2010 Oct;35(5):573-82. **Key Finding:** "Weight loss in response to exercise training and caloric restriction is effective in reducing inflammatory markers, specifically IL-6 and leptin."

Anti-oxidative *and **anti-inflammatory** vasoprotective effects of caloric restriction in **aging**: role of circulating factors and SIRT1.* Csiszar A, Labinskyy N, Jimenez R, et al. Mech Ageing Dev. 2009 Aug;130(8):518-27. **Key Finding:** "Endothelial dysfunction, oxidative stress and inflammation are associated with vascular aging and promote the development of cardiovascular disease. Caloric restriction mitigates conditions associated with aging. Caloric restriction exerts anti-oxidant and anti-inflammatory vascular effects."

Chronic calorie restriction attenuates experimental autoimmune encephalomyelitis. Piccio L, Stark JL, Cross AH. J Leukoc Biol. 2008; 84:940-948. **Key Finding:** "CR induces multiple metabolic and physiologic modifications, including **anti-inflammatory, antioxidant, and neuroprotective effects** that may be beneficial in **multiple sclerosis**. The CR-induced hormonal, metabolic and cytokine changes observed in our studies suggest a combined anti-inflammatory and neuroprotective effect. CR with adequate nutrition and careful medical monitoring should be explored as a potential treatment for MS."

Life extension

*Caloric restriction and **longevity**: effects of reduced body temperature.* Carrillo AE, Flouris AD. Ageing Res Rev. 2011 Jan;10(1):153-62. **Key Finding:** "Caloric restriction causes a reduction in body temperature. Based on current evidence it is concluded that low body temperature plays an integral role in mediating the effects of caloric restriction on health and longevity, and that low body temperature may exert independent biological changes that increase lifespan."

*Dietary interventions to **extend life span** and health span based on calorie restriction.* Minor RK, Allard JS, Younts CM, Ward TM, de Cabo R. J Gerontol A Biol Med Sci. 2010 Jul;65(7):695-703. **Key Finding:** "Using calorie restriction which is well known to improve both health and longevity in controlled studies as their benchmark, gerontologists are coming closer to identifying dietary and pharmacological therapies that may be applicable to aging humans. This review covers some of the more promising interventions targeted to affect pathways implicated in the aging process."

*Glucose restriction can extend normal cell **lifespan** and impair **precancerous cell** growth through epigenetic control of hTERT and p16 expression.* Li Y, Liu L, Tollefsbol TO. FASEB J. 2009 Dec 17 [Epub ahead of print]. **Key Finding:** Restricted calorie diets—specifically in the form of restricted glucose—help human cells live longer. "Cancer cells metabolize glucose at elevated rates and have a higher sensitivity to glucose reduction. We analyzed normal WI-38 and immortalized WI-38/S fetal lung fibroblasts and found that glucose restriction resulted in growth inhibition and apoptosis in WI-38/S cells, whereas it induced lifespan extension in WI-38 cells. Glucose restriction can extend normal cell lifespan and impair precancerous cell growth through epigenetic control of hTERT and p16 expression."

*Long-lived Indy and caloric restriction interact to **extend life span**.* Wang PY, Neretti N, Whitaker R, et al. Proc Natl Acad Sci. 2009 June 9;106(23): 9262-7. **Key Finding:** Caloric restriction (CR) improves health and extends life in a variety of species. We conclude that *Indy* (the Drosophila gene) and CR interact to affect longevity. CR down-regulates Indy expression.

Effect of 6-month calorie restriction on biomarkers of longevity, metabolic adaptation, and oxidative stress in overweight individuals. Heilbronn LK, De Jonge L, Frisard MI, et al. JAMA. 2006 Apr 5; 295(13):1539-48. **Key Finding:** "Our findings suggest that 2 biomarkers of **longevity** (fasting insulin level and body temperature) are decreased by prolonged calorie restriction in humans and support the theory that metabolic rate is reduced beyond the level expected from reduced metabolic body mass."

Delay of T cell senescence by caloric restriction in aged long-lived nonhuman primates. Messaoudi I, Warner J, Fischer M, et al. Proc Natl Acad Sci. 2006 Dec

19; 103(51):19448-53. **Key Finding:** "Our results provide evidence that CR can delay immune senescence in nonhuman primates, potentially contributing to an extended **lifespan** by reducing susceptibility to infectious disease."

*Toward a unified theory of caloric restriction and **longevity** regulation.* Sinclair DA. Mech Ageing Dev. 2005 Sept;126(9):967-1002. **Key Finding:** "Recent data from yeast, worms, flies, and mammals support the idea that CR is not simply a passive effect but an active, highly conserved stress response that evolved early in life's history to increase an organism's chance of surviving adversity."

*Minireview: the role of **oxidative stress** in relation to caloric restriction and longevity.* Gredilla R, Barja G. Endocrinology. 2005;146(9):3713-17. **Key Finding:** Investigations have reported reductions in steady-state oxidative damage to proteins, lipids, and DNA in animals subjected to restricted caloric intake. Several investigations have reported that decreases in oxidative damage are related to a lowering of mitochondrial free radical generation. A decrease in mitochondrial free radical generation has been suggested to be one of the main determinants of the extended **life span** observed in caloric restricted animals.

*Calorie restriction promotes mammalian **cell survival** by inducing the SIRT1 deacetylase.* Cohen HY, Miller C, Bitterman KJ, et al. Science. 2004 July 16;305(5682):390-2. **Key Finding:** "In yeast, caloric restriction (CR) delays aging by activating the Sir2 deacetylase. Here we show that expression of mammalian Sir2 (SIRT1) is induced in CR rats as well as in human cells that are treated with serum from these animals."

*The impact of alpha-lipoic acid, coenzyme Q10 and caloric restriction on **life span** and gene expression patterns in mice.* Lee CK, Pugh TD, Klopp RG, et al. Free Radic Biol Med. 2004 Apr 15; 36(8):1043-57. **Key Finding:** "Our observations suggest that supplementation with LA or CQ results in transcriptional alterations consistent with a state of reduced oxidative stress in the heart, but that these dietary interventions are not as effective as CR in inhibiting the **aging process** in the heart."

How much should we eat? The association between energy intake and mortality in a 36-year follow-up study of Japanese-American men. Willcox BJ, Yang K, Chen R, et al. J Gerontol A Biol Sci Med Sci. 2004 Aug;59(8):789-95. **Key Finding:** Men who consumed 15% below the group mean were at the lowest risk for **all-cause mortality.**

Demography of dietary restriction and death in drosophila. Mair W, Goymer P, Pletcher SD, Partridge L. Science. 2003 Sep 19;301(5640):1731-33. **Key Finding:** "Two days after the application of DR (dietary restriction) at any age for the first time, previously fully fed flies are no more likely to die than flies of the same age that have been subjected to long-term DR. DR of mammals may also reduce short-term risk of death, and hence DR instigated at any age could generate a full reversal of **mortality.**"

*The response to calorie restriction in mammals shows features also common to **hibernation**: a cross-adaptation hypothesis.* Walford RL, Spindler SR. J Gerontol A Biol Sci Med Sci. 1997 Jul;52(4):8179-83. **Key Finding:** "We hypothesize that the response to the calorie restriction regime as studied by gerontologists, rather than being a laboratory artifact, is part of a spectrum of responses to food deprivation which have adaptive value in the wild, and whose triggering mechanism may primarily involve the neuroendocrine system."

Oxidative stress, caloric restriction, and aging. Sohal RS, Weindruch R. Science. 1996 July 5; 273(5271):59-63. **Key Finding:** "Restriction of caloric intake lowers steady-state levels of **oxidative stress** and damage, retards age-associated changes, and extends the maximum **life-span** in mammals."

Multiple sclerosis

Chronic calorie restriction attenuates experimental autoimmune encephalomyelitis. Piccio L, Stark JL, Cross AH. J Leukoc Biol. 2008;84:940-8. **Key Finding:** "CR induces multiple metabolic and physiologic modifications, including **anti-inflammatory, antioxidant, and neuroprotective effects** that may be beneficial in **multiple sclerosis**. The CR-induced hormonal, metabolic and cytokine changes observed in our studies suggest a combined anti-inflammatory and neuroprotective effect. CR with adequate nutrition and careful medical monitoring should be explored as a potential treatment for MS."

Neurodegenerative disorders (in general)

Potential therapeutic targets for **neurodegenerative diseases**: *lessons learned from calorie restriction.* Duan W, Ross CA. Curr Drug Targets. 2010 Oct;11(10):1281-92. **Key Finding**: "This review summarizes the evidence on key biological mechanisms underlying the beneficial effects of caloric restriction based on our current understanding, with particular emphasis on the recent impact of CR on neuroprotection."

A calorie-restricted diet decreases brain iron accumulation and preserves **motor performance** *in old rhesus monkeys.* Kastman EK, Willette AA, Coe CL, et al. J Neurosci. 2010 Jun 9;30(23):7940-7. **Key Finding**: "Our observations suggest that the caloric restriction-induced benefit of reduced iron deposition and preserved motor function may indicate neural protection similar to effects described previously in aging rodent and primate species."

Short-term fasting induces profound neuronal autophagy. Alirezael M, Kemball CC, Flynn CT, et al. Autophagy. 2010 Aug 16;6(6):702-10. **Key Finding**: "Disruption of autophagy—a key homeostatic process in which cytosotic components are degraded and recycled through lysosomes—can cause **neurodegeneration** in tissue culture and in vivo. Upregulation of this pathway may be neuroprotective. One well-recognized way of inducing autophagy is by food restriction, which upregulates autophagy. Our data lead us to speculate that sporadic fasting might represent a simple, safe and inexpensive means to promote this potentially therapeutic neuronal response."

Chronic caloric restriction reduces tissue damage and improves **spatial memory** *in a rat model of traumatic brain injury.* Rich NJ. Van Landingham JW, Figueiroa S, et al. J Neurosci Res. 2010 Oct;88(13):2933-9. **Key Finding**: "Although it has been known for some time that chronic caloric or dietary restriction reduces the risk of neurodegenerative disorders and injury following ischemia, the possible role of chronic restriction in improving outcomes after traumatic brain injury has not been previously studied. In our study using male Sprague-Dawley rats, not only did caloric restriction decrease the size of the cortical lesion after injury, there were marked improvements in spatial memory."

Cellular stress responses: a novel target for chemoprevention and nutritional neuroprotection in aging, neurodegenerative disorders and longevity. Calabrese V, Cornelius C, Mancuso C, et al. Neurochem Res. 2008 Dec;33(12):2444-71. **Key Finding:** "In this review the importance of vitagenes in the cellular stress response and the potential use of dietary **antioxidants** in the prevention and treatment of **neurodegenerative disorders** is discussed."

*Intermittent fasting dissociates beneficial effects of dietary restriction on **glucose metabolism** and **neuronal resistance** to injury from calorie intake.* Anson RM, Guo Z, de Cabo R, et al. Proc Natl Acad Sci. 2003 May 13;100(10):6216-20. **Key Finding:** "Intermittent fasting (in mice) resulted in beneficial effects that met or exceeded those of caloric restriction including reduced serum glucose and insulin levels and increased resistance of neurons in the brain to excitotoxic stress."

Obesity

Do calorie restriction or alternate-day fasting regimens modulate adipose tissue physiology in a way that reduces chronic disease risk? Varady KA, Hellerstein MK. Nutr Rev. 2008 Jun;66(6):333-42. **Key Finding:** This review summarizes the effects of calorie restriction and alternate-day fasting regimens on parameters of adipose physiology which plays a role in **obesity-related disorders**. Both CR and ADF have been shown to decrease the risk of these disorders.

Calorie restriction in biosphere 2: alterations in physiologic, hematologic, hormonal and biochemical parameters in humans restricted for a 2-year period. Walford RL, Mock D, Verdery R, Maccallum T. J Gerontol A Biol Sci Med Sci. 2002 Jun;57(6):8211-24. **Key Finding:** "We conclude that healthy non-obese humans on a low-calorie, nutrient-dense diet show physiologic, hematologic, hormonal, and biochemical changes resembling those of rodents and monkeys on such diets. With regard to the health of humans on such a diet, we observed that despite the selective restriction in calories and marked **weight loss**, all crew members remained in excellent **health** and sustained a high level of physical and mental activity throughout the entire 2 years."

Pain (chronic)

Prolonged fasting as a method of mood enhancement in ***chronic pain*** *syndromes: a review of clinical evidence and mechanisms.* Michalesen A. Curr Pain Headache Rep. 2010 Apr;14(2):80-7. **Key Finding**: "The beneficial claims of fasting are supported by experimental research, which has found fasting to be associated with increased brain available serotonin, endogenous opioids, and endocannabinoids. Fasting-induced neuroendocrine activation and mild cellular stress responses with increased production of neurotrophic factors may also contribute to the mood enhancement of fasting. Fasting treatments may be useful as an adjunctive therapeutic approach in chronic pain patients."

Parkinson's disease

Caloric restriction increases neurotrophic factor levels and attenuates neurochemical and behavioral deficits in a primate model of Parkinson's disease. Maswood N, Young J, Tilmont E, et al. Proc Natl Acad Sci. 2004 Dec 26;101(52):17887-8. **Key Finding:** "We report that a low-calorie diet can lessen the severity of neurochemical deficits and motor dysfunction in a primate model of **Parkinson's disease.**"

CHAPTER FOUR

Nutrient Retention and Health Benefits of Raw vs. Cooked or Processed Vegetables

SINCE 1956, THE HIPPOCRATES HEALTH INSTITUTE and a few other organizations worldwide have maintained that an uncooked, organic, plant-based diet is the most effective path to superior health. Although we have conducted hundreds of our own in-house observational studies on thousands of individuals that affirm this core principle, we are pleased to embrace the scientific data that has now emerged to support our findings.

As our understanding evolves about the destructive nature of high heat on the living cells of plants, we also see the many chemical changes that occur causing dramatic reductions in nutritional levels. There is also accumulating evidence that newly formed toxic compounds created through the cooking process act to weaken the immune systems of people consuming cooked food.

Our ongoing clinical research spotlights the value that unprocessed vegan varieties of fare have on every bodily system. What has emerged is the very real possibility that there are even more elements within these foods that have yet to be identified. Proteins, vitamins, minerals and trace minerals, essential fatty acids, and phytochemicals will someday have additional members added to their illustrious group.

The health benefits of raw foods have been obvious to us since the Hippocrates Health Institute was founded more than a half-century ago. Hundreds of case studies can be cited. Here are two illustrative ones.

In 2006, Anna Lindstrom of Uppsala, Sweden, experienced what at first seemed to be a simple eye infection. Penicillin cleared up the infection within a week, but her health got much worse and she was bedridden for a month. It was severe reactive arthritis, an autoimmune disorder, attacking her immune system and degenerating the cartilage in her joints, even though she was just in her 20s.

For the next two years Anna took steroids and painkillers, yet her symptoms got progressively worse. The paralyzing pain affected her feet to her knees, hip, and back. In March 2007, she decided to try a new approach. She became a vegan, consuming raw living foods, which started relieving her symptoms right away.

As Anna describes it: "I was able to stop taking the prescription drugs. I continued eating raw foods and when my doctors looked at my blood work, they were amazed and impressed by the results. I remember one of my doctors had said that my condition was chronic, and that I would have to increase the dosage of my medication each year. It's now been three years since then and I am medication-free and feel great! Prior to changing my diet, I couldn't do anything physical. Now I can do practically anything again. A diet based on living foods is the main reason I completely eliminated the pain medications and prescriptions drugs."

The second case involves Sherrie Clark, who received a diagnosis of non-Hodgkin, lymphoma in 1998, when she was 22. After removing a five-pound tumor from her abdomen, her physicians told her, "Go home, enjoy your life. Right now it seems we got it all, but it will be back with a vengeance." She was given less than a decade to live.

The cancer returned seven years later. This time, the surgeons who opened up Sherrie's abdomen decided that removing the cancerous tumors was too risky, and they sewed her back up. Over the next few months, the cancer in her abdomen continued to grow. In the face of a grim prognosis, Sherrie decided to try a raw organic diet.

She relates what happened: "After coming home from three weeks at the Hippocrates Health Institute, I adopted this lifestyle and continued to feed my body the raw vegan foods it craves. I had another PET scan two months later. When I received my results, my doctor was speechless. How could I go from having lymphomas all over my body to having all my tumors shrink to half their size and in some areas, be completely gone? My doctor applauded me for making the decision to skip his conventional treatment and go out on my own."

In summarizing the themes of findings described in the studies presented on the following pages, two really good reasons for eating raw (uncooked) plant foods emerge. First, raw food contains much higher levels of nutrients than cooked or processed foods, and higher nutrient levels mean a greater capacity to heal the body and prevent disease. Second, cooked food can create and release toxins harmful to health. Frying foods at high temperatures using vegetable oils or lard, for example, produces fumes that have been labeled "probably carcinogenic" by the International Agency for Research on Cancer. By avoiding these carcinogens in cooked food, and supplying the body with high levels of pure quality nutrients instead, health and healing become more possible.

Nutrient Losses From Cooking and Processing

Effect of different **cooking methods** *on color, phytochemical concentration, and antioxidant capacity of raw and frozen brassica vegetables.* Pellegrini N, Chiavaro E, Gardana C, et al. J Agric Food Chem. 2010 Apr 14;58(7):4310-21. **Key Finding:** "This study evaluated the effect of common cooking practices (i.e., boiling, microwaving, and basket and oven steaming) on the phytochemical contents, total antioxidant capacity, and color changes of three generally consumed brassica vegetables analyzed fresh and frozen. Among cooking procedures, boiling determined an increase of fresh broccoli carotenoids and fresh brussels sprout polyphenols, whereas a decrease of almost all other phytochemicals in fresh and frozen samples was observed. During all cooking procedures, ascorbic acid was lost in great amount from all vegetables. The overall results of this study demonstrate that fresh brassica vegetables retain phytochemicals and total antioxidant capacity better than frozen samples."

Nutritional composition, phenolic compounds, nitrate content in eatable vegetables obtained by conventional and certified organic grown culture subject to thermal treatment. Lima GP, Lopez TVC, Rossetto MRM, Vianello F. Int J Food Sci Tech. 2009 Jun;44:6. **Key Finding:** "Cooking in boiling water seems to have a dramatic effect on phenolic content on both kinds (organic and non-organic) of Chinese cabbage, and, as a consequence, on **antioxidant** activity."

Influence of cooking methods on **antioxidant** *activity of vegetables.* Jimenez-Monreal AM, Garcia-Diz L, Martinez-Tome M, Mariscal M, Murcia MA. J Food Sci. 2009 Apr;74(3):H97-103. **Key Finding:** "The antioxidant activity of vegetables has been evaluated in 20 vegetables. Artichoke was the only vegetable that kept its very high scavenging-lipoperoxyl radical capacity in all the cooking methods. The highest losses of LOO scavenging capacity were observed in cauliflower after boiling and microwaving; pea after boiling; and zucchini after boiling and frying. Beetroot, green bean, and garlic kept their antioxidant activity after most cooking treatments. Swiss chard and pepper lost OH scavenging capacity in all the processes. In short, water is not the cook's best friend when it comes to preparing vegetables."

Effects of different cooking methods on health-promoting compounds of broccoli. Yuan GF, Sun B, Yuan J, Wang QM. J Zhejiang Univ Sci B (Chinese). 2009 Aug;10(8):580-8. **Key Finding:** "The effects of five domestic cooking methods, including steaming, microwaving, boiling, stir-frying and stir-frying followed by boiling, on the nutrients and health-promoting compounds of broccoli were investigated. The results show that all cooking treatments, except steaming, caused significant losses of chlorophyll and vitamin C and significant decreases of total soluble proteins and soluble sugars. Steaming appears the best cooking method in retention of the nutrients in cooking broccoli."

Influence of cooking duration of cabbage and presence of colonic microbiota on the excretion of N-acetylcysteine conjugates of allyl isothiocyanate and bioactivity of phase 2 enzymes in F344 rats. Rungapamestry V, Rabot S, Fuller Z, Ratcliffe B, Duncan AJ. Br J Nutr. 2008 Apr;99(4):773-81. **Key Finding:** "Isothiocyanates have been implicated in the **cancer**-protective effects of brassica vegetables. When cabbage is consumed, sinigrin is hydrolysed by plant or microbial myroinase partly to allyl isothiocyanate, which is mainly excreted as N-acetylcysteine conjugates of AITC in urine. The effect of cooking cabbage on the excretion of NAC of AITC in rat liver and colon was investigated. When plant myrosinase was present, excretion of NAC of AITC/24 h was increased by 1.4 and 2.5 times by the additional presence of microbial myrosinase after consumption of raw and lightly cooked cabbage, respectively. When plant myrosinase was absent, as after consumption of fully cooked cabbage, excretion of the AITC conjugate was almost zero in rats."

Total phenolics, phenolic acids, isoflavones, and anthocyanins and antioxidant properties of yellow and black **soybeans** *as affected by* **thermal processing**. Xu B,

Chang SK. J Agric Food Chem. 2008 Aug 27;56(16):7165-75. **Key Finding**: "As compared to the raw soybeans, all processing methods caused significant decreases in total phenolic content, total flavonoid content, condensed tannin content, monomeric anthocyanin content, free radical scavenging activity, ferric reducing antioxidant power, and oxygen radical absorbing capacity."

Kinetics of changes in glucosinolate concentrations during long-term cooking of white cabbage (Brassica oleracea L. ssp. Capitata f. alba). Volden J, Wicklund T, Verkerk R, Dekker M. J Agric Food Chem. 2008 Mar 26;56(6):2068-73. **Key Finding:** "Cabbage was boiled, resulting in a dramatic decrease of 56% in the total glucosinolate levels within the plant matrix during the first 2 min. After 8-12 min of boiling, the decrease progressed to over 70% loss. Identification of the kinetics of decline of glucosinolates during cooking can aid in designing processing and preparation methods and determining the conditions for the optimal effects of ingestion of brassicaceae toward **cancer** prevention."

*The influence of **processing and preservation** on the retention of health-promoting compounds in **broccoli**.* Galgano F, Favati F, Caruso M, Pietrafesa A, Natella S. J Food Sc. 2007 Mar;72(2):S130-5. **Key Finding:** "When chilled at 6 degrees C and 95% R.H. for 35 d, broccoli showed a vitamin C and sufloraphane loss of about 39% and 29%, respectively. Boiling and steaming caused significant vitamin C losses, 34% and 22%, respectively."

*Effects of **microwave cooking** conditions on bioactive compounds present in **broccoli** inflorescenes.* Lopez-Berenguer C, Carvajal M, Moreno DA, Garcia-Viguera C. J Agric Food Chem. 2007 Nov 28;55(24):10001-7. **Key Finding**: "Cooking considerably affects the health-promoting compounds of brassica vegetables, specifically glucosinolates, phenolic compounds, minerals, and vitamin C studied here. The results of microwave cooking show a general decrease in the levels of all the studied compounds, except for mineral nutrients which were stable under all cooking conditions. Vitamin C showed the greatest losses mainly because of degradation and leaching. The longest microwave cooking time and the higher volume of cooking water should be avoided to minimize losses of nutrients."

*Thermal degradation of **onion** quercetin glucosides under roasting conditions.* Rohn S, Buchner N, Driemel G, Rauser M, Kroh LW. J Agric Food Chem. 2007 Feb 21;55(4):1568-73. **Key Finding**: "In this study, the stability of selected model and onion quercetin glycosides under roasting conditions (180 degrees C) was determined. The thermal treatment led to a degradation of the quercetin glycosides."

Effect of cooking brassica vegetables on the subsequent hydrolysis and metabolic fate of glucosinolates. Rungapamestry V, Duncan AJ, Fuller Z, Ratcliffe B. Proc Nutr Soc. 2007 Feb;66(1):69-81. **Key Finding:** "Isothiocyanates are one of the main groups of metabolites of glucosinolates and are implicated in the preventive effect against **cancer.** During cooking of brassica the glucosinolate-myrosinase system may be modified as a result of inactivation of plant myrosinase, loss of enzymic cofactors such as epithiospecifier protein, thermal breakdown and/or leaching of glucosinolates and their metabolites or volatilization of metabolites. Cooking brassica affects the site of release of breakdown products of glucosinolates, which is the upper gastrointestinal tract following consumption of raw brassica containing active plant myrosinase. After consumption of cooked brassica devoid of plant myrosinase, glucosinolates are hydrolysed in the colon under the action of the resident microflora. Feeding trials with humans subjects have shown that hydrolysis of glucosinolates and absorption of isothiocyanates are greater following ingestion of raw brassica with active plant myrosinase than after consumption of the cooked plant with denatured myrosinase. These sources of variation may partly explain the weak epidemiological evidence relating consumption of brassica to prevention against **cancer**. An understanding of the biochemical changes occurring during cooking and ingestion of brassica may help in the design of more robust epidemiological studies to better evaluate the protective effects of brassica against cancer."

Effect of storage, processing and cooking on glucosinolate content of brassica vegetables. Song L, Thornalley PJ. Food Chem Toxicol. 2007 Feb;45(2):216-24. **Key Finding:** "Bioavailability of glucosinolates and related isothiocyanates are influenced by storage and culinary processing of brassica vegetables. In this work, the content of the 7 major glucosinolates in broccoli, Brussels sprouts, cauliflower and green cabbage and their stability under different storage and cooking conditions is examined. Vegetables shredded finely showed a marked decline of glucosinolate level with post-shredding dwell time, up to 75% over 6 hours. Boiling showed significant losses by leaching into cooking water. Increased bioavailability of dietary isothiocyanates may be achieved by avoiding boiling of vegetables."

Effect of meal composition and cooking duration on the fate of sulforaphane following consumption of broccoli by healthy human subjects. Rungapamestry V, Duncan AJ, Fuller Z, Ratcliffe B. Br J Nutr. 2007 Apr;97(4):644-52. **Key Finding:** "The isothiocyanate, sulforaphane, has been implicated in the **cancer**-protective effects of brassica vegetables. When broccoli is consumed, sulforaphane is released from hydrolysis of glucoraphanin by plant myrosinase and/or colonic microbiota. The estimated yield of sulforaphane in vivo was about 3-fold higher after consumption of lightly cooked broccoli than fully cooked broccoli."

Changes in the content of health-promoting compounds and antioxidant activity of **broccoli** *after domestic processing.* Gliszczyńska-Swiglo A, Ciska E, Pawlak-Lemańska K, et al. Food Addit Contam. 2006 Nov;23(11):1088-98. **Key Finding**: "The effect of water- and steam-cooking on the content of vitamin C, polyphenols, carotenoids, tocopherols and glucosinolates, as well as on the antioxidant activity of broccoli, are reported. The results indicated that steam-cooking of broccoli results in an increase in polyphenols, as well as the main glucosinolates and their total content as compared with fresh broccoli, whereas cooking in water has the opposite effect."

Thermal degradation and leaching of vitamin C from green peas during processing. Lathrop PJ, Leung HK. J Food Sci. 2006;45(4):995-8. **Key Finding:** "Approximately two-thirds of the original vitamin C in fresh peas was lost during processing."

The ascorbic acid content of Nigerian vegetables. Oke OL. J Food Sci. 2006;32(1):85-86. **Key Finding:** "On boiling, 46%-68% of the ascorbic acid of Nigerian vegetables is lost."

Loss of amino acids and water soluble vitamins during potato processing. Sullivan JF, Kozempel MF, Egoville MJ, Talley EA. J Food Sci. 2006;50(5):1249-53. **Key Finding:** Processing potatoes almost totally eradicated ascorbic acid and about 50% of the original amount of riboflavin and niacin.

Effect of soaking temperature on cooking and nutritional quality of beans. Kon S. J Food Sci. 2006;44(5):1329-35. **Key Finding:** "California small white beans were soaked at different temperatures in 10 degree increments, from 20 degrees to 90 degrees. Three water-soluble vitamins (thiamin, riboflavin and niacin) were measured and losses were found to be very small at soaking temperatures up to 50 degrees. An increase in those losses of from three- to fourfold was found when the soaking temperature was raised to 60 degrees Centigrade or above."

*Comparison of the bioactive compounds and antioxidant potentials of fresh and cooked Polish, Ukrainian, and Israeli **garlic**.* Gorinstein S, Drzewiecki J, Leontowicz H, et al. J Agric Food Chem. 2005 Apr 6;53(7):2726-32. **Key Finding**: "It was observed that the bioactive compounds, antioxidant potential, and proteins in garlic decrease significantly after 20 min of cooking at 100 degrees C."

*Investigation of the **antioxidant** properties of tomatoes after processing.* Sahlin E, Savage GP, Lister CE. J Food Comp Analysis. 2004 Oct;17(5):635-647. **Key Finding:** "Boiling and baking has a relatively small effect on the ascorbic, total phenolic, lycopene and antioxidant activity of the two tomato cultivars, while frying significantly reduced the ascorbic, total phenolic and lycopene contents of the two cultivars."

***Antioxidant** capacity and phenolic content in leaf extracts of tree spinach.* Kuti JO, Konuru HB. J Agric Food Chem. 2004;52(1):117-21. **Key Finding:** "Cooking reduced antioxidant activity and phenolic content and resulted in losses of some kaempferol glycoside and quercetin glycoside residues in leaf extracts."

Influence of antioxidant spices on the retention of B-carotene in vegetables during domestic cooking processes. Gayathri GN, Platel K, Prakash J, Srinivasan K. Food Chem. 2004 Jan;84(1):35-43. **Key Finding:** "Considerable amounts of B-carotene were lost during the two domestic methods of cooking commonly used, namely, pressure cooking and open pan boiling, the loss ranging from 27% to 71% during pressure cooking and 16% to 67% during boiling for the four green leafy vegetables examined in this study."

Hydrolysis of glucosinolates to isothiocyanates after ingestion of raw or microwaved cabbage by human volunteers. Rouzaud G, Young SA, Duncan AJ. Cancer Epidemiol Biomarkers Prev. 2004 Jan;13:125-131. **Key Finding:** "Cabbage contains the glucosinolate sinigrin, which is hydrolyzed by myrosinase to allyl isothiocyanate, which are thought to inhibit the development of cancer cells by a number of mechanisms. The effect of cooking cabbage on isothiocyanate production from glucosinolates during and after their ingestion was examined in human subjects. Each of 12 healthy human volunteers consumed three meals, at 48-hr intervals, containing either raw cabbage, cooked cabbage, or mustard, according to a cross-over design. The results indicate that isothiocyanate production is more extensive after consumption of raw vegetables."

*Effects of boiling on the antihypertensive and **antioxidant** activities of onion.* Kawamoto E, Saki Y, Okamura Y, Yamamoto Y. J Nutr Sci Vitaminol (Tokyo). 2004 Jun;50(3):171-6. **Key Finding**: "Our results suggested that the anti-hypertensive activity of onion disappeared during boiling, and the disappearance of the antihypertensive activity of raw onion after boiling might come, in part, from a decrease of the antioxidative activity of onion, with a consequent reduction in the saving of nitric oxide. The antihypertensive effect of boiled onion was not found and the antioxidant activity of it was much weaker than that of raw onion. Raw onion significantly reduced the increase in systolic blood pressure in hypertensive rats and inhibited the increase in thiobarbituric acid-reactive substances."

Influence of cooking process on phenolic marker compounds of vegetables. Andlauer W, Stumpf C, Hubert M, Rings A, Furst P. Int J Vitam Nutr Res. 2003 Mar;73(2):152-9. **Key Finding:** "Until now, little is known about alterations of phenolic compounds content by the cooking process. In the present study, the influence of different volumes of cooking water on the amount of selected phenolic marker compounds resting in the vegetables was assessed. The cooking of zucchini, beans and carrots with smaller amounts of water resulted in significant higher content of phenolic phytochemicals in the vegetables compared to cooking with larger water volumes. For potatoes, which showed great variations in content of phenolic acids after cooking, no significant differences in phenolic acids was observed. It can be concluded from these observations that real intakes of phenolic compounds from cooked vegetables are lower and that the amounts consumed are therefore overestimated."

Health-promoting compounds in **broccoli** *as influenced by refrigerated transport and retail sale period.* Vallejo F, Tomas-Barberan F, Garcia-Viguera C. J Agric Food Chem. 2003 May 7;51(10):3029-34. **Key Finding**: "Results showed major losses of total aliphatic and indole glucosinolates, phenolic compounds, and vitamin C at the end of both periods (transport and cold storage), in comparison to broccoli at harvest. Thus, the respective losses, at the end of cold storage and retail periods, were 71% to 80% of total glucosinolates, 62% to 59% of total flavonoids, 51% to 44% of sinapic acid derivatives, and 73% to 74% caffeoyl-quinic acid derivatives. Distribution and retail periods had minimal effects on vitamin C."

Overview of dietary flavonoids: nomenclature, occurrence and intake. Beecher GR. Am Soc Nutr Sci. 2003 Oct;133:3248-54S. **Key Finding:** "The polyphenolic structure of flavonoids and tannins renders them quite sensitive to oxidative enzymes and cooking conditions."

Nutrient and antinutrient contents in raw and cooked young leaves and immature pods of Moringa oleifera. Gidamis B, Panga JT, Sawatt SV, Chove BE, Shayo NB. Ecol Food Nutr. 2003;42(6):399-411. **Key Finding:** "Cooking caused significant reductions in the contents of crude protein, crude fiber, ether extracts, ash, ascorbic acid, and B-carotene in the leaves and pods."

Potential of commonly consumed green leafy vegetables for their **antioxidant** *capacity and its linkage with the micronutrient profile.* Tarwadi K, Agte V. Int J Food Sci Nutr. 2003 Nov;54(6):417-25. **Key Finding:** "Differences between raw and cooked values were highly significant for all the three indices. The super oxide scavenging ability values exhibited large variation with significantly higher values in the raw state than the cooked state."

The effect of different cooking methods on folate retention in various foods that are amongst the major contributors to folate intake in the UK diet. McKillop DJ, Pentieva K, Daly D, et al. Br J Nutr. 2002;88:681-8. **Key Finding:** "Boiling for typical time periods resulted in only 49% retention of folate in spinach and only 44% in broccoli. Steaming of spinach or broccoli, in contrast, resulted in no significant decrease in folate content."

Effects of processing and cooking on ascorbic acid content of chickpea varieties. Sood M, Malhotra SR. J Sci Food Agric. 2001;82(1):65-68. **Key Finding:** "It was found that the ascorbic acid content of both varieties of chickpea decreased after all treatments (cooking and processing) except germination."

The influence of **heating** *on the* **anticancer properties of garlic.** Song K, Milner JA. J Nutr. 2001 Mar;131(3s):1054-7S. **Key Finding**: "Heating has a negative influence on the beneficial pharmacologic properties of garlic. We recently conducted several studies to investigate the influence of microwave or oven heating on the anticarcinogenesis property of garlic. Our studies showed that as little as 60 seconds of microwave heating or 45 minutes of oven heating can block garlic's ability to inhibit in vivo binding of mammary carcinogen metabolite in rat mammary epithelial cell DNA. These studies suggest that heating destroyed garlic's active allyl sulfur compound formation, which may relate to its anticancer properties."

Disposition of glucosinolates and sulforaphane in humans after ingestion of steamed and fresh **broccoli.** Conaway CC, Getahun SM, Liebes LL, et al. Nutr Cancer. 2000;38(2):168-78. **Key Finding:** "In this study the metabolic fate of glucosinolates after ingestion of steamed and fresh broccoli was compared in 12 male subjects in a crossover design. Results of this study indicate that the bioavailability of ITCs from fresh broccoli is approximately three times greater than that from cooked broccoli. Considering the cancer-chemopreventive potential of ITCs, cooking broccoli may markedly reduce its beneficial effects on health."

Vitamin C *losses in some frozen vegetables due to various cooking methods.* Nursai B, Yucecan S. Nahrung (Turkey). 2000 Dec;44(6):451-3. **Key Finding**: "While boiling **spinach, peas, green beans, and okra** without thawing resulted in 46.5%, 25.2%, 18.2% and 21.6% vitamin C loss in double based stainless steel pan, boiling them in Pyrex pan resulted in 58.5%, 36.0%, 42.1%, and 28.2% vitamin C loss, respectively."

Effect of raw versus boiled aqueous extract of **garlic and onion** *on platelet aggregation.* Ali M, Bordia T, Mustafa T. Prostaglandins Leukot Essent Fatty Acids. 1999 Jan;60(1):43-7. **Key Finding**: "The results of this study show that garlic is about 13 times more potent than onion in inhibiting platelet aggregation and suggest that garlic and onion could be more potent inhibitors of blood platelet aggregation if consumed in **raw** than in cooked or boiled form."

Heating **garlic** *inhibits its ability to suppress 7,12-dimethylbenz(a)anthracene-induced DNA adduct formation in rat mammary tissue.* Song K, Milner JA. J Nutr. 1999 Mar;129(3):657-61. **Key Finding:** This study examined the impact of heating by microwave or convection oven on the protection provided by garlic against DMBA-induced adduct formation. "Microwave heating of garlic for 30 s resulted in a 90% loss of alliinase activity. Heating in a convection oven also completely blocked the ability of uncrushed garlic to retard DMBA bioactivation."

Effect of processing on major flavonoids in processed onions, green beans, and peas. Ewald C, Fjelkner-Modig S, Johansson K, Sjoholm I, Akesson B. Food Chem. 1999 Feb;64(2):231-6. **Key Finding:** "The greatest loss of flavonoids in onion took place during the pre-processing step where the onion was peeled, trimmed, and chopped before blanching. Blanched onion contained 25 mg quercetin and 0.35 mg kaempferol per 100 g edible part. Blanched green beans contained 1.3 mg quercetin and 0.24 mg kaempferol per 100 g. and blanched peas only 0.15 mg quercetin per 100 g. Further cooking, frying or warm-holding for up to 2 h of the blanched vegetables did not influence the flavonoid content."

Evaluation of total carotenoids and B-carotene in carrots during home processing. Pinheiro-Santana HM, Stringheta PC, Brandao CC, Paez HH, Queiroz VMV. *Ciênc* Tecnol Aliment. 1998 Jan/Apr;18(1):39-44. **Key Finding:** "The retention of the analyzed carotenoids ranged from 60.13% to 85.64%; water cooking without pressure promoted higher retention levels of a- and b-carotene and Vitamin A values, while water cooking with pressure promoted higher retention levels of total carotenoids."

Nutrient losses and gain during frying: a review. Fillion L, Henry CJK. Int J Food Sci Nutr. 1998 Mar;49(2):157-68. **Key Finding:** "Some unsaturated fatty acids and antioxidant vitamins are lost due to oxidation during frying, though the high temperature and short transit time of the frying process causes less loss of heat labile vitamins than other types of cooking."

Nutrients and antinutritional factors in faba beans as affected by processing. Vidal-Valverde C, Frias J, Sotomayor C, et al. Zeitschrift fur Lebensmittelunter-suchungund-Forschung A (Germany). 1998 Aug;207(2):140-5. **Key Finding:** "Of all the treatments studied (including cooking and dry-heating) germination appears to be the best processing method to obtain nutritive faba bean flour."

Absorption of lycopene from single or daily portions of raw and processed **tomato.** Porrini M, Riso P, Tesolin G. Br J Nutr. 1998 Oct;80(4):353-61. **Key Finding:** "Plasma total lycopene concentration was higher after the tomato puree intake than after the raw tomato in both the first and second experiments, demonstrating a significant effect of food matrix on absorption."

Effect of traditional processing practices on the content of total carotenoid, B-carotene, a-carotene and vitamin A activity of selected Tanzanian vegetables. Mosha TC, Pace RD, Adeyeye S, Laswai HS, Mtebe K. Plant Foods Hum Nutr. 1997 Sep;50(3):189-201. **Key Finding:** "Conventional blanching and cooking resulted in a significant (p<0.05) increase in the concentration of carotenoids in the cowpea, peanut and pumpkin leaves while in amaranth and sweet potato greens, thermal processing resulted in a significant (p<0.05) decrease in the concentration of these nutrients."

Vitamin retention in cook/chill and cook/hot-hold hospital food services. Williams PG. J Am Dietetic Assoc. 1996 May;96(5):490-8. **Key Finding:** "The vitamins with the greatest losses during the hot-holding of food are vitamin C, folate, and vitamin B-6. Losses of vitamin C and folate can be greater than 30% when food is reheated after storage."

Effect of home processing on ascorbic acid and B-carotene content of spinach and amaranth leaves. Yadaz SK, Sehgal S. Plant Foods for Human Nutrition. 1995 Feb;47(2):125-131. **Key Finding:** "A markedly greater reduction in ascorbic acid and B-carotene was observed in cooked leaves."

Investigations on the effect of traditional food processing, preservation and storage methods on vegetable nutrients: a case study in Tanzania. Lyimo MH. Nyagwegwe S. Mnkeni AP. Plant Foods Hum Nutr. 1991 Jan;41(1):53-7. **Key Finding:** "Traditional cooking method for 90 min for cassava, 50 min for pumpkin and mwage leaves resulted in significant losses in protein, fats and vitamins.

Traditional methods for processing of vegetables cause significant losses of nutrients, an effect that could account for poor nutritional status."

Antinutrients in amphidiploids (black gram, mung bean): varietal differences and effect of domestic processing and cooking. Kataria A, Chauhan BM, Punia D. Plant Foods Hum Nutr. 1989 Sep; 39(3):257-66. **Key Finding:** "Domestic processing and cooking methods, ordinary and pressure cooking of soaked and unsoaked seeds, and sprouting significantly lowered phytic acid, saponin and polyphenol contents of the amphidiploids seeds."

Reversed phase HPLC analysis of alpha- and beta-carotene from selected raw and cooked vegetables. Dietz JM, Sri Kantha S, Erdman JW Jr. Plant Foods Hum Nutr. 1988;38(4):333-41. **Key Finding:** "The vegetables lettuce, spinach and winged bean and carrot root were boiled or steamed. Boiling for 30 minutes resulted in a 53% and 40% loss of beta-carotene from lettuce and carrots, respectively. Full retention or even an increase in beta-carotene content in boiled winged bean leaves and spinach was noted. Steaming resulted in very good retention of alpha- and beta-carotene in all vegetables (83%-139% retention.)"

Retention of vitamins in fresh and frozen broccoli prepared by different cooking methods. Hudson DE, Dalal AA, LaChance PA. J Food Quality. 1985;8(1):45-50 . **Key Finding:** "Fresh and frozen broccoli were analyzed for retention of ascorbic acid, riboflavin and thiamine by semi-automated fluorometry before and after steaming, boiling or microwave cooking for 5 min. Retention of vitamins in general was higher for fresh than for frozen broccoli. Boiled fresh samples retained least riboflavin and ascorbic acid, and microwaved samples the least thiamine."

Losses of vitamin C during the cooking of Swiss chard. Fenton F, Tressler DK, Camp SC, King CG. J Nutr. May 24, 1937: 207. **Key Finding:** "The leaf portion of fresh raw Swiss Chard is a good source of vitamin C. About one-half of the original vitamin C passes into the cooking water by the method of cooking used. The so-called ascorbic acid oxidizing enzyme is very active in Swiss chard. The enzyme is inactivated during the first few minutes of cooking."

Losses of vitamin C during the cooking of peas. Fenton F, Tressler DK, King CG. J Nutr. March 11, 1936: 128. **Key Finding:** "About one-half of the vitamin C passes into cooking water during the cooking of peas. The greatest rate of loss of vitamin C from the peas occurred during the first 2 minutes of cooking."

Factors influencing the vitamin C content of vegetables. Tressler DK, Mack GL, King CG. Am J Pub Health. 1936 Sep; 905-9. **Key Finding:** "Preliminary cooking studies conducted on peas, snap beans, and cabbage indicate that a considerable proportion of the ascorbic acid passes into the water during the boiling of vegetables. In the case of snap beans, approximately one-third of the vitamin C dissolved in the cooking water in 20 minutes time."

Antioxidation

Nutritional composition, phenolic compounds, nitrate content in eatable vegetables obtained by conventional and certified organic grown culture subject to thermal treatment. Lima GP, Lopez TVC, Rossetto MRM, Vianello F. Int J Food Sci Tech. 2009 Jun;44:6. **Key Finding:** "Cooking in boiling water seems to have a dramatic effect on phenolic content on both kinds (organic and non-organic) of Chinese cabbage, and, as a consequence, on **antioxidant** activity."

*Influence of cooking methods on **antioxidant** activity of vegetables.* Jimenez-Monreal AM, Garcia-Diz L, Martinez-Tome M, Mariscal M, Murcia MA. J Food Sci. 2009 Apr;74(3):H97-103. **Key Finding:** "The antioxidant activity of vegetables has been evaluated in 20 vegetables. Artichoke was the only vegetable that kept its very high scavenging-lipoperoxyl radical capacity in all the cooking methods. The highest losses of LOO scavenging capacity were observed in cauliflower after boiling and microwaving; pea after boiling; and zucchini after boiling and frying. Beetroot, green bean, and garlic kept their antioxidant activity after most cooking treatments. Swiss chard and pepper lost OH scavenging capacity in all the processes. In short, water is not the cook's best friend when it comes to preparing vegetables."

Investigation of the **antioxidant** *properties of tomatoes after processing.* Sahlin E, Savage GP, Lister CE. J Food Comp Analysis. 2004 Oct;17(5):635-47. **Key Finding:** "Boiling and baking has a relatively small effect on the ascorbic, total phenolic, lycopene and antioxidant activity of the two tomato cultivars, while frying significantly reduced the ascorbic, total phenolic and lycopene contents of the two cultivars."

Antioxidant *capacity and phenolic content in leaf extracts of tree spinach.* Kuti JO, Konuru HB. J Agric Food Chem. 2004;52(1):117-21. **Key Finding:** "Cooking reduced antioxidant activity and phenolic content and resulted in losses of some kaempferol glycoside and quercetin glycoside residues in leaf extracts."

Effects of boiling on the antihypertensive and **antioxidant** *activities of onion.* Kawamoto E, Saki Y, Okamura Y, Yamamoto Y. J Nutr Sci Vitaminol (Tokyo). 2004 Jun;50(3):171-6. **Key Finding:** "Our results suggested that the anti-hypertensive activity of onion disappeared during boiling, and the disappearance of the antihypertensive activity of raw onion after boiling might come, in part, from a decrease of the antioxidative activity of onion, with a consequent reduction in the saving of nitric oxide. The antihypertensive effect of boiled onion was not found and the antioxidant activity of it was much weaker than that of raw onion. Raw onion significantly reduced the increase in systolic blood pressure in hypertensive rats and inhibited the increase in thiobarbituric acid-reactive substances."

Potential of commonly consumed green leafy vegetables for their **antioxidant** *capacity and its linkage with the micronutrient profile.* Tarwadi K, Agte V. Int J Food Sci Nutr. 2003 Nov;54(6):417-25. **Key Finding:** "Differences between raw and cooked values were highly significant for all the three indices. The super oxide scavenging ability values exhibited large variation with significantly higher values in the raw state than the cooked state."

Chemoprotective *glucosinolates and isothiocyanates of broccoli sprouts: metabolism and excretion in humans.* Shapiro TA, Fahey JW, Wade KL, Stephenson KK, Talalay P. Cancer Epidemiol Biomarkers Prev. 2001 May;10(5):

501-8. **Key Finding:** "Broccoli sprouts are a rich source of glucosinolates and isothiocyanates that induce phase 2 detoxication enzymes, boost **antioxidant** status, and protect animals against chemically induced **cancer**. When metabolized they are collectively designated dithiocarbamates. We studied the disposition of broccoli sprout glucosinolates and isothiocyanates in healthy volunteers. Dosing preparations included uncooked fresh sprouts (with active myrosinase) as well as boiled sprouts that were devoid of myrosinase activity. Dithiocarbamate excretion was higher when intact sprouts were chewed thoroughly rather than swallowed whole. Thorough chewing of fresh sprouts exposes the glucosinolates to plant myrosinase and significantly increases dithiocarbamate excretion."

*The **antioxidant** potential of the Mediterranean diet.* Ghiselli A, Amicis AD, Giacosa A. Eur J Cancer Prev. 1997;6(Suppl 1):S15-19. **Key Finding:** "The preference for fresh fruit and vegetables in the Mediterranean diet will result in a higher consumption of raw foods, a lower production of cooking-related oxidants and a consequent decreased waste of nutritional and endogenous **antioxidants**."

***Antioxidant** status in long-term adherents to a strict uncooked vegan diet.* Rauma AL, Torronen R, Hanninen O, Verhagen H, Mykkanen H. Am J Clin Nutr. 1995;62:1221-7. **Key Finding:** "The present data indicate that the living food diet provides significantly more dietary antioxidants than does the cooked, omnivorous diet, and that the long-term adherents to this diet have a better antioxidant status than do omnivorous control subjects."

Arthritis

*Divergent changes in serum sterols during a strict uncooked vegan diet in patients with **rheumatoid arthritis**.* Agren JJ, Tvrzicka E, Nenonen MT, Helve T, Hanninen O. Br J Nutr. 2001 Feb;85(2):137 9. **Key Finding:** "Serum total and **LDL-cholesterol** and -phopholipid concentrations were significantly decreased by the vegan diet. The levels of serum cholesterol and lathosterol also decreased."

Vegan diet in physiological health promotion. Hanninen O, Rauma AL, Kaartin-
en K, Nenonen M. Acta Physiol Hung. 1999;86(3-4):171-80. **Key Finding:** "We have performed a number of studies including dietary interventions and cross-sectional studies on subjects consuming uncooked vegan
food, called living food, consisting of germinated seeds, cereals, sprouts,
vegetables, fruits, berries and nuts. The subjects eating living food show
increased levels of carotenoids and vitamins C and E and lowered cholesterol concentration in their sera. The **rheumatoid arthritis** patients
eating the living foods diet reported amelioration of their pain and swelling of joints. The **fibromyalgic** subjects eating living foods lost weight
compared to their omnivorous controls. The results on their joint stiffness
and pain, on their quality of sleep, all improved. It appears that the adoption of vegan diet exemplified by the living food leads to a lessening of
several health risk factors to **cardiosvascular diseases** and **cancer**."

*Uncooked, lactobacilli-rich, vegan food and **rheumatoid arthritis**.* Nenonen
MT, Helve TA, Rauma AL, Hanninen OO. Br J Rheumatol. 1998
Mar;37(3):274-81. **Key Finding:** "We tested the effects of an uncooked
vegan diet, rich in lactobacilli, in rheumatoid patients randomized into
diet and control groups. The results showed that an uncooked vegan diet
decreased subjective symptoms of rheumatoid arthritis."

Atherosclerosis

*Shifting from conventional diet to an uncooked vegan diet reversibly alters serum lipid
and apolipoprotein levels.* Ling WH, Laitinen M, Hanninen O. Nutrition Research. 1992 Dec;12(12):1431-40. **Key Finding:** "Eighteen subjects were
randomly divided into test and control groups. In the test group, subjects
adopted the uncooked extreme vegan diet for one month and then resumed a conventional diet for a second month. Controls consumed a conventional diet throughout the study. Total serum cholesterol, triglyceride,
LDL, HDL cholesterol and apoliopoprotein AI as well as B decreased
significantly throughout the period of consuming the vegan diet. The results from this test group suggest that the uncooked extreme vegan diet
causes a significant decrease of the **atherosclerosis** risk factor."

Cancer (bladder, breast, colon, esophageal, gastric, leukemia, oral, pancreatic, thyroid, urothelial)

Dietary factors and the risks of **oesophageal adenocarcinoma** *and Barrett's oesophagus.* Kubo A, Corley DA, Jensen CD, Kaur R. Nutr Res Rev. 2010 Dec;23(2):230-46. **Key Finding**: Epidemiological evidence is strongest for an inverse relationship between intake of vitamin C, B-carotene, fruits and vegetables, particularly raw fruits and vegetables, and the risk of oesophageal adenocarcinoma and Barrett's oesophagus.

Intake of cruciferous vegetables modifies **bladder cancer** *survival.* Tang L, Zirpoli GR, Guru K, et al. Cancer Epidemiol Biomarkers Prev. 2010 Jul;19(7):1806-11. **Key Finding**: "A strong and significant inverse association was observed between bladder cancer mortality and broccoli intake, in particular, raw broccoli intake." The study was based on 239 bladder cancer patients with eight years of follow-up.

Food intake and the occurrence of **squamous cell carcinoma** *in different sections of the esophagus in Taiwanese men.* Chen YK, Lee CH, Wu IC, et al. Nutrition. 2009 Jul-Aug;25(7-8):753-61. **Key Finding:** "We found that intake of vegetables, raw onions and garlic, are significantly protective against esophageal squamous cell carcinoma risk, whereas intake of hot foods (cooked foods) can significantly increase its risk."

Greater vegetable and fruit intake is associated with a lower risk of **breast cancer** *among Chinese women.* Zhang CX, Ho SC, Chen YM, et al. Int J Cancer. 2009 Jul 1;125(1):181-8. **Key Finding:** In this case-control study, 438 cases were matched to 438 controls. Dietary intake was assessed by interviews. Total vegetable and fruit intake (including raw foods) was found to be inversely associated with breast cancer risk. Dark green leafy vegetables, cruciferous vegetables, carrots and tomatoes, banana, watermelon, papaya and cantaloupe were all inversely significantly related to breast cancer risk.

Influence of cooking duration of cabbage and presence of colonic microbiota on the excretion of N-acetylcysteine conjugates of allyl isothiocyanate and bioactivity of phase 2 enzymes in F344 rats. Rungapamestry V, Rabot S, Fuller Z, Ratcliffe B,

Duncan AJ. Br J Nutr. 2008 Apr;99(4):773-81. **Key Finding:** "Isothiocy-anates have been implicated in the **cancer**-protective effects of brassica vegetables. When cabbage is consumed, sinigrin is hydrolysed by plant or microbial myroinase partly to allyl isothiocyanate, which is mainly ex-creted as N-acetylcysteine conjugates of AITC in urine. The effect of cooking cabbage on the excretion of NAC of AITC in rat liver and co-lon was investigated. When plant myrosinase was present, excretion of NAC of AITC/24 h was increased by 1.4 and 2.5 times by the additional presence of microbial myrosinase after consumption of raw and lightly cooked cabbage respectively. When plant myrosinase was absent, as after consumption of fully cooked cabbage, excretion of the AITC conjugate was almost zero in rats."

Consumption of raw cruciferous vegetables is inversely associated with **bladder cancer risk**. Tang L, Zirpoli GR, Guru K, et al. Cancer Epidemiol Bio-markers Prev. 2008 Apr;17(4):938-44. **Key Finding:** "Cruciferous veg-etables contain isothiocyanates, which show potent chemopreventive ac-tivity against bladder cancer in both in vitro and in vivo studies. Cooking can substantially reduce or destroy isothiocyanates and this could account for epidemeliogic study inconsistencies. In this hospital-based case-con-trol study involving 275 individuals with incident primary bladder cancer and 825 individuals without cancer, we examined the usual prediagnostic intake of raw and cooked cruciferous vegetables in relation to bladder cancer risk. We observed a strong and statistically significant inverse asso-ciation between bladder cancer risk and raw cruciferous vegetable intake. There were no significant associations for fruit, total vegetables, or total cruciferous vegetables. These data suggest that cruciferous vegetables, when consumed raw, may reduce the risk of **bladder cancer**."

Kinetics of changes in glucosinolate concentrations during long-term cooking of white cabbage (Brassica oleracea L. ssp. Capitata f. alba). Volden J, Wicklund T, Verkerk R, Dekker M. J Agric Food Chem. 2008 Mar 26;56(6):2068-73. **Key Finding:** "Cabbage was boiled, resulting in a dramatic decrease of 56% in the total glucosinolate levels within the plant matrix during the first 2 min. After 8-12 min of boiling, the decrease progressed to over 70% loss. Identification of the kinetics of decline of glucosinolates during cooking can aid in designing processing and preparation methods and determining the conditions for the optimal effects of ingestion of brassicaceae toward **cancer** prevention."

*Dietary factors and breast **cancer** risk: a case control study among a population in Southern France.* Bessaoud F, Daures JP, Gerber M. Nutr Cancer. 2008;60(2):177-87. **Key Finding:** "One of two methods of measuring dietary intakes found a significant association related to the lowest consumption of raw vegetables and breast cancer risk. Breast cancer risk was also found to increase by 56% for each additional 100 g/day of meat consumption."

*Consumption of raw cruciferous vegetables is inversely associated with **bladder cancer** risk.* Tang L, Zirpoli GR, Guru K, et al. Cancer Epidemiol Biomarkers Prev. 2008 Apr;17(4):938-44. **Key Finding:** "This hospital-based case-control study involved 275 individuals with incent primary bladder cancer and 825 individuals without cancer. These data suggest that cruciferous vegetables, when consumed raw, may reduce the risk of bladder cancer, an effect consistent with the role of dietary isothiocyanates as chemopreventive agents against bladder cancer."

*Randomized comparison of cooked and noncooked diets in patients undergoing remission induction therapy for acute myeloid **leukemia**.* Gardner A, Mattiuzzi G, Faderl S, et al. J Clin Oncol. 2008 Dec 10;26(35):5684-8. **Key Finding:** "One hundred fifty-three patients receiving induction therapy for newly diagnosed acute myeloid leukemia were randomly assigned to a diet containing no raw fruits or vegetables (cooked diet) or to a diet containing fresh fruit and fresh vegetables (raw diet). All patients received antibacterial and antifungal prophylaxis. Twenty-nine percent of patients in the cooked group and 35% of patients in the raw group developed a major infection. Fever of unknown origin occurred in 51% of the cooked group and 36% of the raw group."

Giacomo Castelvetro's salads. Anti-HER2 oncogene nutraceuticals since the 17th century? Colomer R, Lupu R, Papadimitropoulou A, et al. Clin Transl Oncol. 2008 Jan;10(1):30-4. **Key Finding:** "Epidemiological and experimental studies begin to support the notion that 'The Sacred Law of Salads' (i.e., 'raw vegetables…plenty of generous olive oil') originally proposed in 1614 by Giacomo Castelvetro in his book 'The Fruits, Herbs & Vegetables of Italy' might be considered the first (unintended) example of customized diets for **breast cancer** prevention based on individual genetic make-up. A high consumption of raw vegetables and olive oil appears to exert a protective effect mostly confined to the HER2-positive breast cancer subtype. If early 1600s Castelvetro's salads can be used as dietary protocols capable to protect women against biologically aggressive HER2-positive breast cancer subtypes is an intriguing prospect that warrants evaluation in human pilot studies in the future."

Effect of cooking brassica vegetables on the subsequent hydrolysis and metabolic fate of glucosinolates. Rungapamestry V, Duncan AJ, Fuller Z, Ratcliffe B. Proc Nutr Soc. 2007 Feb;66(1):69-81. **Key Finding:** "Isothiocyanates are one of the main groups of metabolites of glucosinolates and are implicated in the preventive effect against **cancer.** During cooking of brassica the glucosinolate-myrosinase system may be modified as a result of inactivation of plant myrosinase, loss of enzymic cofactors such as epithiospheci-fier protein, thermal breakdown and/or leaching of glucosinolates and their metabolites or volatilization of metabolites. Cooking brassica affect the site of release of breakdown products of glucosinolates, which is the upper gastrointestinal tract following consumption of raw brassica containing active plant myrosinase. After consumption of cooked brassica devoid of plant myrosinase, glucosinolates are hydrolysed in the colon under the action of the resident microflora. Feeding trials with humans subjects have shown that hydrolysis of glucosinolates and absorption of isothiocyanates are greater following ingestion of raw brassica with active plant myrosinase than after consumption of the cooked plant with denatured myrosinase. These sources of variation may partly explain the weak epidemiological evidence relating consumption of brassica to prevention against **cancer.** An understanding of the biochemical changes occurring during cooking and ingestion of brassica may help in the design of more robust epidemiological studies to better evaluate the protective effects of brassica against cancer."

Salad vegetables dietary pattern protects against HER-2-positive **breast cancer:** *a prospective Italian study.* Sant M, Allemani C, Sieri S, et al. Int J Cancer. 2007 Aug 15;121(4):911-4. **Key Finding:** "We analyzed 8,861 volunteer women residents of the Varese Province, Italy. The salad vegetables dietary pattern (high consumption of raw vegetables and olive oil) had a protective effect against HER-2-positive cancers. This important finding that a salad vegetables dietary pattern protects mainly against a specific breast cancer subtype indicates that future studies on environmental/dietary risk factors should explicitly take account of the heterogenecity of breast cancer phenotypes."

Dietary factors and **oral cancer:** *a case-control study in Greater Metropolitan Sao Paulo, Brazil.* Marchioni DM, Fisberg RM, Gois Filho JF, et al. Cad Saude Publica (Portugese). 2007 Mar;23(3):553-64. **Key Finding:** "A total of 835 subjects, 366 with histologically confirmed incident cases of oral-cavity or pharyngeal cancer and 469 controls, participated in the study. An inverse association with risk of oral cancer was found for the highest intake of bean or raw vegetables. Positive associations were observed for the highest intake of eggs or potatoes or milk."

Watercress supplementation in diet reduces lymphocyte DNA damage and alters blood anti-oxidant status in healthy adults. Gill CI, Haldar S, Boyd LA, et al. Am J Clin Nutr. 2007 Feb;85(2):504-10. **Key Finding:** "A single-blind, randomized, cross-over study was conducted in 30 men and 30 women. The subjects were fed 85 g raw watercress daily for 8 wk in addition to their habitual diet. Watercress supplementation was associated with reductions in basal DNA damage by 17%, basal plus oxidative purine DNA damage by 23.9%, and in basal DNA damage in response to ex vivo hydrogen peroxide challenge by 9.4%. The results support the theory that consumption of watercress can be linked to a reduced risk of **cancer** via decreased damage to DNA and possible modulation of antioxidant status by increasing carotenoid concentrations."

*Vegetables and fruits and risk of **stomach cancer**.* Zickute J, Strumylaite L, Dregval L, et al. Medicina (Kaunas) (Lithuanian). 2005;41(9):733-40. **Key Finding:** "Higher consumption of raw vegetables, such as cabbage, carrots, garlic and broccoli may decrease a risk of stomach cancer, whereas intake of citrus fruits has no relation with a reduced risk of the disease."

*Dietary patterns and risk of **cancer** of the **oral cavity** and pharynx in Uruguay.* De Stefani E, Boffetta P, Ronco AL, et al. Nutr Cancer. 2005;51(2): 132-9. **Key Finding:** "The stew pattern loaded positively on boiled meat, cooked vegetables, potato and sweet potato; this pattern was directly associated with risk of oral and pharyngeal cancer. The vegetables and fruits factor loaded positively on raw vegetables and citrus fruits; this pattern was inversely associated with risk of oropharyngeal carcinoma."

*Vegetable and fruit intake and **pancreatic cancer** in a population-based case-control study in the San Francisco Bay area.* Chan JM, Wang F, Holly EA. Cancer Epidemiol Biomarkers Prev. 2005 Sep;14(9):2093-7. **Key Finding:** "We conducted a population-based, case-control study with direct interviews of 532 cases and 1,701 age- and sex-matched controls. These results suggest that increasing vegetable and fruit consumption may impart some protection against developing pancreatic cancer." Raw vegetables were found in this study to be more protective than cooked ones.

*Association between diet and **esophageal cancer** in Taiwan.* Hung HC, Huang MC, Lee JM, et al. J Gastroenterol Hepatol. 2004 Jun;19(6): 632-7. **Key Finding:** "Consumption of preserved/pickled vegetables and overheated foods was found to be associated with increased risk of esophageal cancer, whereas intake of fresh fruits, vegetables (raw) and tea was inversely associated with this risk."

*Dietary patterns and risk of **gastric cancer**: a case-control study in Uruguay.* De Stefani E, Correa P, Boffetta P, et al. Gastric Cancer. 2004;7(4):211-20. **Key Finding:** "The individual analysis of food groups showed increased risk of gastric cancer for rice, salted meat, stewed meat, white bread, potatoes, and tubers. On the other hand, raw vegetables, total fruits, legumes, and black tea were inversely associated with risk of gastric cancer."

Dietary patterns and risk of **breast cancer** *in the ORDET cohort.* Sieri S, Krogh V, Pala V, et al. Cancer Epidemiol Biomarkers Prev. 2004 Apr;13(4):567-72. **Key Finding:** "Nutritional data from 8,984 women with an average follow up of 9.5 years was used from an Italian cohort. Four dietary patterns emerged. Only the salad vegetables pattern was associated with significantly lower (34%-35%) breast cancer incidence. These findings suggest that **a diet rich in raw vegetables and olive oil protects against breast cancer.**"

Raw versus cooked vegetables and **cancer** *risk.* Link LB, Potter JD. Cancer Epidemiol Biomarkers Prev. 2004 Sep;13(9):1422-35. **Key Finding**: "This review of the medical literature from 1994 to 2003 summarizes the relationship between raw and cooked vegetables and cancer risk. Twenty-eight studies examined the relationship between raw and cooked vegetables and risk for various cancers. Twenty-one studies assessed raw, but not cooked, vegetables and cancer risk. Most showed that vegetables, raw or cooked, were inversely related to oral, pharyngeal, laryngeal, esophageal, lung, gastric and colorectal cancers. Nine of 11 studies of raw and cooked vegetables showed statistically significant inverse relationships of these cancers with raw vegetables, but only four with cooked vegetables. Both raw and cooked vegetable consumption are inversely related to epithelial cancers, particularly those of the **upper gastrointestinal tract, and possibly breast cancer**; however, these relationships may be stronger for **raw vegetables** than cooked vegetables."

Raw and cooked vegetables, fruits, selected micronutrients, and **breast cancer** *risk: a case-control study in Germany.* Adzersen KH, Jess P, Freivogel KW, Gerhard I, Bastert G. Nutr Cancer. 2003;46(2):131-7. **Key Finding:** "Three hundred ten cases with primary breast cancer were matched to 353 controls with conditions unrelated to diet or endocrine disorders. Intake of raw vegetables, total vegetables and whole-grain products was inversely associated with breast cancer risk. In this population of German women, components of raw vegetables and some micronutrients appear to decrease breast cancer risk."

The influence of dietary patterns on the development of **thyroid cancer**. Markaki I, Linos D, Linos A. Eur J Cancer. 2003 Sep;39(13):1912-9. **Key Find-**

ing: "We conducted a case-control study of 113 persons with histologically verified thyroid cancer and 138 controls. Dietary patterns of fruits, raw vegetables and mixed raw vegetables and fruits led to a reduced risk for all thyroid cancers and similar figures were obtained for papillary thyroid cancers. A dietary pattern of fish and cooked vegetables led to an increased risk of follicular cancer."

*Effect of diet and Helicobacter pylori infection to the risk of early **gastric cancer**.* Lee SA, Kang D, Shim KN, et al. J Epidemiol. 2003 May;13(3):162-8. **Key Finding:** "A hospital-based case-control study was conducted in Korea with 69 patients newly diagnosed as having early gastric cancer and 199 healthy subjects. Decreased risks of early gastric cancer were observed in association with intakes of clear broth, raw vegetables, fruits, fruit or vegetable juices. On the other hand, a high intake of salt-fermented fish and kimchi were associated with an elevated risk of early gastric cancer."

***Oral cancer** in Southern India: the influence of body size, diet, infections and sexual practices.* Rajkumar T, Sridhar H, Balaram P, et al. Eur J Cancer Prev. 2003 Apr;12(2):135-43. **Key Finding:** Frequent consumption of raw green vegetables and cruciferous vegetables decreased oral cancer risk based on a study of 591 incident cases of cancer of the oral cavity and 582 hospital controls.

Self-reported differences in daily raw vegetable intake by ethnicity in a breast screening program. Madan AK, Barden CB, Beech B, et al. J Natl Med Assoc. 2002 Oct;94(10):894-900. **Key Finding:** "There is a substantial difference in the consumption of potentially (**breast cancer**) protective foods among major ethnic groups. There were statistically significant differences between proportions of Caucasian women's and African-American women's consumption of daily raw vegetables (51% versus 29% respectively)."

***Chemoprotective** glucosinolates and isothiocyanates of broccoli sprouts: metabolism and excretion in humans.* Shapiro TA, Fahey JW, Wade KL, Stephenson KK, Talalay P. Cancer Epidemiol Biomarkers Prev. 2001 May;10(5): 501-8. **Key Finding:** "Broccoli sprouts are a rich source of glucosinolates and isothiocyanates that induce phase 2 detoxication enzymes, boost **antioxidant** status, and protect animals against chemically induced **cancer**. When metabolized they are collectively designated dithiocarbamates. We studied the disposition of broccoli sprout glucosinolates and isothiocyanates in healthy volunteers. Dosing preparations included uncooked fresh sprouts (with active myrosinase) as well as boiled sprouts that were devoid of myrosinase activity. Dithiocarbamate excretion was higher when intact sprouts were chewed thoroughly rather than swallowed whole. Thorough chewing of fresh sprouts exposes the glucosinolates to plant myrosinase and significantly increases dithiocarbamate excretion."

*Consumption of vegetables and fruits and **urothelial cancer** incidence: a prospective study.* Zeegers MP, Goldbohm RA, Van den Brandt PA. Cancer Epidemiol Biomarkers Prev. 2001 Nov;10(11):1121-8. **Key Finding: Raw vegetables and raw leafy vegetable** consumption is suggestive of a lower overall risk of urothelial cancer, whereas total vegetable consumption did not appear to be associated with urothelial cancer risk.

*Food groups and **colorectal cancer** risk.* Levi F, Pasche C, La Vecchia C, Lucchini F, Franceschi S. Br J Cancer. 1999 Mar;79(7-8):1283-7. **Key Finding:** Significant associations with colorectal cancer risk were observed for refined grain, red meat, pork and processed meat. Significant protections were observed for whole grain, **raw vegetables** and garlic."These findings in a central European population support the hypothesis that a diet rich in refined grains and red meat increases the risk of colorectal cancer."

Comparison of serum carotenoid responses between women consuming vegetable juice and women consuming raw or cooked vegetables. McEligot AJ, Rock CL, Shanks TG, et al. Cancer Epidemiol Biomarkers Prev. 1999 Mar;8(3):227-31. **Key Finding**: "Study subjects included female **breast cancer** patients. At 12 months, blood samples were collected and analyzed for carotenoid concentrations. Serum concentrations of alpha-carotene and lutein were significantly higher in the vegetable juice group than in the raw or cooked vegetable group. These results suggest that alpha-carotene and lutein appear to be more bioavailable in the **juice form** than in raw or cooked vegetables."

*Risk factors for **breast cancer** in women under 40 years.* Tavani A, Gallus S, La Vecchia C, et al. Eur J Cancer. 1999 Sep;35(9):1361-7. **Key Finding:**

"Cases were 579 women with histologically confirmed, incident breast cancer and controls were 668 women. **Raw vegetable** and beta-carotene consumption were inversely related to breast cancer risk."

Vegetables, fruit, and cancer prevention: a review. Steinmetz KA, Potter JD. J Am Dietetic Assoc. 1996 Oct;96(10):1027-39. **Key Finding:** "The types of vegetables or fruit that most often appear to be protective against **cancer** are raw vegetables, followed by allium vegetables, carrots, green vegetables, cruciferous vegetables, and tomatoes."

*Food habits and **pancreatic cancer**: a case-control study of the Francophone community in Montreal, Canada.* Gahdirian P, Baillargeon J, Simard A, Perret C. Cancer Epidemiol Biomarkers Prev. 1995 Dec;4(8):895-9. **Key Finding:** "The study found an increased risk of pancreatic cancer associated with a high consumption of salt, smoked meat, dehydrated food, fried food, and refined sugar. An inverse association was found with the consumption of food with no preservatives or additives, and raw food."

*Dietary and other environmental risk factors in acute **leukaemias**: a case-control study of 119 patients.* Kwiatkowski A. Eur J Cancer Prev. 1993 Mar;2(2):139-46. **Key Finding:** "Dietary risk factors were studied in 119 adult patients with acute leukaemia in Poland. Rare consumption of raw vegetables resulted in an elevation of risk for acute leukaemia. The risk was also elevated with frequent drinking of milk, frequent consumption of poultry."

Shifting from a conventional diet to an uncooked vegan diet reversibly alters fecal hydrolytic activities in humans. Ling WH, Hanninen O. J Nutr. 1992 Apr;122(4):924-30. **Key Finding:** "Results suggest that this uncooked extreme vegan diet causes a decrease in bacterial enzymes and certain toxic products that have been implicated in **colon cancer** risk."

*Vegetables, fruit, and **cancer**. I. Epidemiology.* Steinmetz KA, Potter JD. Cancer Causes Control. 1991 Sep;2(5):325-57. **Key Finding:** "The epidemiologic literature on the relationship between vegetable and fruit consumption and human cancer at a variety of sites is reviewed systematically. A total of 13 ecologic studies, nine cohort studies, and 115 case-control studies are included. The association is most marked for epithelial cancers, particularly those of the alimentary and respiratory tracts. The association exists for a wide variety of vegetables and fruit with some suggestion that raw forms are associated most consistently with lower risk."

*Nutrition and lifestyle factors in **fibrocystic disease** and cancer of the breast.* Simard A, Vobecky J, Vobecky JS. Cancer Detect Prev. 1990;14(5):567-72. **Key Finding:** "Within a study on diet as a risk factor for fibrocystic disease and **breast cancer**, 68 patients with breast cancer were compared to 340 patients with fibrocystic disease and to 343 controls. The cancer patients consumed significantly more poultry, fish, pastry, margarine and alcohol. The cancer patients consumed less raw vegetables."

*Carotenoid analyses of selected raw and cooked foods associated with a lower risk for **cancer**.* Micozzi MS, Beecher GR, Taylor PR, Khachik F. J Natl Cancer Inst. 1990 Feb 21;82(4):282-5. **Key Finding**: "**Cooking** differentially reduced the lutein content compared with the beta carotene content in green, leafy vegetables. These analyses suggest that consumption of carotenoids in addition to beta carotene may be associated with a lower risk for cancer."

*Study of risk factors in invasive **cancer of the corpus uteri**.* Zemla B, Guminski S, Banasik R. Neoplasma. 1986;33(5):621-9. **Key Finding:** "With the application of the case-control method, 173 patients suffering from invasive cancer of the corpus uteri were analyzed. Incidence risk can be characterized by the high consumption of meat, animal fat and sugar. The lack of raw vegetables in the diet influences the incidence risk of invasive cancer of the corpus uteri."

Cardiovascular disease

Dietary patterns and the risk of acute myocardial infarction in 52 countries: results of the INTERHEART study. Iqbal R, Anand S, Ounpuu S, et al. Circulation. 2008 Nov 4;118(19):1913-4. **Key Finding:** "Diet is a major modifiable risk factor for **cardiovascular disease**. The objectives of the present study were to assess the association between dietary patterns and

acute myocardial infarction globally. The present analysis included 5,761 cases and 10,646 control subjects from 52 countries. We identified 3 major dietary patterns: Oriental (high intake of tofu and soy and other sauces), Western (high in fried foods, salty snacks, eggs and meat), and prudent (high in fruit and vegetables.) We observed an inverse association between the prudent pattern and acute myocardial infarction, with higher (consumption) levels being protective." From unhealthy to protective, the dietary risk score went from meat, salty snacks, fried foods, fruits, green leafy vegetables, cooked vegetables to raw vegetables.

Vegan diet in physiological health promotion. Hanninen O, Rauma AL, Kaartinen K, Nenonen M. Acta Physiol Hung. 1999;86(3-4):171-80. **Key Finding:** "We have performed a number of studies including dietary interventions and cross-sectional studies on subjects consuming uncooked vegan food, called living food, consisting of germinated seeds, cereals, sprouts, vegetables, fruits, berries and nuts. The subjects eating living food show increased levels of carotenoids and vitamins C and E and lowered cholesterol concentration in their sera. The **rheumatoid arthritis** patients eating the living foods diet reported amelioration of their pain and swelling of joints. The **fibromyalgic** subjects eating living foods lost weight compared to their omnivorous controls. The results on their joint stiffness and pain, on their quality of sleep, all improved. It appears that the adoption of vegan diet exemplified by the living food leads to a lessening of several health risk factors to **cardiosvascular diseases** and **cancer**."

Cholesterol

Effects of plant-based diets on plasma lipids. Ferdowsian HR, Barnard ND. Am J Cardiol. 2009 Oct 1;104(7):947-56. **Key Finding:** "Large prospective trials have demonstrated that populations following plant-based diets, particularly vegetarian and vegan diets [which include raw foods], are at lower risk for **ischemic heart disease** mortality. The investigators therefore reviewed 27 randomized controlled and observational trials to determine the effectiveness of plant-based diets in modifying plasma lipid concentrations. Interventions testing a combination diet (a vegetarian or vegan diet combined with nuts, soy, and/or fiber) demonstrated the greatest effects (up to 35% plasma low-density lipoprotein **cholesterol** reduction.)"

Long-term consumption of a raw food diet is associated with favorable serum LDL cholesterol and triglycerides but also with elevated plasma homocystein and low serum HDL cholesterol in humans. Koebuick C, Garcia AL, Dagnelie PC, et al. J Nutr. 2005 Oct;135:2372-78. **Key Finding:** "We investigated the effects of an extremely high dietary intake of raw vegetables and fruits on serum lipids and plasma vitamin B-12, folate and total homocysteine. In a cross-sectional study, 201 adherents to a raw food diet (94 men and 107 women) were examined. This study indicates that consumption of a strict raw food diet lowers plasma total **cholesterol** and triglyceride concentrations, but also lowers serum HDL cholesterol and increases the concentrations due to vitamin B-12 deficiency (of raw food consumers, 38% were vitamin B-12 deficient.)"

Shifting from conventional diet to an uncooked vegan diet reversibly alters serum lipid and apolipoprotein levels. Ling WH, Laitinen M, Hanninen O. Nutri Res. 1992 Dec;12(12):1431-40. **Key Finding:** "Eighteen subjects were randomly divided into test and control groups. In the test group, subjects adopted the uncooked extreme vegan diet for one month and then resumed a conventional diet for a second month. Controls consumed a conventional diet throughout the study. Total serum cholesterol, triglyceride, **LDL, HDL cholesterol** and apoliopoprotein AI as well as B decreased significantly throughout the period of consuming the vegan diet. The results from this test group suggest that the uncooked extreme vegan diet causes a significant decrease of the **atherosclerosis** risk factor."

*Effect of ingestion of raw garlic on serum **cholesterol** level, clotting time and fibrinolytic activity in normal subjects.* Gadkari JV, Joshi VD. J Postgrad Med. 1991 Jul;37(3):128-31. **Key Finding:** "The effect of raw garlic was studied in 50 medical students. The subjects of the experimental group were given 10 gm of raw garlic after breakfast for two months. Fasting blood samples of all the subjects were investigated after two months. In the control group, there was no significant change in any of the parameters. In the experimental group, there was a significant decrease in serum cholesterol and an increase in clotting time and fibrinolytic activity. Hence, garlic may be a useful agent in prevent of **thromboembolic** phenomenon."

Crohn's disease

*Diet and **Crohn's disease**: characteristics of the pre-illness diet.* Thornton JR, Emmett PM, Heaton KW. Br Med J. 1979 Sep 29;2(6193):762-4. **Key Finding:** "Thirty newly diagnosed patients with Crohn's disease were interviewed about their habitual, pre-illness diet and compared with 30 health controls. The patients ate substantially more refined sugar and considerably less raw fruit and vegetables than the controls. A diet high in refined sugar and low in raw fruit and vegetables precedes and may favour the development of Crohn's disease."

Diabetes

*A low-fat vegan diet and a conventional **diabetes** diet in the treatment of type 2 diabetes: a randomized, controlled, 74-wk clinical trial.* Barnard ND, Cohen J, Jenkins DJ, et al. Am J Clin Nutr. 2009 May;89(5):1588S-96S. **Key Finding:** A low-fat vegan diet (which includes raw food) "appeared to improve glycemia and plasma lipids more than did conventional diabetes diet recommendations."

*A low-fat vegan diet improves glycemic control and cardiovascular risk factors in a randomized clinical trial in individuals with **type 2 diabetes**.* Barnard ND, Cohen J, Jenkins DJ, et al. Diabetes Care. 2006 Aug;29(8):1777-83. **Key Finding:** Individuals with type 2 diabetes were randomly assigned to a low-fat vegan diet (which included raw food) or a diet following the American Diabetes Association guidelines. "Both a low-fat vegan diet and a diet based on ADA guidelines improved glycemic and lipid control in type 2 diabetic patients. These improvements were greater with a low-fat vegan diet."

Fibromyalgia

***Fibromyalgia** syndrome improves using a mostly raw vegetarian diet: an observational study.* Donaldson MS. BMC Complement Altern Med. 2001;1:7. **Key Finding:** "Thirty people participated in a dietary intervention using a mostly raw, pure vegetarian diet. This dietary intervention shows that many fibromyalgia subjects can be helped by a mostly raw vegetarian diet."

Vegan diet in physiological health promotion. Hanninen O, Rauma AL, Kaartinen K, Nenonen M. Acta Physiol Hung. 1999;86(3-4):171-80. **Key Finding:** "We have performed a number of studies including dietary interventions and cross-sectional studies on subjects consuming uncooked vegan food, called living food, consisting of germinated seeds, cereals, sprouts, vegetables, fruits, berries and nuts. The subjects eating living food show increased levels of carotenoids and vitamins C and E and lowered cholesterol concentration in their sera. The **rheumatoid arthritis** patients eating the living foods diet reported amelioration of their pain and swelling of joints. The **fibromyalgic** subjects eating living foods lost weight compared to their omnivorous controls. The results on their joint stiffness and pain, on their quality of sleep, all improved. It appears that the adoption of vegan diet exemplified by the living food leads to a lessening of several health risk factors to **cardiosvascular diseases** and **cancer**."

Gastrointestinal disorders

Effect of a 'green' diet on various clinical and metabolic indicators in patients with **gastrointestinal diseases**. Skuia NA, Burmeister MF, Zhikhar L. Vopr Pitan (Russian). 1984 Nov-Dec;(6):22-6. **Key Finding:** "The authors recommend that patients with all chronic diseases of the alimentary organs, particularly with colonic function abnormalities, should receive salads from raw vegetables (100g 3 times a day). The diet containing salad from raw vegetables was received by 93 inpatients with different chronic **diseases of the alimentary tract, gastroduodenal ulcer** included. Pain and meteorism disappeared or were relieved, intestinal evacuation returned to normal in the majority of patients."

Health (in general)

Long-term strict raw food diet is associated with favourable plasma beta-carotene and low plasma lycopene concentrations in Germans. Garcia AL, Koebnick C, Dagnelie PC, et al. Br J Nutr. 2008 Jun;99(6):1293-300. **Key Finding:**

"Dietary carotenoids are associated with a reduced risk of **chronic diseases**. Raw food diets are predominantly plant-based diets that are practiced with the intention of preventing chronic diseases by virtue of their high content of beneficial nutritive substances such as carotenoids. We investigated vitamin A and carotenoid status in raw food diet adherents in Germany in 198 adherents. Long-term raw food diet adherents showed normal vitamin A status and achieve favourable plasma beta-carotene concentrations as recommended for chronic disease prevention, but showed low plasma lycopene levels."

*A dietary pattern rich in olive oil and raw vegetables is associated with lower **mortality** in Italian elderly subjects.* Masala G, Ceroti M, Pala V, et al. Br J Nutr. 2007 Aug;98(2):406-15. **Key Finding:** Overall mortality was reduced by approximately 50% among consumers of an olive oil and salad dietary pattern characterized by high consumption of olive oil and raw vegetables."

Health effects of vegetarian and vegan diets. Key TJ, Appleby PN, Rosell MS. Proc Nutr Sci. 2006 Feb;65(1):35-41. **Key Finding:** "Cross-sectional studies of vegetarians and vegans [which includes raw food diets] have shown that on average they have a relatively low body mass index and a low plasma cholesterol concentration. Cohort studies have shown a moderate reduction in **mortality.**"

Salad and raw vegetable consumption and nutritional status in the adult US population: results from the Third National Health and Nutrition Examination Survey. Su LJ, Arab L. J Am Diet Assoc. 2006 Sep;106(9):1394-404. **Key Finding:** "Nine thousand four hundred-six women and 8,282 men aged 18 to 45 years, and older than 55 years, were examined. The consumption of salads, raw vegetables and salad dressing was positively associated with above-median serum micronutrient levels of folic acid, vitamins C and E, lycopene, and alpha- and beta-carotene."

Heart disease

Raw and processed fruit and vegetable consumption and 10-year coronary heart disease incidence in a population-based cohort study in the Netherlands. Oude Griep LM, Geleijnse JM, Kromhout D, Ocke MC, Verschuren WM. PLoS One. 2010 Oct 25;5(10):e13609. **Key Finding:** Intake of raw fruit and vegetables as well as processed fruit and vegetables were both inversely related with coronary heart disease incidence in a 10-year population-based study in the Netherlands including 20,069 men and women aged 20 to 65 years.

Effects of plant-based diets on plasma lipids. Ferdowsian HR, Barnard ND. Am J Cardiol. 2009 Oct 1;104(7):947-56. **Key Finding:** "Large prospective trials have demonstrated that populations following plant-based diets, particularly vegetarian and vegan diets [which include raw foods], are at lower risk for **ischemic heart disease** mortality. The investigators therefore reviewed 27 randomized controlled and observational trials to determine the effectiveness of plant-based diets in modifying plasma lipid concentrations. Interventions testing a combination diet (a vegetarian or vegan diet combined with nuts, soy, and/or fiber) demonstrated the greatest effects (up to 35% plasma low-density lipoprotein **cholesterol** reduction.)"

Dietary habits and mortality in 11,000 vegetarians and health-conscious people: results of a 17- year follow up. Key TJ, Thorogood M, Appleby PN, Burr ML. BMJ. 1996 Sep 28;313(7060):775-9. **Key Finding:** "In this cohort of health conscious individuals, daily consumption of fresh fruit (raw) is associated with a reduced mortality from **ischaemic heart disease, cerebrovascular disease**, and all causes combined."

The effect of fried versus raw garlic on fibrinolytic activity in man. Chutani SK, Bordia A. Atherosclerosis. 1981 Feb-Mar;38(3-4):417-21. **Key Finding:** "Raw or fried garlic was administered for 4 weeks to 20 patients with **ischaemic heart disease,** and fibrinolytic activity was measured at weekly intervals. It showed a sustained increase, rising to 84.8% at the end of the 28th day when raw garlic was administered. With fried garlic the rise was 72%. Within 6 hours of administration of raw garlic the fibrinolytic activity increased by 72% compared to 63% for fried garlic."

Hypertension

Effects of a raw food diet on **hypertension** *and* **obesity**. Douglass JM. Southern Med J. 1985 Jul;78(7):841-4. **Key Finding:** "We examined responses to cooked and uncooked food in 32 outpatients with essential hypertension; 28 were also overweight. After a mean duration of 6.7 months, average intake of uncooked food comprised 62% of calories ingested. Mean weight loss was 3.8 kg and mean diastolic pressure reduction 17.8 mm Hg, both statistically significant."

Immune system

Raw food and **immunity**. Gaisbauer M, Langosch A. Fortschr Med (German). 1990 Jun 10;108(17):338-40. **Key Finding:** "Uncooked food is an integral component of human nutrition, and is a necessary precondition for an intact immune system. Its therapeutic effect is complex, and a variety of influences of raw foods and its constitutents on the immune system have been documented. Such effects include antibiotic, anti-allergic, tumor-protective, immunomodulatory, and anti-inflammatory actions. In view of this, uncooked food can be seen as a useful adjunct to drugs in the treatment of allergic, rheumatic and infectious diseases."

Obesity

Effects of a raw food diet on **hypertension** *and* **obesity**. Douglass JM. Southern Med J. 1985 Jul;78(7):841-4. **Key Finding:** "We examined responses to cooked and uncooked food in 32 outpatients with essential hypertension; 28 were also overweight. After a mean duration of 6.7 months, average intake of uncooked food comprised 62% of calories ingested. Mean weight loss was 3.8 kg and mean diastolic pressure reduction 17.8 mm Hg, both statistically significant."

Stroke

Raw and processed fruit and vegetable consumption and 10-year stroke incidence in a population-based cohort study in the Netherlands. Griep LO, Verschuren WM,

Kromhout D, Ocke MC, Geleijnse JM. Eur J Clin Nutr. 2011 Mar 23 [Epub ahead of print]. **Key Finding:** "High intake of raw fruit and vegetables may protect against stroke; no association was found between processed fruit and vegetable consumption and incident stroke among 20,069 men and women aged 20-65 years."

Thrombosis (blood clots)

*An evaluation of garlic and onion as **antithrombotic** agents.* Bordia T, Mohammed N, Thomson M, Ali M. Prostaglandins Leukot Essent Fatty Acids. 1996 Mar;54(3):183-6. **Key Finding:** "Garlic and onion should be consumed in a raw rather than cooked form in order to achieve a beneficial effect as antithrombotic agents. Boiling of these plants may cause the decomposition of the potential antithrombotic ingredient present in these herbs."

*Effect of ingestion of raw garlic on serum **cholesterol** level, clotting time and fibrinolytic activity in normal subjects.* Gadkari JV, Joshi VD. J Postgrad Med. 1991 Jul;37(3):128-31. **Key Finding:** "The effect of raw garlic was studied in 50 medical students. The subjects of the experimental group were given 10 gm of raw garlic after breakfast for two months. Fasting blood samples of all the subjects were investigated after two months. In the control group, there was no significant change in any of the parameters. In the experimental group, there was a significant decrease in serum cholesterol and an increase in clotting time and fibrinolytic activity. Hence, garlic may be a useful agent in prevent of **thromboembolic** phenomenon."

Ulcers (peptic)

*Role of the alimentary factor in the genesis and recurrences of **peptic ulcer**.* Budagovskaia VN, Sal'nikova GM. Vopr Pitan (Russian). 1977 May-Jun;(3):54-9. **Key Finding:** "Dietetic history data covering 500 persons with duodenal ulcer was recorded. Patients were characterized by excessive consumption of animal fats with insufficient consumption of raw vegetables and fruits."

CHAPTER FIVE

Studies Contrasting the Nutrients in Organic and Nonorganic Fruits and Vegetables

EVEN AS CONSUMERS PURCHASE INCREASING AMOUNTS of biologically grown organic food each year, corporate nonorganic farming interests continue to insist that there is no nutritional difference between organic and nonorganic plant foods.

Beyond the issue of spraying crops with insecticides, fungicides, and herbicides, known disease causers, nutrient-depleted soil adds another dimension to the problem we face. Over the last century, agricultural experts reported that crop growers had farmed and eroded away at least 75 percent of the nutrients in our soil. This, in turn, strongly reflects how much nutrition will be contained in plants grown and sold to consumers.

With this said, there is accumulating scientific data portraying non-sprayed organic fruits and vegetables, generally grown in nutrient-replenished soil, to be far superior nutrient sources than chemically saturated, commercially grown varieties harvested from virtual wastelands. One of the more significant studies, done in 2007, compared the flavonoid content of organic versus nonorganic tomatoes over a ten-year period. The study demonstrated that organic soils, over time, cumulatively intensify the levels of flavonoids in tomatoes, whereas nonorganic soils produced no such beneficial effect.

The finding that organic soils intensify nutrient levels over time has not been taken into account fully in many subsequent studies. This is especially true with meta-analyses or comparative reviews of studies that purport to examine the differences between organic and nonorganic growing practices. This nutrient difference ultimately shows up in products on grocery store shelves. A ground-breaking study in 1993, for instance, compared the mineral content of five food crops grown organically and conventionally as they were taken from store shelves over a two-year period. Clear gaps in nutrient levels were discovered.

Not long ago, I delved into this important subject by reading, speaking to, and interviewing the world's leading experts on sustainable farming. Those interactions left me even more convinced that organic food, properly grown, builds healthy people.

Eating organic means limiting the levels of synthetic chemicals being absorbed, and so can contribute to a range of health benefits, which I have seen firsthand. Take Rick Metz, for instance, who had been diagnosed with clinical depression. He spent years taking antidepressants and ended up becoming addicted to them.

As Rick told me, "I finally decided to take it upon myself to find the cause of this 'chemical imbalance' instead of simply treating it. After research I found that the chemicals going into my body in my food, as well as personal hygiene products, needed to be examined thoroughly. I gave up all of these products and went organic and vegetarian. While I had some severe withdrawals—incessant itching—the result was far beyond my wildest dreams. I am so happy to be free of medications and to live again without depression."

Michael Lanning is a Vietnam War veteran who embraced a raw organic vegetarian diet after being told in 2006 that he had kidney cancer, which had metastasized to the adrenal and lymph glands and his lungs. He was given only a year or less to live because neither chemotherapy or radiation would help. Resigned to dying, he e-mailed his good-byes to people he loved and respected.

Michael's former battalion commander, a retired major general, convinced him to try a dietary approach to treatment, as a last resort. The recommended diet was raw, organic, and vegan, and consisted mostly of sprouts, greens, onions, wheatgrass and green juices.

Michael picks up his story here: "After the first week I began to detox as more and more dark spots appeared on my body, some with small pus-filled sores. My body was now consuming only good things and was ridding itself of the previous chemical poisons I had taken in. Itching accompanied the detox. I was paying for my past dietary transgressions."

Three months after adopting this diet, Michael went to Houston's MD Anderson Cancer Center for testing. No growth in the tumors was detected. Another year passed and the tumors remained stable. Now, several years past the date when cancer specialists predicted he would be dead, Michael remains not only alive, but vigorously so. "Since my adoption of the raw diet, I have resumed a normal life. I feel better than I did before my diagnosis. Every day that I live is one more day that seven conventional doctors said that I would not. More importantly, my days are as good as they can get."

While eating organic in and of itself can't explain these medical breakthroughs, the purity of the nutrients we absorb are important factors in the synergies that are created, which are a key to health. Simply said, healthy soil equals healthy plants, and that translates into healthy people. Here are the studies, presented in chronological order, lending support to that point of view.

2010

Characterization of phenolic content, in vitro biological activity, and pesticide loads of extracts from white grape skins from organic and conventional cultivars. Corrales M, Fernandez A, Vizoso Pinto MG, et al. Food Chem Toxicol. 2010 Dec;48(12):3471-6. **Key Finding**: "Possibly as a result of higher amounts of quercetin and its derivatives, higher antimicrobial effects against Listeria monocytogenes and Salmonella typhimurium were observed for the organic white grape skin extracts."

Organic foods contain higher levels of certain nutrients, lower levels of pesticides, and may provide health benefits for the consumer. Crinnion WJ. Altern Med Rev. 2010 Apr;15(1):4-12. **Key Finding**: "Studies of the nutrient content in organic foods vary in results due to differences in the ground cover and maturity of the organic farming operation. Nutrient content also varies from farmer to farmer and year to year. However, reviews of multiple studies show that organic varieties do provide significantly greater levels of vitamin C, iron, magnesium, and phosphorus than nonorganic varieties of the same foods. While being higher in these nutrients, they are also significantly lower in nitrates and pesticide residues. In addition, with the exception of wheat, oats and wine, organic foods typically provide greater levels of a number of important antioxidant phytochemicals."

2009

Polyphenol content and antiradical activity of Cichorium intybus L. from biodynamic and conventional farming. Heimler D, Isolani L, Vignolini P, Romani A. Food Chem. 2009 June 1;114(3):765-70. **Key Finding:** Conventional and organic-grown chicory was compared for its polyphenol content and antiradical activity during growing with severe water stress and without stress. Measurements of eight flavonoids found greatest negative changes in the conventional farming crop; antiradical activity was higher for the organic.

Comparison of phenolic acids in organically and conventionally grown pak choi (Brassica rapa L. chinensis). Zhao X, Nechols JR, William KA, Wang W, Carey EE. J Sci Food Agric. 2009;89(6): 940-46. **Key Finding:** In a field experiment, organic fertilization using compost and fish emulsion resulted in "significantly higher phenolic concentrations" compared with conventional chemical fertilization.

Yielding and fruit quality of three sweet pepper cultivars from organic and conventional cultivation. Szafirowska A, Elkner K. Vegetable Crops Research Bulletin (Poland). 2008;69:135-43. **Key Finding:** "The results revealed a good response of bell pepper to organic cultivation system. Pepper fruits obtained from organic cultivation system comprised higher amount of vitamin C, beta-carotene total flavonoids and polyphenols than from the conventional."

Polyphenolic profile and antioxidant activity of five apple cultivators grown under organic and conventional agricultural practices. Valavanidis A, Vlachogianni T, Psomas A, Zovoili A, Siatis V. Int J Food Sci Tech. 2009 June; 44(6):1167-75. **Key Finding:** Polyphenols and total antioxidant activity of five apple cultivators grown by organic and conventional methods were analyzed. Polyphenolic concentrations "do not differentiate significantly between the organic and conventional apples." Organic did show a slight advantage in antioxidant value.

Three-year comparison of the polyphenol contents and antioxidant capacities in organically and conventionally produced apples (Malus domestica Bork. Cultivar 'Golden Delicious'). Stracke BA, Rufer CE, Weibel FP, Bub A, Watzi B. J Agric Food

Chem. 2009 Jun 10;57(11):4598-605. **Key Finding:** "Apples grown under defined organic and conventional conditions were harvested at five comparable commercial farms over the course of three years (2004-06). In 2005 and 2006 the antioxidant capacity was 15% higher in organically produced apples than in conventionally produced fruits. In 2005 significantly higher polyphenol concentrations were found in the organically grown apples. In 2004 and 2006 no significant differences were observed."

Comparison of physiochemical, microscopic and sensory characteristics of ecologically and conventionally grown crops of two cultivars of tomato. Ordonez-Santos L, Arbones-Macineira E, Fernandez-Perejon J, et al. J Sci Food Agric. 2009;89(5):743-49. **Key Finding:** "The statistically significant differences found in this study were mainly between cultivars rather than between tomatoes grown using different management practices."

Nutritional quality of organic foods: a systematic review. Dangour AD, Dodhia SK, Hayter A, Lock AE, Uauy R. Am J Clin Nutr. 2009 Sep;90(3):680-5. **Key Finding:** "From a total of 52,471 articles, we identified 162 studies (137 crops and 25 livestock products); 55 were of satisfactory quality. On the basis of a systematic review of studies of satisfactory quality, there is no evidence of a difference in nutrient quality between organically and conventionally produced foodstuffs. The small differences in nutrient content detected are biologically plausible and mostly relate to differences in production methods."

Environmental stresses induce health-promoting phytochemicals in lettuce. Oh MM, Carey EE, Rajashekar CB. Plant Physiol Biochem. 2009 Jul;47(7):578-83. **Key Finding:** "We have used mild environmental stresses (such a heat shock, chilling or high light intensity) to enhance the phytochemical content of lettuce. In response to these stresses, there was a two- to three-fold increase in the total phenolic content and a significant increase in the antioxidant capacity. The concentrations of two major phenolic compounds in lettuce, chicoric acid and chlorogenic acid, increased significantly in response to all of the stresses. Quercetin-3-0-glucoside and luteolin-7-0-glucoside were not detected in the control plants, but showed marked accumulations following the stress treatments. The results suggest that certain phenolic compounds can be induced in lettuce by environmental stresses. It is possible to use mild environmental stresses to successfully improve the phytochemical content and hence the health-promoting quality of lettuce with little or no adverse effect on its growth or yield."

Antioxidant *and* ***antigenotoxic*** *activities of purple grape juice – organic and conventional – in adult rats.* Dani C, Oliboni LS, Umezu FM, et al. J Med Food. 2009 Oct;12(5):1111-8. **Key Finding:** "The aim of this study was to evaluate the protection of organic and conventional purple grape juices in brain, liver, and plasma from adult Wistar rats against the oxidative damage provoked by carbon tetrachloride. The chemical and analytical determination showed that the highest levels of total phenolic, resveratrol, and catechins were seen in organic purples grape juices. In all treatment groups it was observed that in all tissue and plasma, treatment increased the lipid peroxidation levels. Both grape juices were capable to reduce LP levels in cerebral cortex and hippocampus; however, in the striatum and substantia nigra only the organic grape juice reduced LP level."

Bioavailability and nutritional effects of carotenoids from organically and conventionally produced ***carrots*** *in healthy men.* Stracke BA, Rufer CE, Bub A, et al. Br J Nutr. 2009 Jun;101(11):1664-72. **Key Finding**: "Thirty-six volunteers consumed either organically or conventionally produced blanched carrots or no carrots in a double-blind, randomized intervention study. No statistically significant differences were observed in the total carotenoid contents of organic and conventional carrots."

2008

Health-promoting substances and heavy metal content in ***tomatoes*** *grown with different farming techniques.* Rossi F, Godani F, Bertuzzi T, et al. Eur J Nutr. 2008 August;47(5): 266-72. **Key Finding:** "Organic tomatoes contained more salicylic acid but less vitamin C and lycopene" than conventionally grown tomatoes. "Organic tomatoes had higher Cd and Pb levels but a lower Cu content. Organic fruits had a slightly higher protein content than conventionally cultivated fruits...their higher salicylate content support the notion that organic foodstuffs are more wholesome."

Strawberry (Frafaria x ananassa Duch) fruit quality grown under different organic matter sources. Abu-Zahra TR, Tahboub AA. ISHA Acta Horticulturae 807: International Symposium on Strategies Towards Sustainability of Protected Cultivation in Mild Winter Climate. 2008. **Key Finding:** "Organic source treatments produced fruit with better color, higher dry matter, total phenols, crude fibre and carotene contents as compared to those produced by the control or conventional treatments. Also, the organic source treatments produced fruit with higher total soluble solids percentage and ascorbic acid content than with the conventional or the control treatments."

Rats show differences in some biomarkers of health when eating diets based on ingredients produced with three different cultivation strategies. Lauridsen C, Yong C, Halekoh U, et al. J. Sci Food Agric. 2008;88:720-32. **Key Finding:** Rats were fed diets of vegetables and rapeseed oil from three different cultivation methods—organic, and two methods using pesticides and varying fertilizer inputs. Rats fed from a diet grown with pesticides and high fertilizer use showed lower health-related biomarkers in most categories measured than the organic.

Intake of purple grape juice as a hepatoprotective agent in Wistar rats. Dani C, Pasquali M, Oliveira MR, et al. J Med Food. 2008 March;11(1):127-32. **Key Finding:** "Antioxidant activities were significantly correlated with polyphenol content. Our findings suggest that the intake of purple grape juice, especially of organic juice, induces a better antioxidant capacity when compared to conventional juice."

Antioxidant content in black currants from organic and conventional cultivation. Kazimierczak R, Hallmann E, Rusaczonek A, Rembialkowska E. EJPAU. 2008; 11(2). **Key Finding:** "The obtained results showed that organic black currant had considerably higher levels of compounds with antioxidant properties and higher antioxidant potential compared to fruits produced using conventional methods."

Isoflavonoids, flavonoids, phenolic acids profiles and antioxidant activity of soybean seeds as affected by organic and bioorganic fertilization. Taie H, El-Mergawi R, Radwan S. American-Eurasian J Agric Environ Sci. 2008; 4(2):207-13.

Key Finding: "Adding multi-bioorganic to 50% or 75% compost treatments produce great enhancement effects on total phenolics, total flavonoids, quercetin, genistein and daidzein contents as compared with other treatments." Addition of organic treatments "resulted in 68% and 40% increases in quercetin and genistein, respectively, as compare with inorganic treatment."

Comparison of lycopene, B-carotene and phenolic contents of tomato using conventional and ecologically horticultural practices, and arbuscular mycorrhizal fungi (AMF). Ulrichs C, Fischer G, Buttner C, Mewis I. Agron. Colomb. 2008 Jan/June;26(1). **Key Finding:** "When comparing the cultivation method, no significant differences for the analyzed nutritional parameters were found; only tomatoes grown organically had slightly lower total phenolic contents. Organic grown tomatoes increased B-carotene and total phenolic contents in fruits as a result of the AMF treatment."

The changes of the bioactive compounds in pickled red pepper fruits from organic and conventional production. Rembialkowska E, Hallmann E. J Research and Applications in Agriculture (Poland). 2008;53(4):51-7. **Key Finding:** "The obtained results of fresh red pepper showed that organic fruits contained more vitamin C, rutin, lutein, also dry matter. Conventional pepper contained more beta-carotene and lycopene."

Comparison of polyamine, phenol and flavonoid contents in plants grown under conventional and organic methods. Lima GP. da Rocha SA. Takaki M. Ramos PR. Ono EO. Int J Food Sci Tech. 2008 Oct.;43(10):1838-43. **Key Finding:** Peels of zucchini, squash, banana, potato, eggplant, orange, lime, mango, passion fruit and radish, and leaves and stalks of zucchini, squash, broccoli, carrot, collard, cassava, radish, grape, and spinach were analyzed. "Most analysed vegetables presented higher contents of polyamines and total phenols under organic cropping, contrary to the results obtained for total flavonoids, possibly because of the cultural practices adopted."

Fruit quality, antioxidant capacity, and flavonoid content of organically and conventionally grown blueberries. Wang SY, Chen CT, Sciarappa W, Wang CY, Camp MJ. J Agric Food Chem. 2008 July 23; 56(14):5788-94. **Key Finding:** "Results from this study showed that blueberry fruit grown from organic culture yielded significantly higher sugars (fructose and glucose), malic acid, total phenolics, total anthocyanins, and antioxidant activity (ORAC) than fruit from the conventional culture."

A 3-year study on quality, nutritional and organoleptic evaluation of organic and conventional extra-virgin olive oils. Ninfali P, Bacchiocca M, Biagiotti E, et al. J Am Oil Chem Soc. 2008 Feb.;85(2):151-8. **Key Finding:** "The concentrations of phenols, o-diphenols, tocopherols, the antioxidant capacity and the volatile compounds showed differences in some years and no difference, or opposite differences, in others. Our results showed that organic versus conventional cultivation did not affect consistently the quality of the high quality EVOO considered in this study, at least in the measured parameters. Genotype and year-to-year changes in climate, instead, had more marked effects."

Effects of agricultural practices on instrumental colour, mineral content, carotenoid composition, and sensory quality of mandarin orange juice, cv. Hernandina. Beltran-Gonzalez F, Perez-Lopez AJ, Lopez-Nicholas JM, Carbonell-Barrachina AA. J Sci Food Agric. 2008; 88(10):1731-38. **Key Finding:** "Organic farming of mandarin oranges resulted in juices with higher contents of minerals and carotenoids, and of better sensory quality. For instance, organic juice contained a total concentration of carotenoids of 14.4 mg L compared to 10.2 mg L of conventional juice."

Effect of plant cultivation methods on content of major and trace elements in foodstuffs and retention in rats. Kirstensen M, Ostergaard LF, Halekoh U, et al. J Sci Food Agric2008; 88(2):2161-72. **Key Finding:** "This study does not support the belief that organically grown foodstuffs generally contain more major and trace elements than conventionally grown foodstuffs, nor does there appear to be an effect on the bioavailability of major and trace elements in rats."

Wild and commercial mushrooms as source of nutrients and nutraceuticals. Barros L, Cruz T, Baptista P, Estevinho LM, Ferreira IC. Food Chem Toxicol. 2008 Aug;46(8):2742-7. **Key Finding:** Experiments were performed in wild and commercial species of mushrooms to analyze nutrient and phytochemical levels. Commercial species seemed to have higher concentrations of sugars, while wild species had higher contents of alpha-Tocopherol. Wild also had a higher content of phenols but a lower content of ascorbic acid than commercial species. There was no difference found in the antimicrobial properties of wild and commercial species.

Influence of irrigation and organic/inorganic fertilization on chemical quality of almond (Prunus amygdalus cv. Guara). Sanchez-Bel P, Egea I, Martinze-Madrd MC, Flores B, Romojaro F. J Agric Food Chem. 2008 Nov 12;56(21):10056-62. **Key Finding:** "Among the fertilizing treatments employed, the organic ones have shown the best results related to chemical quality, regardless of the quantity of fertilizer employed. The organic treatments produced almonds with a higher content of sugar, organic acids and fiber and a similar fat content."

2007

Organic vs Conventionally Grown Rio Red Whole Grapefruit and Juice: Comparison of Production Inputs, Market Quality, Consumer Acceptance, and Human Health-Bioactive Compounds. Lester GE. J Agric Food Chem. 2007 May 30;55(11): 4474-80. **Key Finding:** Conventionally grown fruit was higher in lycopene; organic fruit was higher in ascorbic acid and sugars.

Ten-year comparison of the influence of organic and conventional crop management practices on the content of flavonoids in tomatoes. Mitchell A, Hong YJ, Koh E, et al. J. Agric Food Chem. 2007 June 23;55(15): 6154-59. **Key Finding:** "Comparisons of analyses of archived samples from conventional and organic production systems demonstrated statistically higher levels of quercetin and kaempferol in organic tomatoes. Ten-year mean levels of quercetin and kaempferol in organic tomatoes were 79% and 97% higher than those in conventional tomatoes. The levels of flavonoids increased over time in samples from organic treatments, whereas the levels of flavonoids did not vary significantly in conventional treatments."

Quality of plant products from organic agriculture. Rembialkowska E. J Sci Food Agric. 2007 Sep 21;87(15):2757-62. **Key Finding:** "Organic crops contain fewer nitrates, nitrites, and pesticide residues but, as a rule, more dry matter, vitamin C, phenolic compounds, essential amino acids and total sugars than conventional crops. Organic crops also contain statistically more mineral compounds."

Yield and fruit quality response of sweet pepper to organic and mineral fertilization. Del Amor FM. Renew Agr Food Syst. 2007; 22: 233-8. **Key Finding:** "Organic farming increased antioxidant activity but reduced both chlorophylls and B-carotene."

Phenolic content and antioxidant activities of white and purple juices manufactured with organically or conventionally produced grapes. Dani C, Oliboni LS, Vanderlinde R, et al. Food Chem Toxicol. 2007 Dec;45(12): 2574-80. **Key Finding:** "Organic grape juices showed statistically different (p<0.05) higher values of total polyphenols and resveratrol as compared conventional grape juices. Purple juices presented higher total polyphenol content and in vitro antioxidant activity as compared to white juices."

Antioxidant capacity of leafy vegetables as affected by high tunnel environment, fertilization and growth stage. Zhao X, Iwamoto T, Carey E. J Sci Food Agric. 2007;87(14):2692-99. **Key Finding:** "Organic fertilizer markedly increased the antioxidant capacity of pak choi compared with conventional treatment...in contrast to the first trial, organic fertilization did not cause an increase in antioxidant capacity of the leafy vegetables."

Differential effect of organic cultivation on the levels of phenolics, peroxidase and capsidiol in sweet peppers. Del Amor FM, Serrano-Martinez A, Fortea I, Nunez-Delicado E. J Sci Food Agric. 2007 Dec 11;88(5):770-7. **Key Finding:** "Peroxidase activity in organic sweet peppers was higher than in conventional ones, in both maturity stages studied. The level of total phenolics compounds was also higher in organic than in conventional sweet peppers. With respect to the capsidiol activity, it was not affected by the cultivation method at the green mature stage. However, at the red mature stage, organic sweet peppers showed higher capsidiol activity than those grown under the conventional system."

Nutritional quality of organic, conventional, and seasonally grown broccoli using vitamin C as a marker. Wunderlich SM, Feldman C, Kane S, Hazhin T. Int J Food Sci Nutr. 2008 Feb;59(1): 34-45. **Key Finding:** "Although the vitamin C content of organically and conventionally labeled broccoli was not significantly different, significant seasonal changes have been observed. The fall values for vitamin C were almost twice as high as those for spring for both varieties. The seasonal changes in vitamin C content are larger than the differences between organically labeled and conventionally grown broccoli."

A comparative study of composition and postharvest performance of organically and conventionally grown kiwifruits. Amodio ML, Colelli G, Hasey JK, Kader AA. J Sci Food Agric. 2007; 87(7):1228-36. **Key Finding:** "All the main mineral constituents were more concentrated in organic kiwifruits, which also had higher levels of ascorbic acid and total phenol content, resulting in a higher antioxidant activity."

Differential effect of organic cultivation on the levels of phenolics, peroxidase and capsidiol in sweet peppers. Del Amor FM, Serrano-Martinez A, Fortea I, Nunez-Delicado E. J Sci Food Agric. 2007;88(5):770-7. **Key Finding:** "Sweet peppers grown under organic culture have a maturity-related response with high levels of phenolic compounds and peroxidase and capsidiol activity that contribute to disease resistance in organic farming." Organic sweet peppers had higher total phenolics and peroxidase activity and capsidiol activity than those grown under the conventional system.

Effects of agricultural practices on color, carotenoids composition, and minerals content of sweet peppers, cv. Almuden. Perez-Lopez AJ, Lopez-Nicholas JM, Nunez-Delicado E, Del Amor FM, Carbonell-Barrachina AA. J Agric Food Chem. 2007 Oct 3;55(20): 8158-64. **Key Finding:** "Experimental results proved that organic farming provided peppers with the highest (a) intensities of red and yellow colors (b) contents of minerals (c) total carotenoids. The concentrations of total carotenoids were 3231, 2493, and 1829 mg kg (-1) for organic, integrated, and conventional sweet peppers, respectively. Finally, organic red peppers could be considered as those having the highest antioxidant activity of all studied peppers."

2006

*Antioxidant levels and inhibition of **cancer cell proliferation** in vitro by extracts from organically and conventionally cultivated strawberries.* Olsson ME, Andersson CS, Oredsson S, Berglund RH, Gustavsson KE. J Agric Food Chem. 2006 Feb 22;54(4):1248-55. **Key Finding:** "The ratio of ascorbate to dehydroascorbate was significantly higher in the organically cultivated strawberries. The strawberry extracts decreased the proliferation of both HT29 **colon cancer** cells and MCF-7 **breast cancer** cells in a dose-dependent way. The inhibitory effect for the highest concentration of the extracts was in the range of 41%-63% inhibition compared to controls for the HT29 cells and 26%-56% for MCF-7 cells. The extracts from organically grown strawberries had a higher antiproliferative activity for both cell types at the highest concentration than the conventionally grown, and this might indicate a higher content of secondary metabolites with anticarcinogenic properties in the organically grown strawberries."

High-Performance Liquid Chromatography Analysis of Black Currant (Ribes nigrum L.) Fruit Phenolics Grown either Conventionally or Organically. Antonnen MJ. Karjalainen RO. J Agric Food Chem. 2006, 54(20):7530-38. **Key Finding:** "Statistically significant differences between farms were found for almost all phenolic compounds," ranging from 24% to 77% in values, but "it was concluded that the biochemical quality of organically grown black currant fruits does not differ from those grown conventionally."

Antioxidant effectiveness of organically and nonorganically grown red oranges in cell culture systems. Tarozzi A, Hrelia S, Angeloni C, et al. . Eur J Nutr. 2006 April; 45(3):152-8. **Key Finding:** "The organic orange extracts had a higher total antioxidant activity than nonorganic orange extracts (p<0.05). Our results clearly show that organic red oranges have a higher phytochemical content (i.e. phenolics, anthocyanins and ascorbic acid), total antioxidant activity and bioactivity than integrated (nonorganic) red oranges."

Influence of different types of fertilizers on the major antioxidant components of tomatoes. Toor RK, Savage GP, Heeb A. J Food Compost Anal. 2006 Feb;19():20-7. **Key Finding:** "The mean total phenolic and ascorbic acid content of tomatoes grown using chicken manure and grass-clover mulch (organic) was 17.6% and 29% higher, respectively, than the tomatoes grown with mineral nutrient solutions. The mean lycopene content was 40% lower in tomatoes grown with high chloride levels and grass-clover mulch compared with other treatments (chicken manure). The mean antioxidant activity of the ammonium-treated plants was 14% lower compared with other treatments."

2005

Quality of organically and conventionally grown potatoes: four-year study of micronutrients, metals, secondary metabolites, enzyme browning and organoleptic properties. Hajslova J, Schulzova V, Slanina P, et al. Food Addit Contam. 2005 June;22(6): 514-34. **Key Finding:** "The results indicated lower nitrate content and higher vitamin C and chlorogenic acid content to be the parameters most consistently differentiating organically from conventionally produced potatoes."

Extracts from organically and conventionally cultivated strawberries inhibit cancer cell proliferation in vitro. Olsson ME, Andersson SC, Berglund RH, Gustavsson KE, Oredsson S. ISHS Acta Horticulturae 744: International Symposium on Human Health Effects of Fruits and Vegetables. 2005. **Key Finding:** "The strawberry extracts inhibited cell proliferation in colon cancer cells HT29 and breast cancer cells MCF-7 in a concentration dependent way. Extracts from organically grown strawberries inhibited cell proliferation to a higher extent than conventionally grown at the two highest concentrations. The content of ascorbate was 36% higher and the ratio of ascorbate to dehydroascorbate were eight-fold higher in the organically grown strawberries than in the conventionally grown. Ascorbate is suggested to act synergistically with other substances in the extracts."

Sensory quality and mineral and glycoalkaloid concentrations in organically and conventionally grown redskin potatoes (Solanum tuberosum). Wszelaki AL, Delwiche JF, Walker SD, et al. J Sci Food Agric. 2005; 85:720-26. **Key Finding:** "Glycoalkaloid levels tended to be higher in organic potatoes. In tuber skin and flesh, potassium, magnesium, phosphorus, sulfur and copper concentrations were also significantly higher in organic treatments, while iron and manganese concentrations were higher in the skin of conventionally grown potatoes."

Phenolic compounds in some apple (Malus domestica Borkh) cultivars of organic and integrated production. Veberic R, Trobec M, Herbinger K, et al. J Sci Food Agric. 2005 Mar 31;85(10):1687-94. **Key Finding:** "Organically grown apples exhibited a higher content of phenolic substances in the apple pulp compared with the apple cultivars of integrated production. The apple peel contained higher concentrations of identified phenols than the pulp."

Phytochemical phenolics in organically grown vegetables. Young JE, Zhao X, Carey E, et al. Mol Nutr Food Res. 2005;49(12):1136-42. **Key Finding:** "Statistically, we did not find significant higher levels of phenolic agents in lettuce and collard samples grown organically. The total phenolic content of organic pak choi samples as measured by the Folin-Ciocalteu assay, however, was significantly higher than conventional samples."

2004

Nutrients and antioxidant molecules in yellow plums (Prunus domestica L.) from conventional and organic productions: a comparative study. Lombard-Boccia G, Lucarini M, Lanzi S, Aguzzi A, Cappelloni M. J AgricFood Chem. 2004; 52(1): 90-94. **Key Finding:** Ascorbic acid, y-tocopherols, and B-carotene were higher in organic plums grown on soil with natural meadow. Total polyphenols content and quercetin were higher in conventional plums. Myrecitin and kaempferol were higher in organic plums.

Grain mineral concentrations and yield of wheat grown under organic and conventional management. Ryan MH, Derrick JW, Dann PR. J Sci Food Agric. 2004;84(3):207-16. **Key Finding:** Conventional grain had lower Zn and Cu, but higher Mn and P than organic grain. "These variations in grain minerals had nutritional implications primarily favouring the organic grain."

Influence of organic versus conventional agricultural practices on the antioxidant microconstituent content of tomatoes and derive purees; consequences on antioxidant plasma status in humans. Caris-Veyrat C, Amiot MJ, Tyssandier V, et al. J Agric Food Chem. 2004 Oct;52(21):6503-9. **Key Finding:** "In tomato purees, no difference in carotenoid content was found between the two modes of culture, whereas the concentrations of vitamin C and polyphenols remained higher in purees made out of organic tomatoes."

Changes in USDA food composition data for 43 garden crops, 1950 to 1999. Davis DR, Epp MD, Riordan HD. J Am Coll Nutr. 2004;23(6):669-82. **Key Finding:** Statistically reliable declines were found for 6 nutrients (protein, Ca, P, Fe, riboflavin and ascorbic acid). Declines ranged from 6% for protein to 38% for riboflavin. These measurements were taken from nonorganic crops in the 43 crop categories.

2003

Comparison of the total phenolic and ascorbic acid content of freeze-dried and air-dried marionberry, strawberry, and corn grown using conventional, organic, and sustainable agricultural practices. Asami DK, Hong YJ, Barrett DM, Mitchell A. J Agric Food Chem. 2003;51(5):1237-41. **Key Finding:** "Statistically higher levels of total phenolics were consistently found in organically and sustainably grown foods as compared to those produced by conventional agricultural practices." Organically grown corn and marionberries contained up to 65% more phenolic compounds than conventionally grown crops, while organic strawberries contained 19% more.

Organically produced plant foods – evidence of health benefits. Lundegardh B, Martensson A. Agriculturae Scandinavica. 2003;Section B. **Key Finding:** "It is a reasonable assumption that organic foods can strengthen the immune system and other defense systems depending on an interaction between various favourable properties of the organic foods."

Organic food: nutritious food or food for thought? A review of the evidence. Magkos F, Arvaniti F, Zampelas A. Int J Food Sci Nutr. 2003 Sep;54(5):357-71. **Key Finding:** "Although there is little evidence that organic and conventional foods differ in respect to the concentrations of the various micronutrients (vitamins, minerals and trace elements), there seems to be a slight trend towards higher ascorbic acid content in organically grown leafy vegetables and potatoes." Protein concentration is of higher quality in some organic vegetables and "animal feeding experiments indicate that animal health and reproductive performance are slightly improved when they are organically fed."

Effect of diets based on foods from conventional versus organic production on intake and excretion of flavonoids and markers of antioxidative defense in humans. Grinder-Pedersen L, Rasmussen SE, Bugel S, et al. J. Agric. Food Chem. 2003;51:5671-76. **Key Finding:** "The food production method affected the content of the major flavonoid, quercetin, in foods and also affected urinary flavonoids and markers of oxidation in humans." Urinary excretion of quercetin and kaempferol was higher after 22 days on intake of the organically produced diet when compared to the conventionally produced.

2002

Modulation of antioxidant compounds in organic vs conventional fruit (peach, Prunus persica L., and pear, Pyrus communis L.) Carbonaro M, Mattera M, Nicoli S, Bergamo P, Cappelloni M. J Agric Food Chem. 2002; 50(19):5458-62. **Key Finding:** "A parallel increase in polyphenol content and PPO activity of organic peach and pear as compared with the corresponding conventional samples was found. Ascorbic and citric acids were higher in organic than conventional peaches, whereas a-tocopherol was increased in organic pear. These data provide evidence that an improvement in the antioxidant defense system of the plant occurred as a consequence of the organic cultivation practice."

Nutritional quality of organic food: shades of grey or shades of green? Williams CM. Proc Nutr Soc. 2002;61:19-24. **Key Finding:** "There are reasonably consistent findings for higher nitrate and lower vitamin C contents of conventionally produced vegetables, particularly leafy vegetables," compared to organic produce.

2001

Salicylic acid in soups prepared from organically and nonorganically grown vegetables. Baxter GJ, Graham AB, Lawrence JR, Wiles D, Paterson JR. Eur J Nutr. 2001 Dec;40(6):289-92. **Key Finding:** "Organic vegetable soups contained more salicylic acid (almost six times) than nonorganic ones, suggesting that the vegetables and plants used to prepare them contained greater amounts of the phenolic acid than the corresponding nonorganic ingredients. Consumption of organic foods may result in a greater intake of salicylic acid."

Polyphenoloxidase activity and polyphenol levels in organically and conventionally grown peach (Prunus persica L., cv. Regina Bianca) and pear (Pyrus communis L., cv. Williams). Carbonaro M, Mattera M. Food Chem. 2001 March;72(4):419-24. **Key Finding:** "All organic peach samples showed a highly significant (P<0.001) increase in polyphenols compared with conventional peaches, while, of the three organic pear samples, two displayed an increased polyphenol content with respect to the conventionally grown sample. Activity of PPO was significantly higher in most of the organic peach and pear samples."

Organic agriculture: does it enhance or reduce the nutritional value of plant foods? Brandt K, Molgaard JP. J Sci Food Agric. 2001;81(9):924-31. **Key Finding:** "There is ample, but circumstantial, evidence that, on average, organic vegetables and fruits most likely contain more of these compounds (minerals, vitamins, proteins, etc.) than conventional ones, allowing for the possibility that organic plant foods may in fact benefit human health more than corresponding conventional ones."

Nutritional quality of organic versus conventional fruits, vegetables, and grains. Worthington V. J Altern Complement Med. 2001 Apr; 7(2):161-73. **Key Finding:** "Organic crops contained significantly more vitamin C, magnesium, and phosphorus and significantly less nitrates than conventional crops. There appear to be genuine differences in the nutrient content of organic and conventional crops."

Organic Farming, Food Quality and Human Health: A Review of the Evidence. Heaton, Shane. Soil Association Ltd., Bristol (United Kingdom). 2001. Available at http://www.soilassociation.org/LinkClick.aspx?fileticket=cY8kfP 3Q%2BgA%3D&tabid=388. Accessed on 27 May 2011. **Key Finding:** "Viewed collectively the valid and relevant scientific evidence indicates that organically grown foods are significantly different in terms of their safety, nutritional content and nutritional value from those produced by nonorganic farming."

2000

Production of lettuce under different fertilisation treatments, yield and quality. Premuzic Z, Garate A, Bonilla I. ISHA Acta Horticulturae 571: Workshop

Towards Ecologically Sound Fertilisation in Field Vegetable Production. 2000. **Key Finding:** Four fertilizer treatments were applied to lettuce—two organic (vermicompost and biostabilised compost) and two inorganic. "Vermicompost presented the best result, i.e. a high yield, a low nitrate content and a high vitamin C content."

Comparative investigation of concentrations of major and trace elements in organic and conventional Danish agricultural crops. Onions (Allium cepa Hysam) and peas (Pisum sativum Ping Pong). Gundersen V, Bechmann IE, Behrens A, Sturup S. J Agric Food Chem. 2000; 48(12): 6094-102. **Key Finding:** "Comparative statistical tests of the element concentration mean values for each site show significantly ($p<0.05$) different levels of Ca, Mg, B, Bi, Dy, Eu, Gd, Lu, Rb, Sb, Se, Sr, Ti, U and Y between the organically and conventionally grown onions and significantly ($p<0.05$) different levels of P, Gd, and Ti between the organically and conventionally grown peas."

1998

Effect of agricultural methods on nutritional quality: a comparison of organic with conventional crops. V. Worthington. Altern-Ther-Health-Med. 1998 Jan;4(1):58-69. **Key Finding:** "Existing studies show that organic fertilization practices produce crops with higher levels of ascorbic acid, lower levels of nitrate, and improved protein quality compared with conventionally grown crops."

Are organically grown apples tastier and healthier? A comparative field study using conventional and alternative methods to measure fruit quality. Weibel FP, Bickel R, Leuthold S, Alfoldi T. ISHS Acta Horticulturae 517: XXV International Horticultural Congress, Part 7: Quality of Horticultural Products. 1998. **Key Finding:** P-content was 31% higher ($p<0.01$) in organic apples. Content of phenols (mainly flavanols) was 19% and image forming quality 60% higher in organic apples.

Yield, vitamin and mineral contents of organically and conventionally grown potatoes and sweet corn. Warman PR, Havard KA. Agric Ecosyst Environ 1998 April;68(3): 207-16. **Key Finding:** There was no difference between treatments in the vitamin C or E contents of corn. In organically fertilized potatoe plots the P, Ca, Mg and Cu were higher. Mg content was higher in the organic corn.

1997

Yield, vitamin and mineral contents of organically and conventionally grown carrots and cabbage. Warman PR, Havard KA, Agric Ecosyst Environ. 1997 Feb;61(2-3): 155-62. **Key Finding:** "Analysis of the 3 years of data showed that the yield and vitamin content of the carrots and cabbages were not affected by treatments. Five elements in carrot roots (N, S, Mn, Cu, B) and two elements in carrot leaves (S, Na) were influenced by treatments; in cabbages, N, Mn, and Zn were affected."

Historical changes in the mineral content of fruits and vegetables. Mayer AM. British Food Journal. 1997;99(6):20711. **Key Finding:** A comparison of the mineral content of 20 fruits and 20 vegetables grown in the 1930s and the 1980s (published in the UK government's Composition of Foods tables) shows several marked reductions in mineral content. There are statistically signficiant reductions in the levels of Ca, Mg, Cu and Na in vegetables and Mg, Fe, Cu and K in fruit. The only mineral over the 50-year period that showed no significant difference was P. These differences could have been caused by changes in agricultural practices.

A comparison of organically and conventionally grown foods – results of a review of the relevant literature. Woese K, Lange D, Boess C, Bogl KW. J Sci Food Agric. 1997;74:281-93. **Key Finding:** 150 studies comparing organic to conventional were reviewed covering cereals, potatoes, vegetables, fruits, wine, beer, bread, cakes, milk, meat, eggs and honey, as well as products made from them. About 100 of the studies dealt with potatoes, vegetables, fruits and nuts. From among those studies, the following trends were identified—organic potatoes had higher phosphorus and potassium levels than conventionally grown, and some studies showed that organic contained higher vitamin C, while other studies showed no difference. There were clear findings that organic vegetables had a lower nitrate content than conventional; in half of the studies organic vegetables had a higher iron content, otherwise, no differences were observed in the contents of minerals and trace elements between organic and conventional products.

Vitamin C in organic vegetables was found to be higher by roughly half of the studies, while the other half found no major difference. Higher Vitamin C content was particularly noted in organic lettuce, savoy cabbage, spinach, and chard (leaf beet). Few studies addressed qualitative differences between fruit, nuts and oil seeds from organic and conventional cultivation. As a last observation from the studies, "animals distinguish between the foods on offer from the various agricultural systems and almost exclusively prefer organic produce."

1993

Organic foods vs supermarket foods: element levels. Smith BL. J Appl Nutr. 1993;45:35-39. **Key Finding:** Over a two-year period the mineral content of organically and conventionally grown apples, corn, pears, potatoes, and wheat was analyzed in Chicago. "The average elemental concentration in organic foods on a fresh weight basis was found to be about twice that of commercial foods." Organic foods were higher than conventionally grown in these eight mineral categories: calcium 63% higher; chromium 78% higher; iodine 73% higher; iron 59% higher; magnesium 138% higher; potassium 125% higher; selenium 390% higher; and zinc, 60% higher.

Index

Medical conditions and diseases appear in *italicized* typeface; **bold** typeface indicates major discussions of those topics.

1,1-bis(3'-indolyl)-1-(*p*-substituted phenyl)methanes (D-DIMs), *pancreatic cancer* and, 133

1alpha,25-dihydroxyvitamin D3, *leukemia* and, 221

1-cyano-2-dydroxy-3-butene (crambene), 31, 204, 210

2-phenylethylisothiocyanate, as antimicrobial, 205

3,3'-Diindolylmethane (DIM), 17; *cancer* and, 54, 69, 90–91; *breast cancer,* 94, 96; *cervical cancer,* 101, 141; *colon cancer,* 103–4, 219; *pancreatic cancer,* 133; *prostate cancer,* 135–36, 140, 141, 145

5-deoxykaempferol, *skin cancer* and, 149–50

5-fluorouracil, *liver cancer* and, 223

[6]-gingerol, *cancer* and, 68, 74, 79

[6]-paradol, *cancer* and, 79

8-prenylnaringenin, *cancer* and, 69

A

acetic acid, antioxidant activity and, 27

ADHD (attention deficit hyperactivity disorder), 44, 45

aging (ageing), 18–21, 200, 245–50

aglycones, 50, 184

Aiello, Jennifer, nutritional healing and, 11

AITC (allyl isothiocyanate). *See* allyl isothiocyanate (AITC)

alcohol/alcohol abuse/alcohol consumption: *cancer* and, 82, 111, 115, 307; *hypertension (high blood pressure)* and, 269; phytoestrogens and, 99, 118, 161, 185, 191; resveratrol and, 43

alfalfa, cholesterol and, 234

alimentary tract cancer, 86, 213

a-linolenic acid (ALA), 177–78

alkaloids, 25, 150, 174, 176, 177

allergies, 21

allicin, 17, 68

alliin, 17, 232

allium compounds/vegetables, 17, 74, 208, 306, 335

allspices, as antimicrobial, 24, 66

allyl alcohol, *candida* and, 232

allyl isothiocyanate (AITC), 17; as antimicrobial, 205; *cancer* and, 70, 87, 113, 282, 287, 297–98; *obesity* and, 188

allyl methyl trisulfide, 17

almonds/almond skins, 201, 203, 238, 261, 326

alpha-carotene (a-carotene): *cancer* and, 84; *breast cancer,* 98, 305; *colorectal cancer,* 115; *lung cancer,* 128, 129; *prostate cancer,* 143, 144, 230; cooking's effect on, 290, 291, 292, 305; *hypertension (high blood pressure)* and, 181; in raw foods, 312

alpha-cryptoxanthin, *prostate cancer* and, 144

alpha-lipoic acid, *aging (ageing)* and, 249, 274

alpha-tocopherol (a-tocopherol)/a-tocopherol succinate, 23, 95, 132, 326, 333

alternate-day fasting, 257, 258, 263, 265, 277

Alternate Healthy Eating Index score, 265

Alzheimer's disease, 21–23, 251

amaranth leaves, cooking's/processing's effect on, 291

Amelanchier ainifolia (serviceberry), *diabetes* and, 172

American Diabetes Association, 265, 310

amino acids, cooking's effect on, 285

aminoglycosides, as antibiotic, 205

anacardic acid, 17

anethole (fennel), 16, 51, 68

animal fats, 115, 307, 315

anthocyanidins, 13, 57, 96, 120

anthocyanins, 13. *See also* specific types of; *Alzheimer's disease* and, 22; *cancer* and, 28, 46, 53, 66; *breast cancer,* 93; *colon cancer,* 106, 108–9, 113, 220, 225, 231; *oral cancer,* 220, 225, 231; *prostate cancer,* 220, 225, 231; *cardiovascular (coronary/heart) disease* and, 152, 156; cognitive function and, 166, 167; cooking's effect on, in black soybeans, 283; *eye (retinal)* diseases and, 175; *obesity* and, 189; in organic vs. nonorganic fruits/ vegetables, 325, 329

antibacterials, 23–25, 165, 181, 205, 299

anti-inflammatories. *See also* specific types of: *aging (ageing)* and, 18; *Alzheimer's disease* and, 22; *arthritis* and, 40; *cancer* and, 75; natural agents and, 49; phytochemicals and, 64, 65, 69, 75; plant-based foods and, 55, 57, 111; spice ingredients and, 74; sulforaphane and, 56, 218; sulindac and, 109; *neurodegenerative diseases* and, 186–87

antimicrobials, 23–25, 66, 205, 242, 319, 326

antimutagenicity: antioxidant activity and, 70; berries and, 69; beta-carotene (b-carotene) and, 213; cruciferous vegetables and, 177; flavanones/flavones/flavonoids/ flavonols and, 80, 102; green peppers and, 213; green tea and, 177; lycopene and, 46; phytochemicals and, 70; Polynesian diet and, 79; selenium and, 177; tomatoes and, 46; vegetables and, 60, 62; xanthophyll and, 213

antineoplastic agents/effects, *cancer* and, 63, 65, 71

antioxidant response element (ARE), *cancer* and, 28, 31, 34, 73, 116

antioxidants/antioxidant activity. *See also* specific types of: *aging (ageing)* and, 18–19, 20, 21, 22, 26, 83, 200; caloric restriction/fasting and, 246, 262; *Alzheimer's disease* and, 186, 191; antimutagenicity and, 70; *atherosclerosis* and, 159; caloric restriction/fasting and, 251–53, 272, 275; *cancer* and, 100, 129, 149, 169, 174; *cardiovascular (coronary/heart) disease* and: carotenoids and, 170, 171; catechins and, 170; cranberries and, 157; dietary fats and, 169; dietary supplements and, 25; flavanones/flavones/flavonoids/flavonols, 159, 169, 170, 171, 174; fruits/vegeta-

B

bacterial pathogens, cranberries and, 48, 154, 182, 186

baicalein, *eye (retinal)* diseases and, 175

bananas: antioxidant activity and, 37; *cancer* and, 79, 297; *cognitive function/impairment* and, 167; organic vs. nonorganic, 324; oxalic acid in, 17

bay leaves, as antimicrobial, 24, 66

b-carotene. *See* beta-carotene (b-carotene)

b-cryptoxanthin, *hypertension (high blood pressure)* and, 181

beans, 12, 16, 17. *See also* legumes; specific types of; cooking's effect on, 286, 287; *hyper-glycemia* and, 179, 180; *hypertension (high blood pressure)* and, 180; *oral cancer* and, 301

beetroots, cooking's effect on, 282, 293

bell peppers, organic vs. nonorganic, 320. *See also* specific types of

benzo[a]pyrene (BP)/benzo[a]pyrene-3 sulfate, *cancer* and, 50, 70, 91, 100, 126, 222

benzo-gamma-pyrone, reactive oxygen species and, 39

benzyl isothiocyanate/benzyl ICT, *cancer* and, 68, 87

bergamotiin, *gastric cancer* and, 120

berries/berry juice. *See also* specific types of: *aging (ageing)* and, 18, 19, 21; *Alzheimer's disease* and, 22; antimutagenicity and, 69; antioxidant activity and, 202, 203, 211; *cancer* and, 45, 58, 59, 69–70, 75, 186, 203–4; *breast cancer*, 92, 107, 139, 151; *colon cancer*, 53, 106, 107, 108, 109; *esophageal (oesophageal) cancer*, 154; *hepatocellular carcinoma*, 123; *intestinal cancer*, 92, 107, 139, 151; *prostate cancer*, 92, 107, 139, 151; *stomach cancer*, 92, 107, 139; *cardiovascular (coronary/heart) disease* and: antioxidant activity and, 168, 172, 179; cranberries and, 164; efficacy and, 45, 154, 186; living-foods diet and, 308; *diabetes* and, 172; *fibromyalgia* and, 311; *hypertension (high blood pressure)* and, 163, 168, 172, 173, 179; *menopausal symptoms* and, 154; *metabolic syndrome* and, 172; *neurodegenerative diseases* and, 45, 185–86; *rheumatoid arthritis* and, 296; *type 2 diabetes* and, 172

beta-aescin, *liver cancer* and, 223

beta-carbolines, as antimicrobial/antiviral, 25

beta-carotene (b-carotene): antimutagenicity and, 213; *cancer* and, 77, 84, 85, 213; *breast cancer*, 98, 101, 306; *colorectal cancer*, 115; *esophageal (oesophageal) cancer*, 297; *lung cancer*: carotenoids/flavonoids and, 128, 137, 154, 162; fruits/vegetables and, 127, 129–30; low levels and, 85, 90; *pancreatic cancer*, 132; *prostate cancer*, 143, 149, 230; *cardiovascular (coronary/heart) disease* and, 90, 128, 130, 137, 154, 162, 181; *chronic diseases* and, 312; cooking's effect on, 286, 288, 290, 291, 292, 307; *esophageal (oesophageal) cancer* and, 297; *hypertension (high blood pressure)* and, 181; *lung cancer* and, 85, 90; in organic vs. nonorganic fruits/vegetables, 320, 324, 327, 331; in raw foods, 312

beta-catenin, *colon cancer* and, 102, 109, 114, 116

beta-cryptoxanthin, 98, 115

betacyanins, 16

betalains, 16. *See also* specific types of

beta-lapachone (b-lapachone), 144, 182, 230

betanin, 16

beta sitosterol/beta-sitosteryl oleate, 16, 131, 165, 203

betaxanthins, 16

betulinic acid, 16

bilberries, 13, 16; antioxidant activity and, 202, 203, 211; *colon cancer* and, 106, 109, 113

Biosphere 2, caloric restriction/fasting and, 261, 266, 268, 270, 278

bitter gourd, *skin cancer* and, 151

blackberries/blackberry juice, 13, 14, 92, 107, 109, 139, 151

black cumin, 24, 51, 66

black currants/black currant juice: antioxidant activity and, 323; *cancer* and, 92, 107, 139, 151; lignans (phytoestrogens) in, 14; lipids in, 16; organic vs. nonorganic, 323, 329

black raspberries, 109, 131, 210

black soybeans, cooking's effect on, 282–83

black tea, 13, 24, 66, 142, 148, 231, 302

bladder cancer, 86–88, 213

blood lipids: caloric restriction/fasting and, 269; nuts and, 153, 163; soy (soya) and, 44, 99, 118, 152, 161, 191

blueberries/blueberry juice: *aging (ageing)* and, 21, 42, 58; anthocyanins in, 325; antioxidant activity and, 36, 202, 203, 211, 325; *atherosclerosis* and, 42, 58, 193–94; *cancer* and, 42, 58, 69–70, 92, 193; *breast cancer,* 88, 107, 139, 151; *colon cancer,* 109; *intestinal cancer,* 107, 139, 151; *prostate cancer,* 107, 139, 151; *stomach cancer,* 107, 139, 151; health benefits of, 237; *HIV infection* and, 238; *inflammation* and, 42, 58, 183, 194; *ischemic (ischaemic) stroke* and, 42, 58, 194; malic acid in, 325; *neurodegenerative diseases* and, 186–87, 194; organic vs. nonorganic, 324–25; oxidative stress and, 194; *Parkinson's disease* and, 191–92; secoisolariciresinol in, 13; *vascular disease* and, 42, 58

blue flavonoids, 12

blue fruits/vegetables, 13

boiled meat, *cancer* and, 302

bone density/bone density maintenance, 44, 99, 118, 152, 161, 191

botanicals/botanical diversity, 29, 74–75, 116, 201–2

BP (benzo[a]pyrene). *See* benzo[a]pyrene (BP)/benzo[a]pyrene-3 sulfate, *cancer* and

brassica vegetables. *See also* specific types of: antioxidant activity and, 204; *cancer* and, 59, 68, 73, 81, 82, 282, 284; isothiocyanates (ITCs) and, 298, 300; cooking's effect on, 281, 282, 283, 284, 285, 298–99, 300; organic vs. nonorganic, 320; phytochemicals in, 12, 14, 15, 17

breast cancer, 88–101, 214–17

broccoli/broccoli sprouts: antioxidant activity and, 31, 36, 204, 281, 285, 304; *cancer* and: cruciferous vegetables and, 74, 300; glucosinolates and, 294–95, 304–5; green foods and, 159, 192; isothiocyanates and, 289, 294–95, 304–5; raw vegetables and, 302; selenium and, 72; sulforaphane and, 54; types of: *bladder cancer,* 297; *colon cancer,* 117, 219; *lung cancer,* 124; *prostate cancer,* 137, 229; *stomach cancer,* 302; *cardiovascular (coronary/heart) disease* and, 159; cooking's effect on: boiling and, 281, 282; cooking duration and, 285; folate and, 288; microwaving and, 282, 283; preserving and, 283; processing and, 283, 284, 285; steaming and, 282, 289;

stir-frying and, 281; uncooked vs., 295; vitamins and, 292; *gastric disease* and, 222; *Helicobacter pylori infection* and, 176, 222; indoles/glucosinolates in, 17; lignans (phytoestrogens) in, 14; organic vs. nonorganic, 324, 327–28; storing's and transporting's effect on, 284–85, 288

Brussels sprouts, 13, 17; *cancer* and, 73, 159, 192; cooking's/storing's effect on, 281, 284; *hypercholesterolemia (high cholesterol/hyper-cholesterolaemia)* and, 166; nutrient combining and, 204

buffaloberries (Shepherdia argentea), *diabetes* and, 172

Burns, Fiona, raw-food diet and, 244

butyrate, *colon cancer* and, 103–4

C

Ca (citric acid), 27, 332, 333, 335, 336

cabbage. *See also* specific types of: antioxidant activity and, 36; *cancer* and, 62, 302; cooking's effect on, 282, 283, 293, 297–99; indoles/glucosinolates in, 17; organic vs. nonorganic, 336

caffeic acid, 14

calcium, 101, 105, 111, 117, 141, 337

caloric restriction/fasting, 243–45; *aging (ageing)* and, 18, 243, 245–50, 251, 252–53, 259, 266; *cognitive impairment* and, 261–62; *immune system* and, 271; *inflammation* and, 272; *allergies* and, 268; alternate-day fasting, 257, 258, 263, 265, 277; *Alzheimer's disease* and, 251, 268; antioxidant activity and, 251–53, 272, 275, 277; *atherosclerosis* and, 255; *attention-deficity hyperactivity disorder (ADHD)* and, 255, 267; *autoimmune disease* and, 268; blood glucose and, 261, 266, 271; blood lipids and, 269; blood pressure and, 261, 266, 269, 270, 271; body temperature and, 272, 273; Burns, Fiona, and, 244; *cancer* and, 243, 245, 255–60, 268, 273; *lymphoma*, 265; *melanoma*, 260; *prostate cancer*, 259; *cardiovascular (coronary/heart) disease* and: *aging (ageing)* and, 245, 260, 268; alternate-day fasting and, 263, 265; Daniel Fast and, 260; *diastolic dysfunction* and, 269; *inflammation* and, 272; intermittent fasting and, 263; life-long restriction and, 269; in monkeys, 243; oxidative damage/stress and, 260; periodic fasting and, 263; short-term restriction and, 269; *cerebral vascular disease* and, 245; cholesterol and, 261, 265, 266, 270, 271; *cognitive impairment* and, 261–63; *diabetes* and, 264–66; *endothelial dysfunction* and, 266–67, 272; *epilepsy* and, 255, 267; fasting blood sugar and, 266, 270; *fibromyalgia* and, 267–68; fibrosis and, 264; glucose and, 273, 277; hearing loss and, 246, 247; hibernation and, 275; *hypertension (high blood pressure)* and, 258, 261, 265, 266, 269–71; *immune system/immune system disorders* and, 245, 271; *infectious disease* and, 274; *inflammation* and, 245, 252, 262–63, 264, 272, 275; insulin sensitivity and, 264, 269; iron deposits and, 276; *ischemia (ischaemia)* and, 269, 276; leukocyte count and, 261, 266, 271; life extension/ lifespan and, 245, 268, 272–76; *liver disease* and, 245; *metabolic disease* and, 260; mortality and, 268, 275; *multiple sclerosis* and, 252, 262–63, 272, 275–76; muscles/ muscle loss and, 245, 248; *neurodegenerative disorders* and, 276–77; neuroprotection and, 245, 252, 262–63, 272, 275; *obesity* and, 277–78; oxidative damage/

stress and, 264, 266, 269, 272, 273, 274, 275; *pain* and, 278; *pancreatitis* and, 264; *Parkinson's disease* and, 268, 278; *rheumatoid arthritis* and, 253–55, 267; *sarcopenia* and, 245; SIRT1 and, 274; *stroke* and, 268; *type 2 diabetes* and, 245; weight loss and: Biosphere 2 and, 261, 266, 268, 270, 278; *cancer* and, 256, 257; *inflammation* and, 272; vegan/vegetarian diets and, 254; Weintraub, Arnie, and, 244; Weintraub, Arnie, and, 244; white blood cell counts and, 266, 270

Camellia sinensis (green/oolong tea), 25, 51, 200

campesterol, 16

camptothecin, *colon cancer* and, 117

cancer, 45–85, 206–13, 255–60, 297–307. *See also* specific types of

candida, 232

cantaloupe, *breast cancer* and, 297

canthaxanthin, 15, 84

capsaicin (red chili), 14, 51, 68, 74, 153, 188, 189

capsicum, *cancer* and, 211

cardiovascular (coronary/heart) disease: caloric restriction/fasting and, 260, 269; nutrient combining/synergies and, 232–33, 235; phytochemicals and, 152–62, 168–71; raw vs. cooked/processed vegetables and, 307–8, 313

carnitine, 173, 188, 235

carnosine, health benefits of, 237

carnosol, 12

carotene(s), 15, 114, 129. *See also* specific types of

carotenoids, 15. *See also* specific types of; *aging (ageing)* and, 21, 83, 162; as antimutagenic, 213; antioxidant activity and, 28, 32, 39, 162; *brain dysfunction* and, 162; *cancer* and, 156, 162; antioxidant activity and, 39, 83; fruits/vegetables and, 84, 85; phytochemicals and, 24, 53, 54, 64, 66, 78, 80; plant phenols and, 81; types of: *bladder cancer,* 84, 88; *breast cancer,* 89–90, 98, 130, 136–37, 154, 305; *colon cancer,* 84, 117; *colorectal cancer,* 115; *head cancer,* 90, 130, 136–37, 154; *lung cancer,* 84, 85, 128, 129–30, 162; *mouth cancer,* 84; *neck cancer,* 90, 130, 136–37, 154; *pancreatic cancer,* 133; *prostate cancer,* 90, 130, 136–37, 143–44, 154; *skin cancer,* 150, 151; *stomach cancer,* 84; *cardiovascular (coronary/heart) disease* and: antioxidant activity and, 83; astaxanthin and, 155; beta-carotene and, 162; fruits/vegetables and, 89–90, 130, 136–37, 154, 170; green leafy vegetables and, 155; living-foods diet and, 308; lycopene and, 155; nuts and, 53, 156; vitamin A and, 171; *cataracts* and, 162, 233; *chronic diseases* and, 312; cooking's effect on, 285, 289, 290, 291; *eye (retinal) diseases* and, 175; *fibromyalgia* and, 311; *immune-system disorders* and, 162; living-foods diet and, 296; *macular degeneration* and, 89–90, 130, 136–37, 154; nutrient combining and, 238; in organic vs. nonorganic fruits/vegetables, 322, 325, 328, 331; oxidative damage/stress and, 204

carrots, 14, 15; antioxidant activity and, 36; *cancer* and, 62, 106, 117, 297, 302, 306; cooking's/processing's effect on, 287, 289, 290, 291, 292, 322; organic vs. nonorganic, 322, 324, 336

carvacrol, 12

cashews, in vegan diet, 261

cassava, 291–92, 324

colitis, 234–35

collard, organic vs. nonorganic, 331

colon cancer/colorectal cancer, 102–19, 218–21

combining nutrients, 197–200

complex quinines, 25

cooking's/processing's effect on vegetables, 279–81; antioxidant activity and, 293–95; *cancer* and, 297–307; *cardiovascular (coronary/heart) disease* and, 307–8; cholesterol and, 295; *fibromyalgia* and, 296; glucosinolates and, 60; nutrient losses and, 281–93

corn/corn oil, 16, 106, 179, 180, 332, 335–36, 337

Cornell University, 243

coronary/coronary artery disease. See **cardiovascular (coronary/heart) disease**

coumarin(s), 14, 120, 123, 176, 177

coumestans, 13

cowpeas, cooking's/processing's effect on, 291

COX-2 (cyclooxygenase-2)/INOS/NOX: *arthritis* and, 40, 183; *cancer* and, 55, 56–57, 68, 75, 209, 218; *colon cancer,* 104, 109, 114–15; *lung cancer,* 125; *endothelial dysfunction* and, 266; *inflammation* and, 40, 55, 56, 75, 183

crambene (1-cyano-2-hydroxy-3-butene), 31, 204, 210

cranberries/cranberry juice: *aging (ageing)* and, 42, 58; antioxidant activity and, 30, 37, 203, 233; anti-viral activity and, 154, 182, 186; *atherosclerosis* and, 42, 58, 193–94; *bacterial pathogens* and, 48, 154, 182, 186; *cancer* and, 154, 182, 186, 193, 208; flavonoids and, 42, 58; phytochemicals and, 46, 48, 55, 66, 152; types of: *breast cancer,* 53, 93, 95, 107, 139, 151, 215; *colon cancer,* 53, 109, 220, 225, 230, 231; *intestinal cancer,* 107, 139, 151; *lung cancer,* 53; *oral cancer,* 220, 225, 230; *prostate cancer,* 53, 107, 134–35, 139, 151; nutrient combining and, 220, 225, 230; *stomach cancer,* 107, 139, 151; *cardiovascular (coronary/heart) disease* and, 46, 48, 152, 154, 157, 182, 186; nutrient combining and, 233; *dental health/infections* and, 46, 152; *diabetes* and, 235–36, 239; *Helicobacter pylori infection* and, 46, 152, 242; *hypercholesterolemia (high cholesterol/hyper-cholesterolaemia)* and, 164, 235–36; *hypertension (high blood pressure)* and, 157, 235, 236, 239; *infections* and, 46, 152; *inflammation* and: flavonoids and, 42, 58, 194; phytochemicals and, 48, 154, 182, 186, 208; *ischemic (ischaemic) stroke* and, 42, 58, 194; *neurodegenerative diseases* and, 186, 194; neuroprotection and, 154, 182, 186; oxidative damage/stress and, 194; *ulcers* and, 242; *urinary tract infections* and, 46, 152; *vascular disease* and, 42, 58

cruciferous vegetables: antimutagenicity and, 177; antioxidant activity and, 34; *arthritis* and, 40, 183; *cancer* and, 74, 210, 212; antioxidant responsive element (ARE) and, 34, 73; botanicals and, 74; indoles and, 60; isothiocyanates and, 60; methyl-3-indolylacetate and, 61; phytochemicals and, 74, 76–77; sprouts and, 68–69; sulforaphane glucosinolate and, 64; types of: *bladder cancer,* 297, 298, 299; *breast cancer,* 91–92, 100, 297, 306; *cervical cancer,* 101, 141; *colon cancer,* 77, 113, 116; *lung cancer,* 124; *non-Hodgkin's lymphoma,* 130; *oral cancer,* 304; *prostate cancer,* 137, 141; cooking's effect on, 298; detoxification and, 204; *HIV infection* and, 177; *inflammation* and, 40, 183

cryptoxanthin, 15

cucumbers, antioxidant activity and, 36

cucurbitacin, *cancer* and, 71

curcumin(s), 14; *aging (ageing)* and, 18, 246; *Alzheimer's disease* and, 22; antioxidant activity and, 30, 200, 201, 202, 246; *cancer* and: chemopreventive agents and, 68, 74; clinical trials and, 47; DNA damage and, 54; nutrient combining and, 209, 212; phytochemicals and, 24, 57, 61, 66, 69, 79, 209; types of: *breast cancer,* 90–91, 92, 95, 217; *colon cancer:* clinical trials and, 47; COX-2 and, 114–15; NF-kappaB and, 113; quercetin and, 219; resveratrol and, 218; tea and, 221, 223, 225; *colorectal adenomas,* 219; *colorectal cancer,* 102, 112; *duodenal cancer,* 221, 223, 225; *forestomach cancer,* 221, 223, 225; *hepatocellular carcinoma,* 120; *leukemia,* 223, 225; *multiple myeloma,* 47; *oral cancer,* 221, 223, 225–26; *pancreatic cancer,* 47, 226; *prostate cancer,* 139–40, 228, 229–30; *inflammation* and, 18, 240, 241, 246; *obesity* and, 188; *osteoarthritis* and, 241; as proxidant, 37

currants. *See* specific types of

cyanidin, 13, 113

cyanidol, *thrombosis (blood clots)* and, 194

cycloartane, *cancer* and, 71

cyclooxygenase-2. *See* COX-2 (cyclooxygenase-2)/INOS/NOX

cysteine, *atherosclerosis* and, 206

D

daidzein, 13; *cancer* and, 74; *breast cancer,* 90, 99; *colorectal cancer,* 106, 137; *prostate cancer,* 106, 137–38, 142, 146; in organic vs. nonorganic soybean seeds, 323–24; oxidative damage and, 37

dammarane, *cancer* and, 71

Daniel Fast, 260, 269

dark greens/vegetables, 15, 16, 129, 297

DASH diet, 270

D-DIMs (1,1-bis[3'-indolyl]-1-[*p*-substituted phenyl]methanes), *pancreatic cancer* and, 133

dehydroascorbate, 215, 220, 329

delphinidin, 13

DeNardo, Erin, nutritional healing and, 198

denistein, *breast cancer* and, 90–91

diabetes, 171–74, 235–36

diallyl disulfide/diallyl sulfide, 17, 68, 188

diarrhea, 174

dietary restriction. *See* caloric restriction/fasting

diet/nutrition. *See also* specific diets: *Alzheimer's disease* and, 268; *cancer* and, 55, 56, 59, 60–61, 66–67, 79, 80–81; *breast cancer,* 95, 96; *colon cancer,* 114, 116; *colorectal adenomas/cancer,* 103, 111, 115; *prostate cancer,* 143

dihydroflavonols, 13

dill, 12, 15

dillapiole, 12

DIM (3,3'-Diindolylmethane). *See* 3,3'-Diindolylmethane (DIM)

diosgenin (fenugreek), 51

diosmin, *cancer* and, 61, 117

dithiolthiones (isothiocyanates), 17

doxorubicin (DOX), *breast cancer* and, 216

dried fruits, in vegan diet, 261

dry bean intake, *colorectal adenomas* and, 110

E

(E)-2-hexenal, as antimicrobial, 205

echinacea/Echinacea purperea, 14, 77

EGCG (epigallocatechin (-3-) gallate). *See* epigallocatechin (-3-) gallate (EGCG)

eggs, 114, 165, 301, 308, 336

eicosapentaenoic acid (EPA), *colon cancer* and, 218

elderberries, antioxidant activity and, 202, 203, 211

ellagic acid, 14; *arsenic exposure* and, 27; *cancer* and, 68, 110, 220, 222, 223, 224; *vascular health* and, 153

ellagitannins, 109, 153

Emblica officinalis, 151, 206, 240

endothelial dysfunction, 266–67

enterodiol, 106, 137

enterolactone, 106, 137

EPA (eicosapentaenoic acid),*colon cancer* and, 218

(-)-epicatechin, 13, 33, 91, 108, 170

epigallocatechin (-3-) gallate (EGCG), 52; antioxidant activity and, 35, 37; *cancer* and, 50, 64, 79, 212; *breast cancer,* 90–91, 100, 214, 217; *colon cancer,* 107, 108, 219, 220–21; *fibrosarcoma,* 221; *hepatocellular carcinoma,* 120; *lung cancer,* 124; *oral cancer,* 225–26; *osteosarcoma,* 226; *prostate cancer,* 135, 139–40, 147–48, 228, 230; *cardiovascular (coronary/heart) disease* and, 153; *diabetes* and, 173; *eye (retinal)* diseases and, 175; in green tea, 13, 50; *HIV infection* and, 176–77; *obesity* and, 188–89; *periodontal disease* and, 192

epilepsy, 267

equoi, 99, 106, 137, 142

eriodictyol, 12, 175

erucin, *breast cancer* and, 95

essential fatty acids, 173, 279

etoposide, *cancer* and, 63

eugenol. *See* cloves (eugenol)

eye (retinal) diseases, 175

F

faba beans, processing's effect on, 291

farnesol, 115, 134

fasting. *See* caloric restriction/fasting

fatty acids, 65, 105, 140, 164, 290. *See also* specific types of

Fe (iron), 238, 276, 319, 330, 332, 336, 337

fennel (anethole), 16, 51, 68

fenugreek (diosgenin), 51

fermented foods, 27, 304

ferulic acid, 14, 131, 205, 239, 240

fiber (fibre): *aging (ageing)* and, 20; *atherosclerosis* and, 159; *cancer* and, 169, 174; *breast cancer,* 100; *colon cancer,* 114, 116, 119; *colorectal adenoma/cancer,* 103, 111; *cardiovascular (coronary/heart) disease* and, 157, 158, 159, 160, 161, 169, 174; cholesterol and, 308, 313; vegan/vegetarian diet and, 313; cooking's effect on, 288; *diabetes* and, 169, 174; *hypercholesterolemia (high cholesterol/hyper-cholesterolaemia)* and, 174, 179, 238; in organic vs. nonorganic fruits/vegetables, 323, 326; in vegan diet, 261

fibromyalgia, 267–68, 310–11

fibrosarcoma, 221

figs, antioxidant activity and, 30

fisetin, 104, 112, 121, 138, 166, 175

fish, 155, 304, 307, 320

flavan-3-ols, 13, 46, 152. *See also* specific types of

flavanones/flavones/flavonoids/flavonols. *See also* specific types of: *aging (ageing)* and, 19; antimutagenicity and, 80, 102; *arthritis* and, 206; *cancer* and, 50, 82–83, 171, 208; *alimentary tract cancer,* 213; *bladder cancer,* 88; *breast cancer,* 89, 93, 95, 96, 98, 147; *colon cancer,* 113, 117, 220; *colorectal adenomas/cancer,* 102, 104, 105, 106–7, 108, 110; *esophageal (oesophageal) cancer,* 105, 154; *gastric cancer,* 105; *intestinal cancer,* 105; *laryngeal cancer,* 120; *leukemia,* 121; *liver cancer,* 123; *lung cancer,* 124, 125, 126, 127, 128–29; *oral cancer,* 220; *ovarian cancer,* 132; *pancreatic cancer,* 132, 133; *prostate cancer,* 220; *renal cell carcinoma,* 149; *skin cancer,* 150; *cardiovascular (coronary/heart) disease* and: adenosine receptors and, 160; berries and, 154, 163, 168; chronic diseases and, 19; cocoa and, 154, 156; cranberries and, 152; green tea and, 156; intake amounts and, 82, 156, 162, 169, 170, 171, 193; phytochemicals and, 162; quercetin and, 156, 157, 163; soy and, 156; ta and, 154; women and, 159, 170; *central nervous system disorders* and, 160; *cerebrovascular disease* and, 41, 162–63; *chronic diseases* and, 162, 174; cognitive function and, 166; cooking's/transporting's effect on, 283, 288, 290; *diarrhea* and, 174; *eye (retinal)* diseases and, 175; *Helicobacter pylori infection* and, 176; *hepatitis* and, 176, 177; *HIV infection* and, 177; *immune-system disorders* and, 160, 181; *inflammation* and, 182–83, 240; *ischemic (ischaemic) stroke* and, 156, 193; *menopausal symptoms* and, 147, 154; *multiple sclerosis* and, 185; *obesity* and, 187–88; *obstructive pulmonary disease* and, 189; in organic vs. nonorganic fruits/ vegetables, 324, 332–33; apples, 335; bell peppers, 320; blueberries, 324; chicory, 320; soybean seeds, 323–24; tomatoes, 317, 326; *thrombosis (blood clots)* and, 194–95; *type 2 diabetes* and, 41, 173

flaxseed, 24, 66

folate/folic acid. *See under* vitamins

food supplements, *breast cancer* and, 92

friedelane, *cancer* and, 71

fried foods, health and, 281, 308, 313

fruits/vegetables. *See also* cooking's/processing's effect on vegetables; specific types of: *aging (ageing)* and, 19, 20, 21, 22, 42, 58, 83; *Alzheimer's disease* and, 22, 191; anthocyanins in, 106; as antibacterial, 24; antimutagenicity and, 60, 62; antioxidant activity and, 24, 27, 28, 29, 34, 36–37, 237; as antiviral, 24; on British ships, in 18th century, 9; *cancer* and: amount consumed and, 83–84; antioxidant activity and: garlic extract and, 24; oxidative damage and, 83, 162; phytochemicals and, 34, 46, 60–61, 237; reactive oxygen species and, 28; bioactive compounds and, 160; flavonoids and, 82–83; isoprenoids and, 78; nutrient combining/synergies and, 221, 225; oxidative biomarkers and, 201–2; phytochemicals and, 75, 77, 78, 82, 209, 210; types of: *adenomatous polyps,* 116; *alimentary tract cancer,* 306; *bladder cancer,* 83, 84, 86–87; *breast cancer:* carotenoids and, 90, 130, 136–37, 154; intake amounts and, 83, 84, 85, 97; nutrients and, 100; phytochemicals and, 95, 215, 216; raw/cooked vegetables and, 297, 299, 301, 303, 304, 306, 307; *cervical cancer,* 83, 84; *colon cancer,* 83–84; carotenoids and, 84; intake amounts and, 83, 114, 115, 119; phytoestrogens and, 99, 118, 152, 161, 190; *colorectal adenomas,* 103, 110, 116; *colorectal cancer,* 84, 105–6, 116, 125, 303; *endometrial cancer,* 84; *esophageal (oesophageal) cancer,* 83, 84, 85, 86, 297, 302, 303; *gall bladder cancer,* 85; *gastric cancer,* 302, 303, 304; *genital cancer,* 85; *head cancer,* 130, 136–37, 154; *laryngeal cancer,* 84, 85, 303; *leukemia,* 121, 299; *liver cancer,* 85; *lung cancer:* beta-carotene (b-carotene) and, 127, 129; carotenoids and, 84, 129–30; genomics and, 105, 125; intake amounts and, 83–84, 85; phytoestrogens and, 99, 118, 152, 161, 190; raw vs. cooked vegetables and, 303; *melanoma,* 121; *mouth cancer,* 84; *neck cancer,* 90, 130, 136–37, 154; *non-Hodgkin's lymphoma,* 130; *oral cancer/oral cavity cancer,* 83, 84, 130–31, 301, 302, 303; *ovarian cancer,* 83, 84; *pancreatic cancer,* 83, 84, 85, 302; *pharyngeal cancer,* 84, 302, 303; *prostate cancer:* beta-carotene and, 149; carotenoids and, 90, 130, 136–37, 154; intake amounts and, 85; phytoestrogens and, 99, 118, 152, 161, 190, 192–93; *rectal cancer,* 84, 85, 118, 152, 161, 190; *renal cell carcinoma,* 149; *respiratory tract cancer,* 306; *stomach cancer,* 83, 84, 99, 118, 152, 161, 190 (*See also* specific); *thyroid cancer,* 85, 303–4; *upper gastrointestinal cancer,* 303; *urinary system cancer,* 85; *urothelial cancer,* 305; *uterine cancer,* 307; vegetarian diet and, 71; *cardiovascular (coronary/heart) disease* and: antioxidant activity and, 21, 83; carotenoids and, 90, 130, 136–37, 154; diets and, 308; intake amounts and, 155, 159, 160, 161, 162, 168–70; Netherlands' study and, 313; phytoestrogens and, 158–59, 161; raw fruit and, 313; *cataracts* and, 162; *cerebrovascular disease* and, 313; cholesterol and, 309; *chronic diseases* and, 159; cooking's/processing's effect on, 281–82, 299, 302, 303, 305, 313; *Crohn's disease* and, 310; *fibrocystic disease* and, 307; *fibromyalgia* and, 311; *haemorrhagic stroke* and, 194; health/protective effects of, 24, 44, 237; *Helicobacter pylori infection* and, 304; homogenates from, 62; *hypercholesterolemia (high cholesterol/hyper-cholesterolaemia)* and, 24, 165; *hypertension (high blood pressure)* and, 24, 165, 180–81; *ischemic (ischaemic) stroke* and, 194, 313; *macular degeneration* and, 130, 136–37, 154; *metabolic syndrome* and, 172; *neurodegenerative diseases* and, 187; neuronal death and, 22; *obstructive pulmonary disease* and, 189; *Parkinson's disease* and, 191; phytochemicals in, 9; *stroke* and, 160, 194, 314–15; *thrombosis (blood clots)* and, 194; *type 2 diabetes* and, 172; *ulcers* and, 315
fruit vinegars, antioxidant activity and, 27
furanyl compounds, 25

G

galangin, 121, 175

gallic acid, 14, 33, 79, 205

gamma sitosterol, 16

gamma-tocotrienol, 214, 233

garlic/garlic extract/garlic oil: *aging (ageing)* and, 20, 23, 37, 194; *Alzheimer's disease* and, 20, 23, 37, 194; as antimicrobial, 24, 66; antioxidant activity and, 37; *cancer* and: antioxidant activity and, 20, 23, 37, 194; cruciferous vegetables and, 74; heating and, 289; types of: *colon cancer,* 113; *squamous cell carcinoma,* 297; *stomach cancer,* 302; white-green foods and, 159, 192; *candida* and, 232; *cardiovascular (coronary/heart) disease* and, 20, 23, 37, 194, 313; cholesterol and, 309, 315; cooking's effect on, 282, 286, 289–90, 293, 315; *Helicobacter pylori infection* and, 176; *hypercholesterolemia (high cholesterol/hyper-cholesterolaemia)* and, 178; *hypertension (high blood pressure)* and, 180; *liver damage* and, 241; oxidative damage and, 180; *stroke* and, 20, 23, 37, 194; *thrombosis (blood clots)* and, 315

gastric cancer, 119–20, 222

gastrointestinal disorders, 311

gemcitabine, *cervical cancer* and, 218

genistein, 13; *cancer* and: antioxidant activity and, 81; herb-drug interactions and, 61; nutrient combining and, 209, 211, 212; soy foods/supplements and, 50, 74; types of: *breast cancer,* 217; antiestrogenic effect and, 92; DNA damage and, 89, 91; flavonoids/vitamin E and, 95; indole-3-carbinol and, 142; phytochemicals and, 100; plasma and, 90; quercetin and, 93; tamoxifen and, 93, 214; *colon cancer,* 117, 118–19; *colorectal cancer,* 106; *prostate cancer:* beta-lapachone and, 144; combining and, 135; indole-3-carbinol and, 142; nutrient combining and, 227, 228, 230, 231; phytochemicals and, 139–40, 142, 145; phytoestrogens and, 106, 137–38; selenium and, 134; signaling pathways and, 147–48; soy and, 146; *diabetes* and, 235; *infertility* and, 182; *obesity* and, 188–89; in organic vs. nonorganic soybean seeds, 323–24

geraniol, *pancreatic cancer,* 134

Gerson's diet therapy, *melanoma* and, 260

ginger (zerumbone), 12, 15, 17, 51, 75, 79

gingerol, 12. *See also* specific types of

Ginkgo biloba, *eye (retinal)* diseases and, 175

ginseng, 75, 112, 176

glioma, 222

glucosamine, *inflammation* and, 241, 242

glucose, caloric restriction/fasting and, 273, 277

glucosinolates, 17; as antimicrobial, 205; antioxidant activity and, 204; *cancer* and: allyl-isothiocyanate (AITC) and, 70; amounts of and, 81; brassica vegetables and, 82; cooking's effect on and, 60, 294–95, 298–99, 304–5; cruciferous vegetables and, 64; phytochemicals and, 52; types of: *alimentary tract cancer,* 86, 213; *breast cancer,* 100; cooking's effect on: in brassica vegetables, 284–85; in broccoli/broccoli sprouts, 283, 284, 285, 288, 289, 294–95, 304–5; in cabbage, 283, 287, 298–99 glutathione/glutathione oxidation/gluthathione S-transferases (GSTs)/GSTP1: *aging (ageing)* and, 246; antioxidant activity and, 204; *cancer* and, 91, 102–3, 119, 121, 124, 128; cruciferous vegetables and, 204

gluten-free vegan diet, *arthritis* and, 253

glyceollins, *cancer* and, 76

glycitein, 13, 99, 106, 137

glycosides: antioxidant activity and, 39; *cancer* and, 53, 66, 220, 225, 231; cooking's effect on, 284, 286, 294

glycyrrhetinic acid, 53

gooseberries/gooseberry juice (Emblica officinalis), 12, 92, 107, 139, 151

gotu kola, *atherosclerosis* and, 206

grains/whole grains, 14; *atherosclerosis* and, 159; *cancer* and, 70–71, 78, 99, 160, 212, 303, 305; *colon cancer*, 118, 152, 161, 190; *lung cancer*, 118, 152, 161, 190; *prostate cancer*, 118, 152, 161, 190; *rectal cancer*, 118, 152, 161, 190; *stomach cancer*, 99, 118, 152, 161, 190; *cardiovascular (coronary/heart) disease* and, 70–71, 158, 159, 160, 161, 169; *diabetes* and, 70–71; *hypercholesterolemia (high cholesterol/hyper-cholesterolaemia)* and, 159; *hypertension (high blood pressure)* and, 159; *inflammation* and, 159; *obesity* and, 70–71; organic vs. nonorganic, 331; protective effect of, 44; *stroke* and, 160

grapefruit, 15, 37, 128, 326

grapes/grape juice/grape seed extract (GSE)/grape seeds, 12; *Alzheimer's disease* and, 22; antioxidant activity and, 33–34, 37; *cancer* and, 62, 93, 109, 113, 123, 216, 224; *cardiovascular (coronary/heart) disease* and, 157, 169, 232, 233, 235; health benefits of, 236; *inflammation* and, 240–41; melatonin in, 236; *obesity* and, 189; organic vs. nonorganic, 319, 322, 323, 324, 327

green bananas, *cancer* and, 79

green beans, cooking's effect on, 282, 289, 290, 293

green cabbage, cooking's/storing's effect on, 284–85

green foods, *cancer* and, 159, 192

green peppers, 213, 327

greens/green leafy vegetables/green vegetables, 15, 17; *cancer* and, 85, 159, 306, 307; *breast cancer*, 297, 306; *colon cancer*, 112, 117; *kidney cancer*, 318–19; *lung cancer*, 129; *oral cancer*, 304; *cardiovascular (coronary/heart) disease* and, 155, 159, 170, 307, 308; chlorophyll in, 32; *chronic diseases* and, 159; cooking's effect on, 286, 288, 291, 294, 307; *gastrointestinal diseases* and, 311; *hypercholesterolemia (high cholesterol/hypercholesterol-aemia)* and, 261; Lanning, Michael, and, 318; organic vs. nonorganic, 332, 333; in vegan diet, 261; Wigmore, Ann, and, 10

green tea, 13; *aging (ageing)* and, 19; as antimicrobial, 24; as antimutagenic, 177; antioxidant activity and, 35; *arthritis* and, 39–40; *atherosclerosis* and, 206; *cancer* and: capscium and, 211; (-)-epicatechin and, 91; epigallocatechin (-3-) gallate (EGCG) and, 50, 62, 64, 211; phytochemicals and, 74–75; polyphenols and, 59; types of: *bladder cancer*, 213; *breast cancer*, 91, 214, 215, 216, 217; *colon cancer*, 107, 108, 113; *fibrosarcoma*, 221; *hepatocellular carcinoma*, 120; *melanoma*, 224; *pancreatic cancer*, 226–27; *prostate cancer*, 138, 142, 145, 148, 231; *renal cell carcinoma*, 232; *skin cancer*, 150; *testicular cancer*, 232; *cardiovascular (coronary/heart) disease* and, 153, 155, 156; *eye (retinal)* diseases and, 175; glucose control and, 153; health benefits of, 237;

H

I

L

lactic acid, antioxidant activity and, 27

Lanning, Michael, diet and, 318–19

lanosterol, 115

lariciresinol, 14

laryngeal cancer, 120–21

L-carnitine, 188, 235

lectins, *cancer* and, 72

legumes, 13, 15, 16. *See also* specific types of; *cancer* and, 69, 77, 160; *colon cancer,* 44, 99, 118, 152, 161, 190; *gastric cancer,* 302; *lung cancer,* 44, 99, 118, 152, 161, 190; *prostate cancer,* 44, 99, 118, 152, 161, 190; *rectal cancer,* 44, 99, 118, 152, 161, 190; *stomach cancer,* 44, 99, 118, 152, 161, 190; *cardiovascular (coronary/heart) disease* and, 158, 160

lemons, antioxidant activity and, 37

lettuce, 15; antioxidant activity and, 36, 321; *colon cancer* and, 117; cooking's effect on, 292; organic vs. nonorganic, 321–22, 331, 334–35, 337

leukemia, 121–22, 222–23

licorice, 14, 53

life extension/lifespan, caloric restriction/fasting and, 272–76

lignans (phytoestrogens). *See* phytoestrogens (lignans)

lignin, 24, 66, 238

limonene, 15, 79, 212

limonoid triterpenoids, *cancer* and, 71

Lindstrom, Anna, raw-food diet and, 279–80

linseed, 99, 118, 152, 161, 190

lipids, 16. *See also* specific types of

liver cancer/damage, 123, 223, 241

living-foods diet, 254, 267, 295, 296, 308, 311

lovastatin, *breast cancer* and, 95

low-fat diet, 260, 263, 265, 310

low-sodium diet, *melanoma* and, 260

lunasin, *cancer* and, 72

lung cancer, 124–30

lupine, *cancer* and, 71

lutein, 15; antioxidant activity and, 204; *cancer* and, 84; *breast cancer,* 98, 305; *colon cancer,* 117; *colorectal cancer,* 115; *gastric cancer,* 120; *lung cancer,* 128; *prostate cancer,* 144, 149; *cataracts* and, 175, 233; cooking's effect on, 305, 307; *eye (retinal)* diseases and, 175; *hypertension (high blood pressure)* and, 181; *macular degeneration* and, 175; in organic vs. nonorganic red peppers, 324; in vegetable juice vs. raw vegetables, 305

luteolin, 12; *atherosclerosis* and, 43; *cancer* and, 50, 65, 67, 81; *leukemia,* 121; *lung cancer,* 128; *prostate cancer,* 137, 229; *eye (retinal)* diseases and, 175; *inflammation* and, 182; *multiple sclerosis* and, 185; in organic vs. nonorganic lettuce, 321

lycopene, 15; antimutagenicity and, 46; antioxidant activity and, 26, 28, 38, 204; *cancer* and, 46, 68, 78, 84; *alimentary tract cancer,* 86; *breast cancer,* 98, 100; *colon cancer,* 218, 329; *colorectal cancer,* 115; *esophageal (oesophageal) cancer* and, 86, 121, 131; *laryngeal* cancer, 86, 121, 131; *oral cavity cancer,* 86, 121, 131; *pancreatic cancer,* 133; *pharyngeal cancer,* 86, 121, 131; *prostate cancer,* 139–40, 145, 146, 147, 149, 159, 192; caloric restriction/fasting and, 259; nutrient combining and, 228, 229, 231, 242; *skin cancer,* 151; *cardiovascular (coronary/heart) disease* and, 38, 78, 155, 159, 192; *chronic diseases* and, 312; cooking's effect on, 286, 291, 293; *eye (retinal) diseases* and, 175; in organic vs. nonorganic fruits/vegetables, 322, 324, 326, 329; in raw foods, 312

lysine, nutrient combining and: antiviral activity and, 205; *atherosclerosis* and, 206; *cancer* and: *bladder cancer,* 213; *breast cancer,* 215; *colon cancer,* 220–21; *fibrosarcoma,* 221; *melanoma,* 224; *osteosarcoma,* 226; *pancreatic cancer,* 226–27; *prostate cancer,* 230; *renal cell carcinoma,* 232; *testicular cancer,* 232

M

magnesium (Mg): *attention hyperactivity disorder (ADHD)* and, 44; *autism* and, 45; in organic vs. nonorganic fruits/vegetables, 319, 330, 334, 336, 337; *prostate cancer* and, 140

Maitake mushroom D-fraction, *cancer* and, 207

maize, 14, 15, 16, 179, 180

malic acid, 27, 325

malvidin, 13

mandarin oranges/mandarin orange juice, 172, 325

mangoes/mango juice, 13, 15, 17, 30, 63, 79, 324

marine algae, *cancer* and, 82

marionberries, organic vs. nonorganic, 332

matairesinol, 14

meat. *See also* specific types of: Aiello, Jennifer, and, 11; *cancer* and, 46, 105–6, 299, 307; *cardiovascular (coronary/heart) disease* and, 308; health problems and, 8; organic vs. nonorganic, 336

meciadonol, *thrombosis (blood clots)* and, 195

medicinal plants, 34, 40, 78, 174, 176, 177, 183

Mediterranean diet/Mediterranean-style diet, 155, 158, 237, 262, 295

melanoma, 224

melatonin, health benefits of, 236

menopause/menopausal symptoms, 184–85

metabolites: *aging (ageing)* and, 247; antioxidant activity and, 27; *atherosclerosis* and, 41; *cancer* and, 80, 86, 91, 97, 150, 213; *cardiovascular (coronary/heart) disease* and, 156; cooking's effect on, 284, 300; in organic vs. nonorganic foods, 329, 330

metformin, *hypoglycemia* and, 240

methionine, 105, 111, 245

methyl-3-indolyacetate, 61

methyl methanesulfonate, *cancer* and, 70

Metz, Rick, diet and, 318

Mg (magnesium). *See* magnesium (Mg)

micronutrients: antimutagenicity and, 78; *atherosclerosis* and, 206; *cancer* and: *alimentary tract cancer,* 213; *alminentary tract cancer* and, 86, 213; *breast cancer,* 90, 97, 100–101, 303;

colon cancer, 114, 116; *colorectal cancer,* 105, 111; *lung cancer,* 129; nutrient combining and, 238; in organic foods, 330, 332; in raw/cooked vegetables, 288, 294, 303, 312; vegan diets and, 265

milk, *oral cancer* and, 301

minerals: *atherosclerosis* and, 159; *cancer* and, 208; *cardiovascular (coronary/heart) disease* and, 157, 159, 169; cooking's effect on, in broccoli, 283; in organic vs. nonorganic fruits/vegetables, 317, 325, 328, 332

miso soup, *colorectal cancer* and, 106

monophenols, 12. *See also* specific types of

monoterpenes, 15. *See also* specific types of

moronic acid, 16

mulberries/mulberry juice, *HIV infection* and, 238

multiple myeloma, 224–25

multiple sclerosis, 185, 275–76

mung beans/mung bean sprouts, 80, 292

mushrooms, 23, 98, 180, 214, 325–26. *See also* specific types of

mustard, 14, 17, 24, 66, 287

mwage leaves, cooking's/processing's effect on, 291–92

myricetin, 12; *cancer* and, 41, 50, 127, 132, 133, 163, 174; in organic vs. nonorganic yellow plums, 331; *type 2 diabetes* and, 127, 163, 174

myrosinase: *cancer* and, 305; cooking's effect on, 282, 284, 285, 287, 295, 298, 300–301

N

n-3 fatty acids, 155, 194

N-acetylcystein (NAC/NAC-ITC), 87, 103, 147, 282, 297–98

naringenin, 12, 37; *asthma* and, 41, 127, 163, 174; *atherosclerosis* and, 43–44, 147; *cancer* and, 61; *breast cancer,* 43–44, 92, 95, 98, 147; *prostate cancer,* 43–44, 98, 141, 146–47; *cerebrovascular disease* and, 41, 127, 162, 174; *prostate cancer* and, 98

naringin, 95, 128

National Cancer Institute, 9

natural agents/compounds/extracts/products: *aging (ageing)* and, 20; *cancer* and, 47, 48, 61, 68, 100, 209; *prostate cancer,* 137; *skin cancer,* 150; cognitive function and, 167; health benefits of, 237; *inflammation* and, 49; *neurological diseases* and, 49

NDGA (nordihydroguaiaretic acid), antioxidant activity and, 37

neck cancer, 130

neobetanin, 16

neohesperidin, *cancer* and, 79

neurodegenerative diseases/disorders, 185–87, 276–77

neuroprotection/neuroprotective effects: antioxidant activity and, 252, 277; caloric restriction and, 245, 252, 262–63, 272, 275, 276; cranberries and, 48, 154, 182, 186; polyphenols and, 185

neurosporene, 15

niacin, 25, 200, 285, 286

Nigerian vegetables, cooking's effect on, 285

nitric oxide: caloric restriction and, 35, 266–67; *cancer* and, 48–49, 70, 75, 125; cooking's effect on, 287, 294; green tea and, 35; *inflammation* and, 48–49, 70; nutrient combining and, 211

nobiletin, 42, 120

non-Hodgkin's lymphoma, 130

non-nutritive compounds, 81, 117

nordihydroguaiaretic acid (NDGA), antioxidant activity and, 37

nutraceuticals: *aging (ageing)* and, 18, 245; *cardiovascular (coronary/heart) disease* and, 157; Castelvetro, Giacomo, and, 299; human stem cells and, 237; mushrooms and, 23, 325–26; nutrient combining and, 29, 61, 209, 237

nutrient combining/synergies, 197–200; *aging (ageing)* and, 197; antioxidant activity and, 200–204, 211; antiviral/antibacterial activities and, 205; *arthritis* and, 205–6; *atherosclerosis* and, 206; *cancer* and, 206–13; *alimentary tract cancer,* 213; *bladder cancer,* 213; *breast cancer,* 214–17, 219; *cervical cancer,* 218; *colon cancer,* 218–21; *duodenal cancer,* 221; *fibrosarcoma,* 221; *forestomach cancer,* 221; *gastric cancer,* 222; *glioma,* 222; *leukemia,* 222–23; *melanoma,* 224; *oral cancer,* 220, 221, 225–26; *osteosarcoma,* 226; *pancreatic cancer,* 226–27; *prostate cancer,* 220, 227–31; *renal cancer,* 232; *testicular cancer,* 232; *candida* and, 232; *cardiovascular (coronary/heart) disease* and, 232–33, 235; *cataracts* and, 233; cholesterol and, 234; *colitis* and, 234–35; *diabetes* and, 235–36; health benefits of, general, 236–38; *HIV infection* and, 238; *hypercholesterolemia (high cholesterol/hyper-cholesterolaemia)* and, 238–39; *hypertension (high blood pressure)* and, 239; *hypoglycemia* and, 239–40; *inflammation* and, 205, 206, 208, 240–41; *liver damage* and, 241; *osteoarthritis* and, 241–42; *prostate health* and, 242; *ulcers* and, 242

nutritional science, 197, 199

nuts/nut butter/nut milk, 12, 16, 17. *See also* specific types of; antioxidant activity and, 25; *arthritis* and, 206, 240; blood lipids and, 153, 163; *cancer* and, 52–53, 156, 160; *cardiovascular (coronary/heart) disease* and: cholesterol and, 308, 313; intake amounts and, 160, 163, 168, 171, 179; living-foods diet and, 308; phytochemicals and, 52–53, 153, 156, 158; vegan/vegetarian diet and, 313; cholesterol and, 308, 313; *diabetes* and, 163, 168, 171, 179; *fibromyalgia* and, 311; *hypercholesterolemia (high cholesterol/hyper-cholesterolaemia)* and, 153, 163, 168, 172, 179, 261; *hypertension (high blood pressure)* and, 163, 168, 172, 173, 179; *inflammation* and, 163, 168, 172, 179, 240; organic vs. nonorganic, 336, 337; oxidative stress and, 163, 172, 179; *rheumatoid arthritis* and, 296; *stroke* and, 160; vegan diet and, 296, 308, 311, 313

O

oat phenolics, cholesterol and, 234

obesity, 187–89, 277–78, 314

obstructive pulmonary disease, 189

Ocimum gratissimum L., as antibiotic, 205

O-desmethylangolensin, 99, 106, 137–38

Okinawan diet, *aging (ageing)* and, 248–49

okra, cooking's effect on, 289

oleanane, *cancer* and, 71

oleanolic acid, 16

oleocanthal, 14

oleuropein, 14

oligomeric proanthocyanidins, 32, 53

olive oil, 14, 237, 299–300, 301, 303, 312, 325

olive vegetation water, *inflammation* and, 241–42

oltipraz, *hepatocellular carcinoma* and, 120

omega-3, 6, 9 fatty acids, 16, 44, 45, 157, 169, 183, 237

onions, 12, 17; antioxidant activity and, 33, 36, 39; *cancer* and, 74, 83, 108, 128, 297; *cardiovascular (coronary/heart) disease* and, 170, 171; cooking's effect on, 284, 287, 289–90, 294, 315; flavonoids in, 170; *hypertension (high blood pressure)* and, 287; Lanning, Michael, and, 318; organic vs. nonorganic, 335; raw, 297, 315; *thrombosis (blood clots)* and, 315

oolong tea (Camellia sinensis), 25, 51, 200

oral cancer, 130–31, 225–26

orange carotenes, 15

oranges/orange juice, 14, 15, 17. *See also* specific types of; antioxidant activity and, 37; *cancer* and, 94–95, 117; cognitive function and, 167; organic vs. nonorganic, 324, 325, 329; oxidative damage/stress and, 167

orange vegetables, 15, 129, 130

oregano, 12, 14, 16; 227, 235, 239, 242

organic acids, 17, 326

organic vs. nonorganic fruits/vegetables, 317–19. *See also* specific types of; amino acids in, 326; antioxidant activity and, 293, 332; ascorbic acid in, 335; biomarkers and, 323; cooking's effect on, 293; flavonoids in, 320, 324, 332–33; immune system and, 332; iron (Fe) in, 319, 336, 337; kaempferol in, 333; Lanning, Michael, and, 318–19; magnesium (Mg) in, 319, 334, 336, 337; major/trace elements in, 325, 332, 336; Metz, Rick, and, 318; minerals in, 327, 332, 334, 336; nutritional quality and, 321, 334; phenols/phenolic compounds in, 324, 326; phosphorous in, 319; polyphenols in, 320; potassium (K) in, 336, 337; quercetin in, 333; riboflavin in, 332; selenium in, 337; sugars in, 327; vitamins in, 319, 326, 332, 334; zinc in, 337

organosulfides, 17

Oriental diet, 308

osteoarthritis, 241–42

osteoporosis, 189–91

osteosarcoma, 226

ovarian cancer, 132

oxalic acid, 17

oxidative damage/stress: *aging (ageing)* and, 162, 247, 249, 250, 251, 272; almond skins and, 202; *Alzheimer's disease* and, 186, 191; *atherosclerosis* and, 206; blueberries and, 194; *brain dysfunction* and, 21, 83, 162; caloric restriction/fasting and: *aging (ageing)* and, 251–52, 266–67, 272, 274, 275; *diabetes* and, 264; *hypertension (high* blood pressure) and, 269; longevity and, 252, 273, 274; *cancer* and, 162; *cardiovascular (coronary/heart) disease* and, 162, 260; *cataracts* and, 21, 162; cognitive function and, 166; cranberries and, 194; fruits/vegetables and, 201–2; green leafy vegetables and, 294; *immune-system disorders* and, 21, 83, 162; *neurodegenerative diseases* and, 186; nut consumption and, 168; *Parkinson's disease* and, 18, 22, 186, 191; purple grape juice and, 322; turmeric and, 202–3

oxyresveratrol, antioxidant activity and, 200

oxysterols, 38

P

P (phosphorous), 319, 330, 335, 336

pac choi, organic vs. nonorganic, 320, 327, 331

pain, 278

pancreatic cancer, 132–34, 226–27

papaya, *breast cancer* and, 297

Parkinson's disease, 191–92, 278

parsley, 12, 62

Paullinia cupana (guarana), 25, 200

pawpaw, *cancer* and, 79

peaches, 13, 15, 37, 333, 334

peanuts, 12, 13, 14, 15, 16; *cancer* and, 52–53, 86, 123, 156; *cardiovascular (coronary/heart) disease* and, 52–53, 156; cooking's/processing's effect on, 291

pears, 13, 14, 15; antioxidant activity and, 37, 333; *asthma* and, 41; organic vs. nonorganic, 333, 334, 337

peas, 282, 285, 289, 290, 293, 335

PEITC (phenethyl isothiocyanate). *See* phenethyl isothiocyanate (PEITC)/phenethyl ITC

PEL (pelargonidin), 13, 57–58

pelargonidin (PEL), 13, 57–58

peonidin, 13

peppers, cooking's effect on, 282, 293. *See also* specific types of

Perilla frutescens, *allergies* and, 21

perillyl alcohol, 15, 134

periodontal disease, 192

persimmon, 16, 31

petunidin, 13

phenethyl isothiocyanate (PEITC)/phenethyl ITC: *cancer* and, 57, 69, 87; *colon cancer,* 113; *lung cancer,* 133; *pancreatic cancer,* 133; *prostate cancer,* 136, 145, 228, 229–30; *inflammation* and, 240

phenolics/phenolic compounds/phenols. *See also* specific types of: as antimicrobial, 205; antioxidant activity and, 27, 32, 37; *cancer* and, 67, 78, 79, 81, 107–8, 156; *oral cancer,* 131; *prostate cancer,* 149; *cardiovascular (coronary/heart) disease* and, 152, 156; in cherries, 166; cognitive function and, 166, 167; cooking's effect on, 281, 282–83, 286, 287–88, 293, 294; *diabetes* and, 179; *hyperglycemia* and, 179; *hypertension (high*

probetanin, 16

probiotics, *Helicobacter pylori infection* and, 176

processed meat, *cancer* and, 46, 111, 305

processing's effect on vegetables. *See* cooking's/processing's effect on vegetables

procyanidins, 33, 54, 113

proline, nutrient combining and: antiviral activity and, 205; *atherosclerosis* and, 206; *cancer and: bladder cancer,* 213; *breast cancer,* 215; *colon cancer,* 220–21; *fibrosarcoma,* 221; *melanoma,* 221, 224; *osteosarcoma,* 226; *pancreatic cancer,* 226–27; *prostate cancer,* 230; *renal cell carcinoma,* 232; *testicular cancer,* 232

prostate cancer/health, 134–49, 192–93, 227–31, 242

protodioscin, *sexual dysfunction* and, 193

provitamin A, 84, 85

prunes, 15, 16, 178–79

Prunus virginiana (chokecherry), *diabetes* and, 172

psyllium, *hypercholesterolemia (high cholesterol/hyper-cholesterolaemia)* and, 178

pterostilbene, 15, 102, 200

pumpkins, 14, 15, 17, 179, 180, 291–92; cooking's/processing's effect on, 291–92

punicalagin(s), 15, 109, 110–11, 220

purified vs. whole food compounds, *cancer* and, 54, 56, 208

purple corn, *colon cancer* and, 106

purple flavonoids, 12

purple fruits/vegetables, 13

purple grape juice, organic vs. nonorganic, 322, 323

Q

quercetin, 12; *Alzheimer's disease* and, 22; antioxidant activity and, 200, 201, 202; *asthma* and, 41, 127, 162, 174; *atherosclerosis* and, 41–42, 43–44, 98, 147, 206; *cancer* and, 50, 61, 65, 81, 209; *breast cancer:* apple extracts and, 214; catechol-O-methyltransferase activity and, 96; cell lines and, 97; estrogen and, 92; genistein and, 93; hormones and, 43–44, 98, 147; *colon cancer,* 97, 112, 114, 219; *colorectal adenomas/cancer,* 104, 108, 112, 219; *gastric cancer,* 120; *leukemia,* 121; *liver cancer,* 123; *lung cancer,* 41, 125, 126, 127, 128, 162, 174; *pancreatic cancer,* 132, 133; *prostate cancer,* 43–44, 98, 135, 146–47, 228; *cardiovascular (coronary/heart) disease* and, 41, 127, 156, 157, 170; *cerebrovascular disease* and, 163; cooking's effect on, 284, 286, 290, 296; *eye (retinal)* diseases and, 175; *glioma* and, 222; *hypercholesterolemia (high cholesterol/hyper-cholesterolaemia),* 41–42; *ischemic (ischaemic) stroke* and, 162, 174; *leukemia* and, 222, 223; in organic vs. nonorganic fruits/vegetables, 319, 321, 323–24, 326, 333; *thrombosis (blood clots)* and, 194; *type 2 diabetes* and, 41, 127, 163, 174

quinic acid, 27, 288

quinines/quinine methides/quinine reductase, 25, 71, 201, 204

R

radishes, 106, 324

raspberries/raspberry juice, 13. *See also* specific types of; antimutagenic activity and, 69–70; antioxidant activity and, 36, 202, 203, 211; *cancer* and, 92, 107, 139, 151

raw (fresh) foods/raw-food diet. *See also* specific types of: *alimentary tract diseases* and, 311; *allergies* and, 314; Burns, Fiona, and, 244; *cancer* and, 300–301, 303, 304–5, 306–7, 314; *bladder cancer,* 297, 298, 299; *breast cancer,* 297, 299–300, 301, 303, 304, 305–6; *colon cancer,* 306; *colorectal cancer,* 305; *esophageal (oesophageal) cancer,* 297, 302; *gastric cancer,* 302, 304; *leukemia,* 299, 306; *melanoma,* 260; *oral cancer/oral cavity cancer,* 301, 302, 304; *pancreatic cancer,* 302, 306; *stomach cancer,* 302; *thyroid cancer,* 303–4; *urothelial cancer,* 305; *uterine cancer,* 307; *cardiovascular (coronary/heart) disease* and, 308, 313; cholesterol and, 308–9; *chronic diseases* and, 312; Clark, Sherrie, and, 280; *Crohn's disease* and, 310; *diabetes/types 2 diabetes* and, 310; *fibrocystic disease* and, 307; *fibromyalgia* and, 310–11; *gastroduodenal ulcers* and, 311; *gastrointestinal disorders* and, 311; as healing/health benefits of, 10–11, 198–99, 279, 280–81, 311–12; *Helicobacter pylori infection* and, 304; *hypertension (high blood pressure)* and, 314; immune system and, 314; *infectious diseases* and, 314; *inflammation* and, 314; Lindstrom, Anna, and, 279–80; *mortality* and, 312; *obesity* and, 314; *rheumatic diseases* and, 314; *stroke* and, 314–15; *thrombosis (blood clots)* and, 315; *ulcers* and, 315; Weintraub, Arnie, and, 244

red cabbage, *cancer* and, 62, 73

red chili (capsaicin), *cancer* and, 14, 51, 68, 74, 153, 188, 189

red currants/red currant juice, *cancer* and, 92, 107, 139, 151

red flavonoids, 12

red foods, lycopene in, 192

red fruits/vegetables, 13

red grapefruit, organic vs. nonorganic, 326

red grapes, antioxidant activity and, 37

red meat, *cancer* and, 46, 112, 114, 115, 119, 305

red oranges, 329

red peppers, 15, 36, 324, 327, 328

redskin potatoes, 330

red wine, 39, 41, 43

refined foods, 38, 119, 269, 305, 306, 310

religious fasting, 260, 269

renal cell carcinoma, 149, 232

resveratrol, 12, 15; *Alzheimer's disease* and, 22; antioxidant activity and, 30, 34, 200, 201, 202, 203; *atherosclerosis* and, 43–44, 98, 147; *cancer* and, 48, 68, 69, 76; *breast cancer,* 43–44, 98, 147, 214; *colon cancer,* 105, 113; *gastric cancer,* 222; *hepatocellular carcinoma,* 120, 123; *leukemia,* 122; *melanoma,* 224; *prostate cancer,* 43–44, 98, 139–40, 146–47, 228; *cardiovascular (coronary/heart) disease* and, 232–33; *eye (retinal) diseases* and, 175; *hypercholesterolemia (high cholesterol/hyper-cholesterolaemia)* and, 43; *inflammation* and, 241; in organic vs. nonorganic fruits/vegetables, 322, 327; *osteoarthritis* and, 241 retinoids, *cancer* and, 56, 128

retinol, *cancer* and, 85, 90, 127

retinolic acid, *cancer* and, 221, 223, 225

rhamnetin, *cancer* and, 79

Rhodiola rosea, *diabetes* and, 235, 239

rho iso-alpha acids, *cardiovascular (coronary/heart) disease* and, 155

riboflavin, 285, 286, 332

rice, 14, 16, 79, 302

rocaglamides, *inflammation* and, 183–84

rosemarinol, 12

rosemary, 12, 24, 66, 235, 237, 239

rosmarinic acid, 21, 227

rubixanthin, 15

rutin, 12; *atherosclerosis* and, 206; *cancer* and, 79, 95, 112; cholesterol and, 234; in organic vs. nonorganic red peppers, 324; *thrombosis (blood clots)* and, 194

S

saffron, 24, 66

sage (Salvia officinalis), 25, 200, 237

salads, diseases and, 299–300, 301, 303, 311, 312

salicylic acid, 14, 322, 333

S-allyl cysteine, *cancer* and, 68

salted meat, *gastric cancer* and, 302

Salvia officinalis (sage), 25, 200, 237

saponins, 16, 176, 177, 292

Satsuma mandarin fruit, *diabetes* and, 172–73

saturated fat, *cancer* and, 128, 230

Se (selenium). *See* selenium (Se)

sea buckhorn/sea buckhorn juice, *cancer* and, 92, 107, 139, 151

secoisolariciresinol, 14

seeds, 12, 14, 292, 296, 308, 311, 337. *See also* specific types of

selenium (Se): antimutagenicity and, 177; *cancer* and, 72, 77, 129, 134, 145, 227; *HIV infection* and, 177; in organic vs. nonorganic foods, 337

sepsis, 193

serviceberries/serviceberry juice (Amelanchier ainifolia), 92, 107, 139, 151, 172

sesquiterpenoid, *colitis* and, 235

Seventh-Day Adventist diet, 261

sexual dysfunction, 193

Shepherdia argentea (buffaloberry), *diabetes* and, 172

shikimic acid, *cancer* and, 79

short chain fatty acids, *colorectal cancer* and, 105

silibinin, 39, 87, 88, 120, 125, 127, 145

silybin, 12

strawberries/strawberry juice: *aging (ageing)* and, 19, 20, 21; antioxidant activity and, 37, 202, 203, 211, 328–29; *cancer* and, 19, 69–70, 92, 107, 167; *breast cancer,* 139, 151, 215, 219–20, 329, 330; *colon cancer,* 109, 215, 219–20, 329, 330; *intestinal cancer,* 139, 151; *prostate cancer,* 139, 151; *stomach cancer,* 139, 151; cognitive function and, 167, 187; flavonoids (polyphenols) in, 12, 13; hydroxycinnamic acids in, 14; lignans (phytoestrogens) in, 14; *neurodegenerative diseases* and, 187; organic vs. nonorganic, 215, 219–20, 323, 328–29, 330, 332; phenolic acids in, 14; secoisolariciresinol in, 14

streptomycin, nutrient combining and, 205

stroke, 193–94, 314–15. *See also* **cardiovascular (coronary/heart) disease;** specific types of

Strong, David, nutritional healing and, 199

sugar(s): Aiello, Jennifer, and, 11; *cancer* and, 119, 306, 307; cooking's effect on, 282; *Crohn's disease* and, 310; in mushrooms, 23, 326; in organic foods, 325, 326, 327

sulfides, *cancer* and, 80

sulforaphane, 17; as antimicrobial, 222; antioxidant activity and, 30, 31; *cancer* and, 79, 212; broccoli and, 53–54, 285; Chinese cabbage and, 64; molecular basis and, 56, 60; Phase 2 enzyme induction and, 82; phLP-DNA adduct repair and, 71; phytochemicals and, 56, 69; types of: *bladder cancer,* 87; *breast cancer,* 95; *colon cancer,* 219; *gastric cancer,* 222; *lung cancer,* 124; *prostate cancer,* 144, 147; cooking's effect on, 283, 285, 289; *Helicobacter pylori infection* and, 222; *inflammation* and, 240; nutrient combining and, 208, 218, 219, 222; *osteoporosis* and, 189–90

sulindac, *colon cancer* and, 108–9, 113

survivin, 88, 91, 104, 136

sweet cherries, cognitive function and, 166–67

sweet peppers, organic vs. nonorganic, 327, 328

sweet potatoes, cooking's/processing's effects on, 291, 302

Swiss chard, cooking's effect on, 282, 292, 293

syn-propanethial-S-oxide, 17

T

TA, 52, 154

Tamogi-take mushroom, *hypertension (high blood pressure)* and, 180

tamoxifen, *breast cancer* and, 93, 214, 217

tannic acid, 14

tannins: *arthritis* and, 206; *cardiovascular (coronary/heart) disease* and, 153; *colon cancer* and, 220; cooking's effect on, 283, 288; *diarrhea* and, 174; *hepatitis* and, 176, 177; *HIV infection* and, 177; *inflammation* and, 240; *obesity* and, 189; in sorghum, 158, 189; *Staphylococcal infections* and, 23–24

Tanzanian vegetables, cooking's/processing's effect on, 291–92

taro leaves, *cancer* and, 79

tartaric acid, 17, 27

ulcers, 242
University of Wisconsin, 243
unsaturated fats, *cardiovascular (coronary/heart) disease* and, 169
ursane, *cancer* and, 71
ursolic acid, 16, 68
UV radiation, 150, 151

V

vanillic acid, *cancer* and, 79
vanillin, 14, 79
vanilloids, 72, 79
vegan/vegetarian diets: *atherosclerosis* and, 296, 309; body affected by, 279; caloric restric-
    tion/fasting and, 253, 265, 267–68, 270; *cancer* and: efficacy and, 40, 46, 158,
    167, 173, 180, 190; living foods and, 296, 311; phytochemicals and, 71; *prostate
    cancer,* 228; *cardiovascular (coronary/heart) disease* and: cholesterol and, 208; efficacy
    and, 40, 158, 167, 173, 180, 190; living foods and, 296, 308, 311; *mortality* and,
    313; cholesterol and, 261, 296, 308, 309, 311; cognitive function and, 167; *demen-
    tia* and, 40, 158, 167, 173, 180, 190; *diabetes* and: caloric restriction/fasting and,
    265; efficacy and, 40, 158, 167, 173, 180, 190; low-fat vegan diet and, 310; *diver-
    ticular disease* and, 40, 158, 167, 173, 180, 190; *fibromyalgia* and, 267–68, 310–11;
    gallstones and, 40, 158, 167, 173, 180, 190; *hypertension (high blood pressure)* and, 40,
    158, 167, 173, 180, 190; Lanning, Michael, and, 318–19; low-fat, 253, 265, 310;
    Metz, Rick, and, 318; *mortality* and, 312; nuts and, 296; *osteoporosis* and, 40, 158,
    167, 173, 180, 190; *renal disease* and, 40, 158, 167, 173, 180, 190; *rheumatoid arthritis*
    and: antioxidant activity and, 253–54, 267; efficacy and, 158, 167, 173, 180, 190;
    fasting and, 253, 254, 255; gluten-free vegan diet and, 253; living foods and, 311;
    low-fat vegan diet and, 253; uncooked vegan diet and, 254, 295–96; Seventh-Day
    Adventists and, 261; *thrombosis (blood clots)* and, 194; Weintraub, Arnie, and, 244
vegetables. *See* fruits/vegetables; specific types of
vegetarian diet. *See* vegan/vegetarian diets
Viburnum trilobum (cranberry), *diabetes* and, 172
vitamins: *atherosclerosis* and, 159; *attention deficit hyperactivity disorder (ADHD)* and, 44, 45; *au-
    tism* and, 44, 45; *cancer* and, 66–67, 77, 114, 208; *breast cancer,* 95, 101; *cardiovascular
    (coronary/heart) disease* and, 157, 159, 169; cooking's effect on, 285, 290, 291, 292;
    diabetes and, 173; *immune-system disorders* and, 181; in organic vs. nonorganic fruits/
    vegetables, 332, 336; types of: folate/folic acid: *cardiovascular (coronary/heart) disease*
    and, 160, 169, 174; cholesterol and, 309; *colorectal cancer* and, 105, 111; cooking's
    effect on, 288, 291, 294; *hypercholesterolemia (high cholesterol/hyper-cholesterolaemia)* and,
    309; in raw foods, 312; niacine, 25, 200, 285, 286; riboflavin, cooking's/soaking's
    effect on, 285, 286, 292; thiamine, 25, 200, 286, 292; vitamin A, 129, 171, 290,
    291, 312; vitamin B$_6$, 169, 291; vitamin B$_{12}$, 169, 309; vitamin C (ascorbic acid),
    9; *Alzheimer's disease* and, 22; antioxidant activity and, 26, 204; as antiviral, 23,
    205; *atherosclerosis* and, 206; *cancer* and, 77; *bladder cancer,* 213; *breast cancer,* 215; *colon*

cancer, 114, 220, 221; *esophageal (oesophageal) cancer,* 297; *fibrosarcoma,* 221; *lung cancer,* 128, 129; *melanoma,* 224; *osteosarcoma,* 226; *pancreatic cancer,* 226, 227; *prostate cancer,* 230; *renal cell carcinoma,* 232; *testicular cancer,* 232; *cardiovascular (coronary/heart) disease* and, 155, 169, 170, 308; *cataracts* and, 233; cholesterol and, 234; cooking's/processing's/transporting's effect on, 285, 286, 288, 289, 291, 292, 293; in amaranth leaves, 291; in broccoli, 282, 283, 285, 288; in cabbage, 293; in chickpeas, 289; in green beans, 289; in hospital food services, 291; in leaves/pods, 288; in okra, 289; in peas, 285, 289, 293; in snap beans, 293; in spinach, 289, 291; in Swiss Chard, 292; in tomatoes, 286, 329; *fibromyalgia* and, 311; *HIV infection* and, 238; *hypertension (high blood pressure)* and, 181; *inflammation* and, 240; living-foods diet and, 296, 308; loss of, during cooking, 281; in mushrooms, 23, 326; nutrient combining and, 201, 203, 206, 207; in organic vs. nonorganic fruits/vegetables, 319, 332, 335, 337; broccoli, 328; chard, 337; corn, 335; green leafy vegetables, 333; kiwifruits, 328; lettuce, 334, 337; mushrooms, 326; peaches, 333; pears, 333; potatoes, 330, 335, 336; red grapefruit, 326; red oranges, 329; red peppes, 324; savoy cabbage, 337; spinach, 337; strawberries, 323; sweet peppers, 320; tomatoes, 322, 329, 331; yellow plums, 331; in raw foods, 312; vitamin D, *colorectal cancer* and, 105, 111; vitamin D3, nutrient combining and, 221, 237; vitamin E: *cancer* and, 77, 95, 114, 128, 129, 229; *cardiovascular (coronary/heart) disease* and, 169, 308; *cataracts* and, 233; cognitive function and, 167, 187; *fibromyalgia* and, 311; living-foods diet and, 296, 308; *neurodegenerative diseases* and, 187; nutrient combining and, 201, 203; in organic vs. nonorganic fruits/vegetables, 335; in raw foods, 312
vulgaxanthin, 16

W

walnuts, 12, 14, 53, 156
watercress, 79, 301
watermelon, 15, 97, 297
water-only fasting, *hypertension (high blood pressure)* and, 270
Wedelia chinensis, *prostate cancer* and, 229
wedelolactone, *prostate cancer* and, 229
weight management, green tea and, 153
Weintraub, Arnie, caloric restriction and, 244
Western diet, 308
white beans, soaking's effect on, 286
white bread, *gastric cancer* and, 302
white cabbage, *cancer* and, 298–99
white currants/white currant juice, *cancer* and, 92, 107, 139, 151
white grapefruit, *lung cancer* and, 128
white grapes, organic vs. nonorganic and, 319
white-green foods, *cancer* and, 159, 192
whole grains. *See* grains/whole grains
Wigmore, Ann, nutritional healing and, 10
winged beans, cooking's effect on, 292

X

xanthophylls, 15, 213. *See also* specific types of

Y

yellow-orange vegetables, *lung cancer* and, 129–30
yellow peppers, organic vs. nonorganic, 328
yellow plums, organic vs. nonorganic, 331
yellow xanthophylls, 15
yerba mate tea, *oral cancer* and, 131
y-terpinene, 206, 234
y-totoctrienol, *cardiovascular (coronary/heart) disease* and, 232–33
Yucca schidigera, 40, 183

Z

zeaxanthin, 15, 143, 144, 175, 230, 233
zerumbone (ginger), 12, 15, 17, 51, 75, 79, 234–35
zinc, 44, 45, 238, 337
zingeroen, *obesity* and, 188
zucchini, 282, 287, 293, 324

About the Author

Dr. Brian R. Clement has directed the renowned Hippocrates Health Institute for more that three decades. He is internationally recognized for his relentless pursuit of complimentary health methods that support recovery and prevention of disease. For more than four decades, Dr. Clement has been personally involved in clinical research on a daily basis with the hundreds of thousands of people who have been through the program he developed and maintains. Research partners have included universities, physicians, and co-workers at the Institute itself. Many whole food supplement companies partner with Dr. Clement and Hippocrates in their pursuit to research the benefits of the products they offer. On several occasions, pioneering efforts have grown out of Clement's passionate pursuit for excellence

Dr. Clement employs his mission statement, to unify the vast world of health professions, to set a round table and encourage discussion among his peers and adversaries. He believes it is time to put the person/patient first and stop perpetuating narrow perceptions and condemnation of what we do not understand as professionals. As the incidence of disease increases, Clement's determination equals it. His observation that catastrophic disorders are now affecting the youngest among us has him acutely concerned. When recently addressing a medical conference, he stated, "Disease is surmountable once we are willing to reengage sincere observation and utilization of the biological world that surrounds us." Dr. Clement hopes this three-volume series, *Food IS Medicine*, will make both patients and practitioners aware of the large quantity of scientific data that documents how the food we eat can either be our best friend or our worst foe.